371.9 Noonan, Mary Jo.
NOO Teaching Young Children
     with Disabilities in
     Natural Environments

6/2014

Children with Disabilities in Natural Environments

ST. MARY PARISH LIBRARY
FRANKLIN, LOUISIANA

ST. MARY PARISH LIBRARY
FRANKLIN, LOUISIANA

Teaching Young Children with Disabilities in Natural Environments

Second Edition

by

Mary Jo Noonan, Ph.D.

College of Education
University of Hawai'i at Mānoa
Honolulu, Hawai'i

and

Linda McCormick, Ph.D.

College of Education
University of Hawai'i at Mānoa
Honolulu, Hawai'i

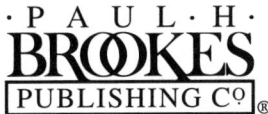

Baltimore • London • Sydney

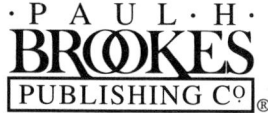

Paul H. Brookes Publishing Co.
Post Office Box 10624
Baltimore, Maryland 21285-0624
USA

www.brookespublishing.com

Copyright © 2014 by Paul H. Brookes Publishing Co., Inc.
All rights reserved.
Previous edition copyright © 2006.

"Paul H. Brookes Publishing Co." is a registered trademark
of Paul H. Brookes Publishing Co., Inc.

Typeset by Cenveo Publisher Services, Columbia, Maryland.
Manufactured in the United States by
Sheridan Books, Inc., Chelsea, Michigan.

Purchasers of *Teaching Young Children with Disabilities in Natural Environments, Second Edition*, are granted permission to download, print, and/or photocopy Appendix 10.1 for educational purposes. This may not be reproduced to generate revenue for any program or individual. *Unauthorized use beyond this privilege is prosecutable under federal law.* You will see the copyright protection notice at the bottom of the form.

Library of Congress Cataloging-in-Publication Data
Noonan, Mary Jo.
  [Early Intervention in Natural Environments]
  Teaching young children with disabilities in natural environments / by Mary Jo Noonan, Ph.D., and Linda McCormick, Ph.D. — Second edition.
     pages   cm
  Includes bibliographical references and index.
  ISBN 978-1-59857-256-8 (alk. paper) — ISBN 1-59857-256-3 (alk. paper)
  1. Children with disabilities—Education (Preschool) 2. Children with disabilities—Rehabilitation. 3. Children with disabilities—Services for. I. McCormick, Linda.

LC4019.3.M66 2013
371.9—dc23   2013018058

British Library Cataloguing in Publication data are available from the British Library

2017 2016 2015 2014 2013

10   9   8   7   6   5   4   3   2   1

Contents

About the Downloadable Materials vii
About the Authors ix
Foreword   *Mary Beth Bruder, Ph.D.* xi
Preface xiii

1   Perspectives, Policies, and Practices
    Linda McCormick, Ph.D. 1

2   Culture, Teaming, and Partnerships
    Linda McCormick, Ph.D. 27

3   Assessment and Planning: The Individualized
    Family Service Plan and Individualized Education
    Program
    Linda McCormick, Ph.D. 47

4   Naturalistic Curriculum Model
    Mary Jo Noonan, Ph.D. 75

5   Planning and Monitoring
    Linda McCormick, Ph.D. 99

6   Instructional Procedures
    Mary Jo Noonan, Ph.D. 117

7   Specialized Instructional Strategies
    Linda McCormick, Ph.D. 149

8	Designing Culturally Relevant Instruction *Mary Jo Noonan, Ph.D.* 177
9	Teaching Children with Autism *Mary Jo Noonan, Ph.D.* 205
10	Challenging Behavior *Mary Jo Noonan, Ph.D.* 233
11	Small-Group Instruction *Mary Jo Noonan, Ph.D.* 263
12	Interventions to Promote Peer Interactions *Linda McCormick, Ph.D.* 283
13	Environmental Arrangements, Adaptations, and Assistive Technologies *Mary Jo Noonan, Ph.D.* 299
14	Transitions *Linda McCormick, Ph.D.* 331

Index 345

About the Downloadable Materials

Attention instructors! A free Instructor's Guide is available to help you teach a course using *Teaching Young Children with Disabilities in Natural Environments, Second Edition*. Please visit **www.brookespublishing.com/faculty** to access the following materials for each chapter:

- Review questions
- True/false and multiple-choice test items
- Short answer discussion questions
- Individual/team and class activities

Purchasers of this book may download, print, and/or photocopy Appendix 10.1 for educational use at **www.brookespublishing.com/noonan/eforms.**

About the Authors

Mary Jo Noonan, Ph.D., College of Education, University of Hawai'i at Mānoa, 3357 Anoai Place, Honolulu, HI 96822

Dr. Noonan coordinates the teacher preparation programs for students with severe disabilities and the Ph.D. in Exceptionalities program at the University of Hawai'i at Mānoa. She is also the lead faculty member in developing a blended early childhood/early childhood special education undergraduate teacher education program. She has been the principal investigator on numerous grants and has consulted extensively throughout the Pacific Basin region.

Linda McCormick, Ph.D., College of Education, University of Hawai'i at Mānoa, 1350 Ala Moana Blvd., PH4, Honolulu, HI 96814

Dr. McCormick focuses on professional development, collaborative teaming, and inclusion in early intervention and early childhood special education. She is the author of numerous articles and textbooks and has provided courses and workshops in the Pacific Basin and Taiwan.

Foreword

It has been 20 years since the first methods text was published by Mary Jo Noonan and Linda McCormick and 7 years since the last revision of their book *Teaching Young Children in Natural Environments*. When I read this latest edition, I felt as though I was experiencing anew the systematic iterations of service delivery practices that have evolved over this time.

When the first edition of this book was published in 1993, it was a bold departure from previous texts in early childhood intervention. This was not because the content differed very much from others but because its organizational framework examined the learning needs of infants and young children with disabilities within and across the contexts in which they lived and learned. Rather than organize the book by addressing the separate developmental domains that are traditionally used in early childhood assessments and curricula, the frame used by Noonan and McCormick focused on the integration of developmental domains through learning in everyday child-focused activities. The text highlighted intervention practices that cross both developmental domains and the various environments in which infants and young children spend their time.

This latest edition continues to lead the field as it examines new challenges and opportunities within well-established principles of early childhood intervention. In fact, there are many other dichotomies that can be used to describe the contents of this book, as I will illustrate. These contradictory yet complementary themes are but one way to illuminate the contribution this book will make to our growing field—a field of practice that continues to expand through both the numbers and complexities of the children and families who are in need of compensatory and remedial intervention services.

Timeless and Timeliness

The content in this book is timeless in that there are well-established principles of early childhood intervention that form its foundation. These principles include developmental theories for learning, family partnerships, and team-based service delivery—none of which has changed in the past 20 years. The first chapter lays these principles out under the title "Perspectives, Policies, and Practices," which includes a history of the field and the legislative mandates that govern services for children and adults with disabilities. This chapter is followed by one that emphasizes the well-established practices of teaming and partnerships in the context of cultural diversity and sensitivity for the changing population demographics of families who participate in early childhood intervention. The methods chapters also include information on early childhood interventions that have proven to be effective over many years (e.g., milieu teaching, prompting systems, and continuous monitoring of progress through data-based decisions). Yet the book also includes updated information on more recent intervention models such as response to intervention, positive behavior supports, social competence, and assistive technology. In addition, the growing population of young children identified as having autism is addressed thoroughly with a review of promising and recommended interventions for these young children. There is little doubt that the adoption and use of these new and recommended practices will contribute to more effective and efficient services for young children and their families.

Comprehensive and Detailed

The book's comprehensiveness and level of detail continue to impress me. The details are what make it exceptional. Each chapter contains objectives, study questions, and references that specify and emphasize important intervention concepts. These concepts are underscored by examples of interventions, practices, and lesson plans that focus on children and family learning. Chapters 2, 3, 5, 6, 7, and 8, for example, illustrate both the broad and specific applications of intervention. In this way the authors model principles of teaching and learning for us to apply both within our personal preparation programs and among the children and families we serve.

Inclusive and Specialized

Teaching Young Children with Disabilities in Natural Environments provides an ecological lens through which to design and implement intervention. The authors have broadened the content of the book to address the continuum of child needs. Chapters cover information on such topics as naturalistic curriculum models (Chapter 4); environmental arrangements, adaptations, and assistive technologies (Chapter 13); and transitions (Chapter 14) to enable all children to benefit from teaching routines in inclusive and natural settings. More specialized chapters provide focused information to benefit high-need children (see Chapters 9–12). By including the range of child needs and settings in which children are served through early intervention (e.g., home, child care, Head Start, schools), the authors have provided both the context and intervention tools needed to ensure successful learning by all infants, young children, families, and service providers.

Grateful and Impatient

In closing, I want to thank Mary Jo and Linda for leaving me with the dichotomy of being grateful for their work as elucidated in this book yet so very impatient in seeing the principles and practices they describe applied to all infants, young children, and families in need of early childhood intervention. This book tells us how to do this, and now the field has the opportunity and challenge to make it happen.

Mary Beth Bruder, Ph.D.

Preface

The previous edition of *Teaching Young Children with Disabilities in Natural Environments* was published by Paul H. Brookes in 2006. Its target audience is undergraduate and graduate students preparing to be early childhood special education teachers. The text is unique among early childhood texts, with foci on natural and inclusive environments, assessment, teaching methods, and a noncategorical approach to intervention. Perspectives on early childhood issues and research-based procedures have been updated by integrating the research and intervention practices that have become available since the previous edition.

Chapter 1, "Perspectives, Policies, and Practices," includes an update to legislation: No Child Left Behind Act; Individuals with Disabilities Education Act, Parts B and C; and Head Start. It also addresses implications of the No Child Left Behind Act, standards-based education, and international perspectives. The discussion of inclusion models has been expanded to include blended teacher preparation (special education and general early childhood). Several recommended practices—assistive technology, research-based practices, and response-to-intervention—have been added. These practices are addressed in more detail in subsequent chapters. Chapter 2, "Culture, Teaming, and Partnerships," reviews communication skills that are essential to effective professional partnerships, teaming, and collaboration. Discussion of the teacher-consultation intervention approach has been added to the section focused on professional partnerships. The second half of the chapter describes characteristics of culturally respectful and effective family partnerships with emphasis on cultural values in parenting, the culture of special education, and the cultural reciprocity approach to establishing effective and collaborative relationships with families. Chapter 3, "Assessment and Planning: The Individualized Family Service Plan and Individualized Education Program," describes norm-referenced, criterion-referenced, and alternative assessment. Coverage of alternative assessment has been expanded, and the topic of standards-based assessment has been added. The components of the IFSP and IEP are reviewed and compared. The chapter concludes with practical information and examples on developing and writing goals and objectives.

Chapter 4, "Naturalistic Curriculum Model," is the theoretical foundation for the remainder of the text. It begins with an overview of curriculum models in early intervention and early childhood special education. A theoretical basis for a naturalistic curriculum is presented, followed by the components and implementation steps of the naturalistic curriculum model. The topic of natural environments has been updated and expanded. Ecological planning and assessment for the ecological curriculum model is presented in Chapter 5, "Planning and Monitoring." This chapter provides step-by-step procedures for conducting ecological assessment, with examples to illustrate each of the steps. A discussion of curriculum-based assessment measures has been added. The chapter concludes with a discussion of related assessment approaches (including portfolio assessment).

Chapter 6, "Instructional Procedures," describes behavioral instructional methods in teacher-friendly terms, such as *providing assistance*. The instructional planning process includes an explanation of how to link early learning standards to instruction in inclusive or blended classrooms. Data-based monitoring approaches conclude the chapter. Approaches to maximizing the features of natural environments in the instructional process are described in Chapter 7, "Specialized Instructional Strategies." The emphasis is on how to use milieu teaching, activity-based instruction, and embedded instruction to provide instruction in the course of typically occurring activities and routines in homes and early intervention and early childhood settings. The chapter also addresses specific adaptations in natural settings for children with motor and sensory disabilities.

Chapter 8, "Designing Culturally Relevant Instruction," reviews research-based instructional strategies and modifications for young children with disabilities from diverse cultural and language backgrounds. The second half of the chapter includes an overview of the typical stages of second-language acquisition and concludes with specific strategies to facilitate language and other learning among young children who are English language learners. The chapter has been substantially updated with current research-based intervention strategies. Given the recent exponential rise in the identification of young children with autism and autism spectrum disorders, and the distinctive characteristics and needs of these children, Chapter 9, "Teaching Children with Autism," is included in this otherwise noncategorical book. The introduction to the chapter describes the unique developmental and learning characteristics of children with autism. This section has been expanded with current research on characteristics such as joint attention, theory of mind, and communication development. The remainder of the chapter focuses on intervention procedures—first, general instructional procedures shown to be effective across a range of children's learning characteristics, and second, instructional procedures developed specifically to address the special learning characteristics and needs of children with autism. The chapter concludes with an expanded review of model programs for young children with autism and autism spectrum disorders. Chapter 10, "Challenging Behavior," focuses on the positive behavior support model as a research-based and recommended practice for decreasing challenging behavior. This chapter has been updated to include the program-wide model of positive behavior support, describing primary, secondary, and tertiary levels of interventions. Detailed procedures are also described for implementing tertiary level supports, including conducting functional assessments and developing individualized positive behavior support plans. A complete example of an individualized positive behavior support plan is included as an appendix to the chapter.

Some families and professionals mistakenly believe that the "best" early intervention–early childhood special education is that which is provided intensely in a one-to-one instructional arrangement. Chapter 11, "Small-Group Instruction," describes the rationale, benefits, and instructional strategies for providing group instruction. Characteristics and types of group instruction are defined, as are group participation skills for young children. The chapter concludes with a discussion and examples of using the context of small groups to support the instructional process. The special group instruction approach of cooperative learning is also described.

The essential topic of promoting peer interactions in inclusive and blended classrooms is the focus of Chapter 12, "Interventions to Promote Peer Interactions." The chapter begins with a discussion of social skills and provides details on how to implement classroomwide and large-group interventions to facilitate social skill development. Social skill and social-communication interventions focused on individual children and social integration activities are also described. This revision elaborates on the roles of parents and teachers in facilitating children's friendships. Chapter 13, "Environmental Arrangements, Adaptations, and Assistive Technologies," discusses adaptations and strategies that support young children to be as independent as possible in natural environments. Adaptations and functionally equivalent responses are defined and explained through numerous examples addressing a range of children's needs, including physical, communication, and self-help needs.

Finally, Chapter 14, "Transitions," presents legal mandates, definitions, and issues associated with early childhood transitions. The chapter focuses on strategies to facilitate smooth and successful early childhood transitions, including home to hospital, infant program to preschool program, and preschool to kindergarten. Curricular aspects of transition (essential skills for the next environment) are also addressed.

This revised text is updated by integrating what we have learned in the past decade about teaching young children effectively in inclusive community settings. We provide practical guidance for determining what to teach and how to teach with methods that fit into naturally occurring activities and routines. As with the previous edition the question that has been uppermost in guiding this second edition is, "What do teachers who work with young children need to know and need to be able to do?"

1

Perspectives, Policies, and Practices

Linda McCormick

●●●●●●●●●●●●●●●●●● **FOCUS OF THIS CHAPTER** ●●●●●●●●●●●●●●●●●●

- History of concern for the needs of young children
- European and American contributors
- Transactional perspectives
- Legislation
- Promising practices

Early intervention (EI) is an array of services for children with disabilities from birth to age 3. These services are designed to meet the developmental needs of the child and the needs of the family as they relate to enhancing the child's development. Early childhood special education (ECSE) provides for the unique needs of children with disabilities from age 3 until the age of eligibility for public school.

This chapter offers a brief overview of the values and beliefs that drive EI and ECSE policies and laws, followed by a description of the practices and services that derive from these values and beliefs. The recommended practices that are introduced in this chapter are elaborated on in the remainder of *Teaching Young Children with Disabilities in Natural Environments*.

HISTORY OF CONCERN FOR THE NEEDS OF YOUNG CHILDREN

The roots of EI and ECSE can be traced to general early childhood education, compensatory education, and special education for school-age children as well as psychology, human development, nursing, and sociology. Innumerable people in these fields committed their professional careers to understanding and affecting the course of development of young children. We briefly summarize the contributions of some of these individuals to give some sense of the beginnings of ECSE.

EUROPEAN AND AMERICAN CONTRIBUTORS

The underpinnings of ECSE can be found in the work of European and American contributors. Europeans, the earliest contributors, were mostly physicians who explored how children learn. The Americans who followed studied the effects of the environment on early development.

European Contributions

Itard, Montessori, and Piaget are probably the best known of the European progenitors of ECSE. Jean-Marc Itard (1775–1838), a French physician and authority on diseases of the ear, is credited with developing and implementing the first intervention procedures for children with disabilities. Itard theorized that learning potential is affected by both the environment and physiological stimulation, an extremely radical idea for his time. He had an opportunity to test his theory and his sensory-training approach with a child who was found wandering around the outskirts of a village in the province of Aveyron, France. The child (later named Victor) was naked, his face and neck were heavily scarred, and he neither spoke nor responded to speech.

Refusing to accept the idea that the boy's condition was incurable and irreversible, Itard devoted the next 5 years to an intensive one-to-one education program (similar to what would be described in a present-day individualized education program, or IEP, for Victor). His goals for the boy were

- To interest him in a social life

- To improve his awareness of environmental stimuli

- To encourage development of new concepts
- To teach him to speak
- To teach him to communicate with symbols such as pictures and written words (Itard, 1962)

Victor did not make the progress that Itard had hoped for. After 5 years he could carry out only simple commands, and he could read and speak only a few words. He demonstrated affection for his caregivers, but his behavior did not approach typical behavior. Itard maintained that his sensory-training approach would have been successful if Victor had been a few years younger. Indeed this may have been the case, but many modern readers of Itard's personal account of his work with Victor conclude that the child most likely had an intellectual disability or autism (French, 2000).

What is important about this effort is that it was the first attempt to provide an enriched environment to compensate for severe developmental delays. It did away with the paralyzing sense of hopelessness and inertia that kept the medical profession and everyone else from trying to do anything constructive for children with significant developmental delays (Kanner, 1967). Edouard Sequin, Itard's student, later improved on and extended Itard's sensory-training approach, earning fame in Europe and elsewhere for his nonverbal intelligence test, which had its roots in Itard's work.

A century later in Italy, another physician, Maria Montessori (1870–1952), drew on the work of Itard, Sequin, and others. Her earliest work was with children who had intellectual disabilities and lived in an institution in Rome. She provided these children with mental stimulation, meaningful activities, and opportunities to develop self-esteem. Many of the children were able to pass standardized tests for sixth-grade students in the Italian public schools. Somewhat later she opened a nursery school called Children's House (Casa del Bambini) for young children living in Rome's tenements.

Montessori's method, which she called a *prepared environment*, stresses the development of initiative and self-reliance. Children are encouraged to pursue independently the things that interest them. She believed that children pass through a series of sensitive periods when they are especially attuned to a particular aspect of learning. She designed learning activities and materials to match these sensitive periods. Montessori's method continues to be used in programs throughout the United States and elsewhere in the world.

Jean Piaget (1896–1980), a Swiss philosopher and psychologist, spent much of his wide-ranging and prolific career listening to and watching children. At the core of Piaget's work is the belief that looking carefully at how knowledge develops in children will elucidate the nature of knowledge in general. Fields of science that grew out of his work include developmental psychology, cognitive theory, and genetic epistemology. Although Piaget was not an educator, his influence on education has been profound and pervasive.

Piaget's work provided new insights into children's thinking processes and products. Among his most important contributions was the notion that the thinking and reasoning processes of children are not quantitatively different from those of adults; rather, they are *qualitatively* different. From infancy, children are "little scientists" who constantly create and then test their theories of the world in every interaction.

Although it is not always acknowledged, early childhood programs in this country draw on Piaget's ideas. The most important are the notions that 1) qualitative shifts occur in children's thinking over time, 2) children gradually move in the direction of greater logic and less egocentrism with age, 3) learning comes through assimilation and accommodation, and 4) learning is necessarily an active process that results from questioning and exploring.

American Contributions

Toward the middle of the 20th century, Americans began to consider the possible effects of the environment on children's cognitive development, thus stimulating concern for services for young children with special needs. It began with a classic research study in Iowa in the 1930s that came about as a result of an unforeseen event (Skeels & Dye, 1939). Harold Skeels, a psychologist, was asked by the superintendent of an orphanage to find a placement for two little girls, ages 18 months and 2 years. Born out of wedlock to mothers with intellectual disability, their IQs were 35 and 46, respectively. The state found temporary space for the girls on wards with women identified as mentally deficient in a state institution. Life on the wards was very different from life in the orphanage, where there had been only minimal attention to children's physical concerns and little contact with adults. To the amazement of the professional community, the little girls showed dramatic IQ gains when they were retested 2 years later: Their intellectual functioning was near typical. They were subsequently placed in foster homes.

Skeels and his colleague Harold Dye were intrigued. They arranged to move 13 more children from the orphanage to the state institution. These children were under the age of 3, and all but two were classified as having intellectual disability. (Their average IQ was 64; classification criteria were less stringent then.) Each child was placed on a ward with adolescent women who had intellectual disability and assigned a surrogate mother out of this group. The teenage "mothers" were trained how to hold, feed, talk to, and play with the children and given toys and educational materials for them. When retested 18–36 months later, the children who had been assigned to the surrogate mothers had made a mean gain of 27.5 IQ points. All of these children were subsequently adopted. A comparison group of 12 children remained in the orphanage. All but two of these children functioned in the typical range. The average IQ of these two children was 86. When they were retested 18 to 36 months later, the children who remained in the orphanage showed a mean loss of 26.2 IQ points.

If these findings had been taken seriously at the time, EI efforts might have begun in the 1940s. However, because of the strong belief at that time in the importance of nature over nurture, the findings were largely ignored. Sadly, many of the most influential psychologists of the time even ridiculed the study, arguing that children suffering from an irreversible condition such as intellectual disability could not possibly show IQ gains and that the data "obviously" reflected a statistical rather than an educational phenomenon (Goodenough & Maurer, 1961).

Skeels's follow-up data, collected some 25 years later, were as remarkable as his earlier findings. Eleven of the thirteen children in the experimental group had married, and only one of the marriages had ended in divorce. The 10 "intact" marriages had produced 9 children, all of typical intelligence. The group's median educational level was 12th grade, and some of them had attended college. All were employed in business or domestic service or working as homemakers. Of the children who remained in the orphanage, one had died and four others were still institutionalized. Their median educational level was third grade. All but 1 of the 7 adults who were not institutionalized were working as skilled laborers.

Other American researchers in the 1940s who tipped the scales in the direction of recognizing the importance of a stimulating environment were Rene Spitz, William Goldfarb, Samuel Kirk, J. McVicker Hunt, and Benjamin Bloom. Spitz (1945) compared infants from a foundling home in which there was little stimulation of or social attention paid to infants in a nursery attached to a reformatory for delinquent girls. The infants in the nursery environment were cared for by their mothers, who were described in reformatory records as, for example, "socially maladjusted," "mentally retarded," "physically disabled," "psychopathic," or "criminal." The infants in the foundling home showed progressive declines in developmental abilities (from a mean developmental quotient [DQ] of 131 to a mean DQ of 72) over a period of 8 to 10 months, as well as weight loss, withdrawal, excessive crying, and an extreme susceptibility to infection. The mean DQ of the infants in the reformatory nursery remained at approximately the same level despite their having what Spitz described as undesirable genetic backgrounds.

William Goldfarb (1945, 1949, 1955) also compared groups of infants in two different environments: those institutionalized for a few months and those institutionalized for the first 3 years of life. Those institutionalized for their first 3 years showed delays in virtually all aspects of development. They were socially immature and unpopular with peers, and they demonstrated hyperactivity, short attention spans, and poor academic performance. Children who were institutionalized for only a few months appeared to develop typically.

Samuel Kirk (1958) initiated an important research study that looked at the impact of EI on children with disabilities. Specifically, he measured the effect of 2 years of preschool experience on the social and cognitive development of 43 institutionalized children with IQs ranging from 40 to 85. His results showed gains of between 10 and 30 points for the experimental group who attended either preschool or nursery school and substantial losses for children in the control group who received no intervention. These differences between the groups were maintained over a period of years. None of the control group left the institution, but almost half of the experimental children were placed in foster homes.

In addition to this early research, two books by respected writers strengthened arguments for the benefits of EI. J. McVicker Hunt (1961) published *Intelligence and Experience,* an extensive review of the accumulated research by Spitz, Goldfarb, and others. Hunt's two major recommendations, which would be accepted as common sense today, were greeted with surprise when the book was published. They were 1) to focus intervention on the early years, because these years are the most critical for later development, and 2) to optimize young children's interactions with the environment to accelerate intellectual development.

Benjamin Bloom's classic 1964 work *Stability and Change in Human Characteristics* presented an extensive review of longitudinal studies in human development. He agreed with Hunt that the data supported several conclusions regarding the role of early experience. First, human characteristics are shaped by early experiences. Second, environment and early experiences are critical because human development is cumulative. Third, initial learning is easier than attempting to replace inappropriate behaviors, once learned, with new ones.

TRANSACTIONAL PERSPECTIVES

What has emerged since the 1960s is a transactional perspective that stresses the bidirectionality of influences in child–adult interactions (Sameroff & Chandler, 1975). Developmental outcomes at any point in time are seen as a result of a continuous dynamic interplay among a child's behavior, adult responses to the child's behavior, and environmental variables that may influence both the child and the adult. A change in the child will trigger a change in the environment, which in turn will affect the child, and so forth.

Another transactional perspective arguing that developmental processes and outcomes are determined by multiple factors is the *ecological model* (Bronfenbrenner, 1979). Developmental processes and outcomes are viewed as a joint function of the characteristics of the environment and of the developing organism. Urie Bronfenbrenner's notions about early development place the emphasis on ecological systems, specifically, the interdependence of the many formal and informal social subsystems (e.g., the immediate family, the extended family, networks of friends and neighbors, churches, agencies, policy-making groups) in a child's life and how they affect one another and the child. Children's behavior and development are considered to be highly influenced by the different subsystems in which children are participating members and the relations among the subsystems (Bronfenbrenner, 1992). Ecological theory has influenced the design of EI programs for children at risk as well as children with disabilities, both nationally and internationally. Table 1.1 provides a summary of the contributions described.

This brief history of influences on ideas and approaches to EI shows how the field has moved beyond appreciation of the effects of both nature and nurture to concern for their interactions with each other. Research on brain development builds on the tradition of the transactional perspective, providing new and provocative data concerning nature and nurture (Shonkoff & Phillips, 2000). Thanks to technological advances in imaging neuroscience, we can literally see that experience affects the very structure of the growing child's brain. These findings further strengthen arguments for EI and support for infants and their caregivers (Shonkoff & Phillips, 2000; Thompson, 2001).

LEGISLATION

Public policy is government action that reflects the current values and concerns of the people. It is interpreted and enforced by legislative actions and

Table 1.1. Historical contributions to early intervention concepts

1800s		Jean-Marc Itard Demonstration: Intervention with Victor First systematic instruction
		Edouard Sequin Demonstration: Extension of Itard's work Argued for training of sensory and motor skills
Early 1900s		Maria Montessori Demonstration: Prepared environment Stimulating/meaningful learning activities and materials to match sensitive periods
Middle 1900s		Jean Piaget Theory: Cognitive theory and genetic epistemology Insights regarding children's learning processes/products
		Harold Skeels Research: IQ gains resulting from early stimulation Attention to the importance of nurture in the nature-nurture debate
		Rene Spitz Research: IQ and other benefits of early stimulation Effects of lack of stimulation on physical and mental development
		William Goldfarb Research: IQ and other developmental benefits of early stimulation Effects of lack of stimulation on social and adaptive development
		Samuel Kirk Research: Preschool versus no early intervention Effects of preschool experience on IQ
		J. McVicker Hunt Book: *Intelligence and Experience* Importance of early years and optimizing early interactions as critical
		Benjamin Bloom Book: *Stability and Change in Human Characteristics* Initial learning easier than trying to replace inappropriate behaviors
		Arnold Sameroff Research/theory: Transactional model Bidirectional influences—a change in the child triggers a change in the environment
Late 1900s		Urie Bronfenbrenner Theory: Ecological model Need to focus intervention on the environment as well as the child

the judicial system. Public policy ultimately stimulates and guides services. Federal education legislation since the 1970s—beginning with the 1972 amendments to the Head Start legislation—reflects the shift of attitudes about the effects of both biological and environmental factors on children's overall development and the growing body of knowledge documenting the effects of EI for children with disabilities. The following summarizes the most significant legislation for young children with disabilities (listed in Table 1.2).

Handicapped Children's Early Education Assistance Act

The efforts of many parents and professionals paid off in 1968 when the Handicapped Children's Early Education Assistance Act (PL 90-538) was passed into

Table 1.2. Major legislation affecting services for young children with special needs

Year	Legislation
1968	PL 90-538, the Handicapped Children's Early Education Assistance Act (HCEEAA) established the Handicapped Children's Early Education Program (HCEEP).
1972	PL 92-424 amended the Economic Opportunity Act to extend Head Start services to children with disabilities.
1975	PL 94-142, the Education for All Handicapped Children Act, was passed, establishing Preschool Incentive Grants and state grant awards that could include 3- through 5-year-olds.
1986	PL 99-457 amended PL 94-142, requiring states to provide a free and appropriate public education to preschoolers (Section 619) and providing incentives for serving infants and toddlers and their families (Part H).
1990	PL 101-476 renamed the Education for All Handicapped Children Act as the Individuals with Disabilities Education Act (IDEA).
1990	PL 101-336, the Americans with Disabilities Act (ADA), was signed into law giving all individuals with disabilities (including infants and preschoolers) the right to equal access and reasonable accommodations in public and private services.
1991	PL 102-119 reauthorized and amended IDEA Part H (services for infants and toddlers and their families) and Section 619 of Part B for preschool children.
1997	PL 105-17 reauthorized IDEA, restructuring it into four parts: Part H was redesignated to Part C and all services for preschoolers were included in Part B.
2004	PL 108-446 reauthorized IDEA and authorized Local Education Agencies to use up to 15 percent of IDEA funds for supportive services to help students who have not yet been identified with disabilities but who require additional academic and behavioral supports to succeed in general education settings.

law. The appropriation accompanying the law provided funds for demonstration projects to identify effective procedures and models for serving infants and young children with disabilities and their families. Initially these projects were called the Handicapped Children's Early Education Program or First Chance Projects; they are now the Early Education Programs for Children with Disabilities. These projects developed and disseminated a variety of intervention procedures across the country, providing a much-needed knowledge base for services and practices for families with infants and young children with disabilities.

Head Start Legislation

The pioneering efforts of early researchers and writers were catalysts for attitudinal changes and substantial later research that provided the roots for the compensatory education movement that began in the 1960s. Head Start was funded under the Elementary and Secondary Education Act passed in 1965. The program was conceived by the Kennedy and Johnson administrations in the early 1960s as a part of the War on Poverty campaign. As one of several compensatory education programs, it was designed to prepare children for success in school by providing stimulating education programs; improving children's nutrition, health care, and social and emotional development; and improving parental attitudes toward education. Head Start was originally a summer program, but it was soon expanded to year-round programming. In its first summer, more than 561,000 children were enrolled.

The original Head Start legislation made no mention of young children with disabilities. In 1972, amendments to the legislation established a requirement that Head Start programs reserve at least 10% of their enrollments for preschoolers with disabilities. The Head Start Act was reauthorized in 2007 with the signing of the Improving Head Start for School Readiness Act (PL 110-134).

Education for All Handicapped Children Act

Passage of the Education for All Handicapped Children Act of 1975 (PL 94-142) marked the beginning of an unprecedented alliance of professionals and parents. Part B of this law mandates a free appropriate public education (FAPE) for all children with disabilities from ages 3 to 21. Educational services are to be provided in the least restrictive environment (LRE), and an IEP must be in effect for all eligible children. Although this legislation was an important milestone in the history of education for children with disabilities, it left some gaping loopholes. The law allowed an exception to the FAPE requirements for 3- through 5-year-olds if children without disabilities in this age range were not served by the state's public schools. Schools were required to identify and evaluate young children with suspected disabilities, but if providing services ran counter to state law or judicial ruling regarding services for preschoolers, then the schools did not have to develop services for these preschoolers with disabilities. Many states used this loophole to avoid serving this population.

Education of the Handicapped Act Amendments of 1986

Passage of the Education of the Handicapped Act Amendments of 1986 (PL 99-457) was a major achievement for proponents of ECSE. It amended and extended Part B of the Education for All Handicapped Children Act to rectify the shortcomings concerning preschoolers, and it established a new program (Part H) that provided for comprehensive services for infants and toddlers with special needs and their families. Although state participation in the Part H program for infants and toddlers at risk for and with disabilities was not mandatory, the monetary incentives were so strong that every state, the District of Columbia, Puerto Rico, and the U.S. territories indicated an intention to develop the recommended EI system. The funds supported planning, development, and implementation of services for children from birth to age 3 who were identified as developmentally delayed. Because the definition of *developmentally delayed* was left to the discretion of the states and other governmental entities, the populations of children eligible for service varies from state to state.

Part H required that each child be given a multidisciplinary assessment. If the child was determined to be eligible for services, an individualized family service plan (IFSP) would be required before the child and family could begin receiving services.

Individuals with Disabilities Education Act

The Individuals with Disabilities Education Act (IDEA) of 1990 (PL 101-476) reauthorized the Education for All Handicapped Children Act. The term *handicapped* was replaced by the term *disabilities,* and "people first" language (e.g., "children with disabilities," "woman with mental retardation") was used to show greater respect and sensitivity for individuals with disabilities and their families. In 1991, there was another reauthorization (PL 102-119) that changed the specific language in Part B and Part H with respect to eligibility, related services, IFSPs for preschoolers, LRE, and funding.

In 1997, IDEA was reauthorized once again and signed into law as PL 105-17. This was the most substantial revision of IDEA since 1975. There was no equivocation or weakening of the strong congressional preference for "full inclusion" of children with disabilities in general education early childhood classrooms. The 1975 mandates were reaffirmed, and federal statutory requirements for inclusion were strengthened. Schools now were accountable not only for conducting an IEP and a placement process that fairly considered placement in a general class but also for providing services in the general education class that would make inclusion effective. The specific mandate for EI programs was that services must—to the maximum extent appropriate—be provided in natural environments, including home and community settings in which children with disabilities participate.

In the 1997 reauthorization, Congress recognized that IDEA had been successful in ensuring FAPE and improved education results for students with disabilities. The need for improvement in some areas was also recognized, resulting in important changes:

- Giving students greater access to the general education curriculum
- Strengthening roles and opportunities for parents to participate in their children's education
- Providing special education and related services, aids, and supports in general education classrooms "whenever appropriate"
- Providing incentives to help children before they become labeled
- Giving the child's regular education teacher a central role in the IEP process
- Reducing paperwork requirements that do not improve educational results

Almost all publicly funded programs have eligibility criteria, and EI programs are no exception. IDEA recognizes three groups of infants and toddlers as potentially eligible to receive EI services: 1) children who have a developmental delay, 2) children who have a diagnosed physical or mental condition that has a high probability of resulting in a developmental delay, and 3) children who are at risk of experiencing substantial delays if not provided with EI.

The 1997 IDEA amendments provided a notable change in the age limit for an eligibility requirement, namely, the possibility of using the eligibility category *developmental delay* as an alternative to a specific disability label for children through age 9 (previously this eligibility category was applicable only for 3- through 5-year-olds). States therefore have the option of continuing to use the categories designated for children ages 6 through 21, or they may choose to serve children who they deem to be "developmentally delayed." If they choose the eligibility category of developmental delay, they must formulate a definition for eligibility in this category and determine the age population for which it will be used (only for preschoolers or for children through ages 6, 7, 8, or 9). Most states define *developmental delay* in terms of standard deviation or delay expressed as a percentage of the chronological age. Some states allow qualitative criteria and "professional judgment."

IDEA requires that, to the maximum extent appropriate, EI services must be provided in natural environments (IDEA, 1997). Initially, many educational agencies thought that the LRE requirement of IDEA did not apply to preschool children. Others thought that simply locating one or more preschool classrooms for children with special needs in general elementary schools was sufficient to meet the LRE requirement for preschools. In the past decade, the LRE requirement has been revised and clarified.

The IFSP, as required by Part C of IDEA, must identify the natural environment in which special services are to be provided and justify the extent, if any, to which the services will not be provided in the natural environment. An exception occurs only when the IFSP team determines that the child's goals and objectives cannot be achieved through intervention in inclusive settings. Part B of IDEA 2004 (PL 108-446) uses the term LRE to refer to inclusive environments. The law and the regulations take into account the significant differences between services for 3- through 5-year-olds and those for school-age children. The IEP for a preschool child must state how the disability affects the child's participation in appropriate activities and describe the child's participation in community-based settings with same-age peers who are developing typically.

Examples of natural environments include those that provide children with opportunities such as playing in a sandbox, splashing in a puddle or pool of water, making mud pies, constructing a fence with blocks, and watching a parade, to name just a few. Services are provided in a variety of community settings (e.g., storytime at the library, playgroups at the park, children's gyms) as well as child care programs and nursery schools that include peers without disabilities. Program locations are selected on the basis of their compatibility with the family's cultural values, the intensity of services that the child needs, and geographical accessibility for the family. Inclusive practices are interventions, practices, and supports that are implemented in natural environments.

The new section of Part B states that any preschool child who is eligible for special education and related services is entitled to all the rights and protections guaranteed to school-age children. These rights and protections include FAPE, placement in the LRE, multidisciplinary evaluation, procedural safeguards, due process, and confidentiality of information.

IDEA was amended again in 2004 (PL 108-446). These amendments updated the agenda for young children and aligned it with the requirements of the No Child Left Behind Act. They focused attention on the documented benefits of EI and preschool services and the role of families not only in the development of their children but also in policy development. Specifically they stated the following:

- The family's EI program (Part C) service coordinator (or other representative of the EI program) is to be invited to participate in the IEP meeting to facilitate a smooth transition from Part C to Part B services. (Chapter 14 discusses transition planning and implementation.)

- The IEP team must consider the materials described in the IFSP when developing the IEP for a child transitioning from an EI program to kindergarten.

- Parents whose child is served under Part B and the child's teacher may agree to make minor changes in the child's IEP during the school year without reconvening the IEP team.

In 2011 the U.S. Department of Education updated regulations to clarify some of the requirements of IDEA. Specifically there were the following clarifications to Part C requirements:

- The multidisciplinary team as required by the IFSP must include the parent and two or more individuals from separate disciplines or professions, one of whom is designated as the service coordinator.

- The transition plan must be included in the IFSP, rather than provided as a separate document.

- There must be a clear differentiation of prereferral, referral, and postreferral IFSP activities such as screening, evaluations, assessment, and IFSP development.

Americans with Disabilities Act

The Americans with Disabilities Act (ADA) of 1990 (PL 101-336) is civil rights legislation for people with disabilities. It was patterned on Section 504 of the Rehabilitation Act of 1973. This legislation, passed in 1990, ensures the right of people with disabilities to participate in society and to have the same access to facilities and information as people without disabilities. The provisions of ADA have special relevance to young children with disabilities and their families. The law guarantees that children with disabilities cannot be excluded from "public accommodations" because they have a disability. "Public accommodations" include private preschools, child care centers, school-age child care programs, after-school programs, and family child care.

ADA is essentially a mandate for inclusion. The basic requirements are straightforward:

- Child care homes and centers must make reasonable modifications to their policies and practices to include children with disabilities unless doing so would constitute a fundamental alteration of the program. The phrase *reasonable modifications* means changes that can be carried out without much difficulty or expense. Examples of such modifications are changing policies and/or procedures, removing physical barriers, training staff, and providing adaptive equipment.

- Centers must provide auxiliary aids and services as needed for effective communication with children with disabilities when doing so would not constitute an undue burden. *Auxiliary aids and services* include devices or services to help children communicate (e.g., sign language, interpreters, large-print books). *Undue burden* means changes that would result in significant difficulty or expense to the program.

- Centers cannot exclude children with disabilities from their programs unless their presence would pose a direct threat to the health or safety of others or require a fundamental alteration of the program. *Direct threat* means that the child's condition poses a significant threat to the health or safety of other children or the staff. Child care providers must evaluate children on an individual basis; they cannot determine risk based on their own personal assumptions about a child.

By opening the doors of community child care and recreational programs, ADA gave young children with disabilities opportunities similar to those available to children without disabilities. If children with disabilities can participate with reasonable accommodations, they may not be denied access solely on the basis of their disability.

PROMISING PRACTICES

Practices are the actualization of values and beliefs: the methodologies to achieve our broad goals. When there are substantial data supporting the success of a practice, it may be referred to as an *evidence-based practice* or a *research-based practice*. Practices that have emerged over the past several decades as showing positive and desirable outcomes for the delivery of quality services to infants and young children with disabilities are the following: 1) culturally competent and relevant services, 2) family-centered intervention, 3) ecological assessment, 4) inclusion, 5) response to intervention, 6) positive behavioral support, and 7) transition planning. The common thread in all of these practices is individualization. The focus of this book is to describe the essential elements of these practices and the procedures (specific ordered steps) to implement each one in the classroom, home, and/or community.

Culturally Competent and Relevant Services

The term *culture* refers to the many different factors that shape our sense of group identity: race, ethnicity, religion, geographic location, income status, gender, and occupation. The way individuals think, feel, perceive, and behave reflects their cultural group membership. Professionals must give careful thought and intensive effort to assessment, intervention, and instructional procedures when they do not share the same worldviews, expectations, values, and behaviors as the families and children they serve. While no individual can truly be competent in the culture of another, professionals can work toward an appreciation and understanding of another person's culture. To meet the needs of culturally diverse families, professionals must know how to interact respectfully with them and how to effectively incorporate their unique beliefs, practices, and values in service delivery.

Culture (the ideas of their social world) affects children as well as adults. It affects how they learn and solve problems (as well as the kinds of problems they will solve), how they organize their environment, which language they learn, and how they spend their leisure time. Children from different cultures achieve the same developmental milestones though the precise behaviors with which they demonstrate these achievements vary across cultures. Culture also affects the views and the behavior of parents and teachers. It affects child-rearing practices and beliefs concerning education and disability.

Recognizing each child as a unique individual and each family as a unique family—and being as accepting and responsive to differences in language, social class, heritage, ethnic origins, geographic location, and religion as to the differing abilities and interests of children and their families—is the first and most important requirement for culturally relevant interventions (Hanson, Gutierrez, Morgan, Brennan, & Zercher, 1997; Hanson et al., 1998). Culturally relevant interventions are described and discussed in Chapter 8, but the concept is embedded in discussions of instructional practices and procedures throughout this book.

Family-Centered Intervention

Family systems theory shifts the focus of attention from the child in isolation to the child as one element of a system—the family system. Turnbull, Summers, and Brotherson (1983) integrated the tenets of this theory into practice. They suggested the following attitudes for professionals working with families: 1) view each family as unique in terms of membership characteristics, culture, and style; 2) recognize that families are systems with constantly shifting components and boundaries; 3) be aware that families and their individual members fulfill many and varied functions to support the continued growth and development of the child; and 4) understand that families experience many changes that produce different amounts of stress for each family member.

EI professionals made significant progress in the 1990s in the conceptualization and implementation of family-centered practices (Dunst, Johanson, Trivette, & Hamby, 1991; Turbiville, Turnbull, Garland, & Lee, 1996). These practices focus on enhancing the well-being of the family as a whole in addition to the well-being of the child. They include 1) treating families with dignity and respect, 2) being sensitive to family cultural and socioeconomic diversity, 3) providing families with choices that defer to their priorities and concerns, 4) ensuring that families have the information they need to make decisions, 5) introducing a range of informal community resources as parenting and family supports, and 6) using helpful practices that empower parents and enhance their competency (Dunst et al., 1991).

The assumptions underlying family-centered intervention are that families should be the decision makers where their children are concerned and that the goals and priorities they identify should drive the intervention process. These assumptions are now basic tenets guiding practices in EI and redefining parent-professional relationships. Professionals in EI programs work continuously to improve their understanding of cultural diversity, human relations, and communication and to put that understanding into practice. In addition to basic responsibilities for conducting assessment and providing and evaluating intervention, professionals must be able to build trust, resolve conflicts, and actively participate in planning with families (especially in helping them link up with needed services). Family-centered intervention is specifically discussed in Chapter 2.

Ecological Assessment

It has been almost 4 decades since Brown et al. (1979) described procedures drawn from ecological theory that could be used to generate functional goals and objectives for students with severe and multiple disabilities. They called this assessment approach *ecological inventory*. Since that time, it has been widely used with children of all ages and disabilities.

The ecological inventory process considers the congruence between the child's behavior and the demands of the routines, activities, and social interactions in the child's natural environments. It is essential for 1) generating functional goals and objectives, 2) individualizing instruction, and 3) planning adaptations. It differs from traditional assessment in that it considers the child's behavior in relation to environmental expectations (rather than in relation to the performance of the population used in standardizing the test). The ecological inventory process answers the following questions:

- What are appropriate intervention goals and objectives?
- Where should intervention be provided?
- How should intervention be provided?
- When should intervention be provided?
- How can intervention be evaluated?

Ecological assessment is equally applicable for identifying goals and objectives for intervention with infants and toddlers as for planning for preschool-age children. The environments in which the infant or young child is expected to function are examined to determine what needs to be taught and what adaptations need to be made to maximize participation. The product of an ecological assessment is a list of functional goals and objectives for the child's specific environments (e.g., home, family child care setting, community recreation site, preschool) and ideas for necessary adaptations of activities and/or materials. For children with more severe disabilities, skill objectives may then be listed in a task analysis for task analytic assessment. Task analytic assessment allows evaluation of the child's performance on each component of the skill. Instructions for implementing ecological assessment and other types of authentic assessment are provided in Chapter 5.

Inclusion

It has been well over a decade since Strain, McGee, and Kohler (2001) pointed out the myths concerning inclusion for young children with autism. While specifically concerned with young children with autism, the case these authors made for inclusion applies equally well to all infants and young children with disabilities. Educational myths argued that children with autism should be served in segregated environments. The authors maintained that arguments in favor of segregated services are baseless because they 1) have no empirical support, 2) often contradict the available data, and 3) are based on the misconception that any success (even when using inappropriate practices) demonstrates the superiority of segregation. The only reason these myths had become institutionalized was that they appeared in the writings of respected professionals and were reflected in outdated funding patterns and service delivery policies and practices.

The myths used to keep young children with disabilities out of inclusive environments include the following:

- *The need for readiness training:* The contention is that children with disabilities (particularly those with severe disabilities) need to achieve certain developmental milestones and learn to comply with simple motor-imitation tasks before they can be successful in inclusive settings.

- *The need for tutorial, one-to-one instruction for acquisition of important developmental skills:* The contention is that direct instruction is the only way to teach developmental skills.

- *The need for distraction-free environments:* The contention is that typical general education environments have too many distractions—that young children with disabilities can learn only in settings with reduced (uninteresting?) stimuli.

- *The need for behavior control procedures that can be provided only in segregated settings:* The contention is that interventions directed toward reducing challenging behaviors cannot be implemented in inclusive environments.

Since 2000 there has been a body of research countering these myths. There is now broad recognition that infants and young children with and without disabilities (including those with autism) can learn together in natural environments—homes, early childhood programs, child care centers, and neighborhoods, to name but a few.

In 2009 the Division for Early Childhood of the Council for Exceptional Children and the National Association for the Education of Young Children released a joint position statement on inclusion (DEC/NAEYC, 2009). This document is the culmination of 2 years of dedicated collaboration between the two organizations and an extensive national validation process to improve early childhood services for all children throughout the United States. Recognizing that high-quality inclusion cannot be achieved without a common understanding of what inclusion means, this document defines it as the "desired results of inclusive experiences for children with and without disabilities and their families" (DEC/NAEYC, 2009, p. 2). The three defining features of inclusion are 1) access, 2) meaningful participation, and 3) system-level supports. Though by no means yet sufficient, there is an ever-increasing body of rigorous research supporting specific practices that are central to these features of quality inclusion.

Access Inclusion takes many forms and it occurs in many environments (e.g., homes, Head Start, family or center-based child care, preschool, public and private prekindergarten, blended early childhood education/ECSE programs). Access means removing physical barriers and providing multiple and varied instructional formats and activities to maximize the development and learning in all of these environments. Access is also important for families, who must feel that they are valued and welcome in their child's educational experience. Examples of practices that support access are universal design for learning (UDL) and assistive technology (AT).

UDL is a concept that generates principles and practices to enable access for all and to all aspects of the individual's physical, social, and instructional environments (National Center on Universal Design for Learning, n.d.). The idea for universal design grew out of a concern for designing buildings and outdoor environments (e.g., power doors, curb cuts, handrails, automatic water faucets) to make then accessible for persons with disabilities. It soon became obvious that all members of the community were using and appreciating these design features and that including them in the initial design of the environments was less costly than making later adaptations and additions.

The implications of universal design for inclusion of young children with disabilities in home, school, and other community environments are readily apparent. UDL provides a conceptual framework for removing physical and structural barriers and developing curricula with varied instructional formats, alternative presentation possibilities, and multiple response modes to support the individual needs of every child. There are three essential principles of UDL (CAST, 2011). A universally designed curriculum must have:

- *Multiple means of representation:* This means that instruction, questions, expectations, and learning opportunities are provided in different formats and at different levels of complexity, addressing a range of ability levels and visual, auditory, and kinesthetic needs.

- *Multiple means of engagement:* There must be many opportunities for eliciting children's attention, curiosity, and motivation and addressing a wide range of interests. Once the child is engaged, engagement is maintained by providing different types of scaffolding and repetition.

- *Multiple means of expression:* Children must have a variety of formats for responding, demonstrating what they know, and for expressing ideas, feelings, and preferences. There must also be a range of options for using resources, toys, and materials in order to address each child's strengths, preferences, and abilities.

There is a reciprocal relationship between UDL and AT. Universal design provides tools for planning; AT provides tools for making necessary adaptations. AT includes both high-tech and low-tech devices, ranging from pens and papers and inexpensive adaptations of toys, books, and eating utensils to computer-based literacy tools, voice output communication aids, speech generating devices, hearing aids, powered scooters, and custom-fitted wheelchairs. AT services directly assist the selection, acquisition, and use of AT devices. The challenges associated with AT—what to get, where to get it, how to use it, how to pay for it, how to evaluate its effectiveness—are not nearly as complicated as they were in the past, because the majority of AT options are now readily available to early childhood practitioners and families (Sadao & Robinson, 2010).

Consideration of whether AT devices or services are provided is part of the IEP or IFSP process. All children eligible for EI or for special education and related services are entitled to receive AT if the devices and services are needed in order to increase access to natural environments. Procedures for providing AT for infants, toddlers, and preschoolers with disabilities are discussed throughout this book, but especially in Chapter 13.

Participation The second defining feature of inclusion is participation. This refers to the use of individualized supports and accommodations to ensure the child's full engagement in play and learning activities in all of his or her environments (DEC/NAEYC, 2009). IDEA mandates delivery of services in children's natural environments—places that do not isolate the child with disabilities or his or her family from mainstream community life. Part C of IDEA 1997 also calls for a shift from discipline-specific assessment and intervention provided in clinics or rehabilitation facilities to family-centered, team-based services to facilitate participation in natural environments.

What occurs in natural environments makes a significant contribution to the quality of life of infants and young children with disabilities. Children develop a range of important and enduring relationships from participating in family and neighborhood life. The routines and events in natural environments provide the context for implementing the specialized instructional procedures that are the focus of this book. Specialized instructional procedures to address developmental and learning goals in inclusive settings include milieu teaching procedures (Kaiser, 1993; Kaiser, 2000; Hawkings & Schuster, 2007); activity-based intervention (Losardo & Bricker, 1994); embedded instruction and distributed time delay (Wolery, 2001); scaffolding (Berk & Winsler, 1995); integrated therapy (McWilliam, 1996); tiered instructional models (Fox, Carta, Strain, Dunlap, & Hemmeter, 2009); high-probability procedures (Santos, 2001); and adaptations and modifications (Campbell, Milbourne, & Wilcox, 2008; Hamm, Mistrett, & Ruffino, 2006). Later chapters provide specific guidelines and tools for using these procedures with young children with disabilities.

System-Level Supports The third defining feature of inclusion is supports (DEC/NAEYC, 2009). An infrastructure of system-level supports that can sustain and further the efforts of individuals and organizations serving young children with disabilities and their families is essential. This infrastructure includes professional development, multiple opportunities for collaboration, and incentives for inclusion.

The goals of preservice and continuing professional development are to provide practitioners, specialists, administrators, and family members with the knowledge, skills, and dispositions to meet the needs of infants and young children with varying types of disabilities and levels of severity. Preservice students in the key EI disciplines should have direct experience working with families and on transdisciplinary teams before they graduate. Families have a valuable role in preparing students in ECSE and related fields at the university level, as understanding of both general and specific priorities and concerns is indispensable for high-quality EI/ECSE services.

From the first days and weeks of implementing the initial legislation for children with disabilities, it was clear that collaboration and communication were the keystones of effective intervention and successful programs. Professional-professional and family-professional collaboration and communication build and strengthen both family and professional capacities. This basic requirement for effective services has been referred to as the *collaboration imperative* (McCormick, 2003). Effective collaboration and communication requires frequent face-to-face interactions and a mutual "we are all in this together" feeling of positive interdependence. Further, it requires small-group interpersonal skills such as trust building, communication, leadership, creative problem solving, decision making, and conflict management and a commitment to set aside time regularly to assess and discuss goals for improving relationships and accomplishing tasks more effectively (Thousand & Villa, 2000). To be good family partners, practitioners must be skilled in human relationships and able to communicate confidently, effectively, and confidentially with families from different cultures who have different worldviews and different expectations for their children (Park, Turnbull, & Park, 2001).

A variety of approaches have been developed over the past several decades to support ongoing communication and collaboration. These include technical assistance, consultation, coaching, mentoring, collaborative problem solving, communities of practice, and teaming.

The teaming approach that has evolved as the best organizational structure for collaboration and communication is the transdisciplinary team model, in which practitioners and families work closely together on a continuous basis to plan, implement, and evaluate interventions.

Response to Intervention

Response to intervention (RTI) is a proactive problem-solving model designed to prevent delays in learning and behavior (Burns, Appleton, & Stehouwer, 2005; Fox, Carta, Strain, Dunlap, & Hemmeter, 2009). It evolved from the growing recognition that identifying students with learning difficulties by documenting the discrepancy between a child's aptitude and achievement before providing intervention and support was not working: children should not have to experience school failure before their learning difficulties are addressed. RTI is a tiered intervention model that links assessment with intervention and organizes instruction from least to most intensive depending on the level of involvement of the teacher. The procedures in RTI models are not new. They derive from applied behavior analysis, precision teaching, curriculum-based assessment, prereferral intervention, data-based decision making, and team-based problem solving (Sugai, 2007). What is new since the turn of the century is the alignment of these concepts into a comprehensive intervention framework. Also significant is the inclusion of RTI as a requirement of special education policy (IDEA, 2004).

RTI is intended to reduce unnecessary referrals to special education by helping teachers provide strategic support and individualized interventions at the first signs of learning and behavior difficulties. The objectives are threefold: 1) early and effective response to learning and behavior difficulties, 2) instructional intensity matched to level of need, and 3) frequent data-based decision making. The critical components of RTI are as follows (Fox et al., 2009):

- *Universal screening:* All students are evaluated to determine if they are making adequate progress, are at some risk of failure if not provided with extra assistance, or are at high risk of failure if not provided with specialized supports.

- *Continuous monitoring of progress:* There is regular and frequent monitoring of student progress to determine when the level of instructional support should be increased.

- *Continuum of interventions:* There are three levels of interventions that vary in intensity or level of support: 1) a core curriculum for all students, 2) modifications of the core for students who are not progressing at an adequate pace, and 3) individualized intensive curricula for those who do not progress with the modified curriculum.

- *Data-based decision making and problem solving:* Most critical to the RTI approach is continuous data-driven instructional decision making.

- *Implementation fidelity:* There is regular documentation of whether all aspects of the model are being implemented accurately and consistently according to plan.

The early RTI studies focused on instructional practices in academic areas with school-aged children. However, the years since the turn of the century have produced a substantial body of research considering provision of the RTI model in early childhood programs. The assumptions inherent in RTI parallel beliefs in EI and ECSE that all young children should participate and learn in the same environments and that interventions should be designed to match child and family needs. There are three RTI models currently available for 3- to 5-year olds: The Pyramid Model (Fox, Dunlap, Hemmeter, Joseph, & Strain, 2003); Recognition & Response (R&R) (Coleman, Buysse, & Neitzel, 2006); and Building Blocks (Sandall & Schwartz, 2008).

Positive Behavior Support

Positive behavior support (PBS) is the application of positive behavioral interventions and procedures to reduce problem behaviors and replace them with socially adaptive behavior. Initially developed as an alternative to aversive interventions used with students who engaged in extreme forms of self-injurious behavior and aggression, it is now used with a wide range of students in a variety of contexts (Sugai, Horner, & Sprague, 1999). The 1997 amendments of IDEA identified PBS as the preferred strategy for dealing with challenging behaviors of students with disabilities. The IEP team may consider other strategies in addition to PBS, but the regulations state that PBS must be considered when a child's behavior is judged to impede his or her learning or that of others. The Division for Early Childhood concurs with the importance of using PBS procedures (Division for Early Childhood, 1999). PBS practices have been thoroughly researched and validated (e.g., Carr, 1977; Carr & Durand, 1985; Repp & Horner, 1999).

PBS relies on a multitiered model to provide a continuum of behavioral supports in home, school, and community environments (Benedict, Horner, & Squires, 2007; Hemmeter, Fox, Jack, & Broyles, 2007). While the three tiers of intervention build on one another, each has a specific focus and different strategies. At the broadest (schoolwide) level are program-level interventions such as classroom and playground rules ("take turns on the swings") and program organization strategies (play areas clearly marked). A second (classwide) tier of intervention provides support when more instruction and structure than what is provided at the first level are needed. Intervention is provided to an entire class or group of children. The purpose of these interventions (e.g., teaching specific social skills) is to prevent behavior problems. Finally, at the third level there are more intense and individualized interventions, the design of which is based on thorough understanding of the function of the challenging behavior and the relevant contributing factors. There is a subset of procedures common to all applications at the third tier: They all begin with a functional behavioral assessment (FBA). The purpose of FBA procedures (informant assessment, observations, and experimental analysis) is to identify the events that are causing and maintaining the challenging behavior and thereby determine the function of the behavior. At this level, PBS emphasizes decision making based on analysis of data collected through a range of procedures and from a variety of sources. In addition to analysis of observable behaviors, intervention design considers a multitude of cognitive, biophysical, developmental, and physical/environmental variables that have the potential to affect the current functioning of the child.

Implementation of PBS varies according to the age of the child, the context of intervention, and the nature of the challenging behavior. Procedures common to PBS applications include 1) environmental arrangement (manipulation of antecedent conditions to reduce or prevent the likelihood that the problem behaviors will occur), 2) teaching new social and communication skills so that the child will no longer need to use the challenging behaviors to obtain desired outcomes, and 3) careful redesign of existing consequences to eliminate the events that are maintaining the challenging behaviors and to replace them with more acceptable social and communication behaviors. The focus is on adjusting social and environmental variables (e.g., routines, responses, instructions) and improving learning environments. Procedures to implement PBS are described in Chapter 10.

Transition Planning

Transitions are times of change. As change is inevitable, so is the need for planning to ensure that transitions will be successful. The important transition periods for infants and young children with disabilities are those 1) from the hospital (e.g., the neonatal intensive care unit) to community-based EI services; 2) from EI services to preschool; and 3) from preschool to kindergarten. Each provides different challenges as well as a set of common experiences. Prominent among the challenges are the interactions between professionals and families, potential differences in concerns and preferences, and issues related to cross-cultural communication. The focus of transition planning is on 1) ensuring continuity of service, 2) minimizing disruption of the family system, and 3) promoting children's functioning in their next environments (Division for Early Childhood Task Force, 1993).

A major goal in EI is to provide a continuity of services, sometimes referred to as a *seamless system of services delivery*. All guidelines for transition emphasize family involvement, child preparation for new environments, information exchange among professionals, continuity between settings, and compliance with federal, state, and other legal mandates. The challenges in providing a seamless system are immense. Legislative mandates related to transition services (e.g., eligibility differences for children from birth to age 3 years and for children ages 3 through 6 years) present a challenge, as do differences in the regulatory systems of the involved programs and services. In many states, responsibility for services for children from birth to age 3 years and responsibility for services for 3- through 6-year-olds reside with different governmental departments. This means that transition difficulties for families are often multiplied because there is more involved than just movement from one program to another: Transitions are across departments and agencies with very different philosophies and separate operating structures. A related issue is differences in the theoretical orientation, preparation, and experience of staff. Planning significantly reduces families' feelings of vulnerability and the disruptions for children. The issues surrounding preschool transitions, factors affecting transitions, and competencies for transition planning and coordination are described in Chapter 14.

SUMMARY

This chapter has provided an introduction to the history of EI and polices affecting services for infants and young children with disabilities and their families. The skills and knowledge that make up the competency base in EI and ECSE are previewed as promising practices. As noted earlier in the chapter, while all of these practices are not yet supported by as extensive a body of rigorous research as might be desired, there is adequate evidence to know that they produce positive and desirable outcomes. Thus, they comprise the competency base for EI and ECSE professionals.

STUDY QUESTIONS

1. Enumerate the significant European and American precursors of the field of early intervention.
2. What are the key tenets of transactional perspectives?
3. Describe the policies and laws that have had the most profound effect on services for infants and young children with disabilities and their families.
4. Differentiate the eligibility criteria for Part C and Part B of IDEA.
5. Describe the relevance of ADA to inclusion of young children with disabilities.
6. What characteristics serve to define *culturally competent and relevant services*?
7. Describe *family-centered intervention*.
8. How does *ecological assessment* differ from traditional assessment?
9. Discuss the myths that have been used to keep young children with severe disabilities out of inclusion environments.
10. Why is the joint position statement set forth in 2009 by DEC and NAEYC so important?
11. What are the basic requirements of a *universally designed curriculum*?
12. What is the role of the *collaboration imperative* in EI and ECSE?
13. Describe the critical components of the RTI model.
14. When and how is PBS used with young children with disabilities?
15. Describe the challenges inherent in the important transitions in infancy and early childhood.
16. Describe the elements of a *seamless system* of services delivery in ECSE.

REFERENCES

Americans with Disabilities Act (ADA) of 1990, PL 101-336, 42 U.S.C. §§ 12101 *et seq.*

Benedict, E.A., Horner, R.H., & Squires, J.K. (2007). Assessment and implementation of positive behavior support in preschools. *Topics in Early Childhood Special Education, 27*(3), 174–192.

Berk, L.E., & Winsler, A. (1995). *Scaffolding children's learning: Vygotsky and early childhood education*. Washington, DC: National Association for the Education of Young Children.

Bloom, B. (1964). *Stability and change in human characteristics*. New York, NY: Wiley.

Bronfenbrenner, U. (1979). *The ecology of human development: Experiments by nature and design*. Cambridge, MA: Harvard University Press.

Bronfenbrenner, U. (1992). Ecological systems theory. In R. Vasa (Ed.), *Six theories of child development: Revised formulations and current issues* (pp. 187–248). Philadelphia: Kingsley, PA.

Brown, L., Branston, M.B., Hamre-Nietupski, S., Pumpian, L., Certo, N., & Gruenewald, L. (1979). A strategy for developing chronological age-appropriate and function curricular content for severely handicapped adolescents and young adults. *Journal of Special Education, 13*, 81–90.

Burns, M.K., Appleton, J.J., Stehouwer, J.D. (2005). Meta-analytic review of responsiveness-to-intervention research: Examination-based and research implemented models. *Journal of Psychoeducational Assessment, 23*, 381–394.

Campbell, P., Milbourne, S., & Wilcox, M. (2008). Adaptation interventions to promote participation in natural settings. *Infants and Young Children, 21*(2), 94–106.

Carr, E.G. (1977). The motivation of self-injurious behavior: A review of some hypotheses. *Psychological Bulletin, 84*, 800–816.

Carr, E.G., & Durand, V.M. (1985). Reducing behavior problems through functional communication training. *Journal of Applied Behavior Analysis, 18*, 111–126.

CAST. (2011). *Universal Design for Learning Guidelines version 2.0*. Wakefield, MA: Author.

Coleman, M.R., Buysse, V., & Neitzel, J. (2006). *Recognition and response: An early intervening system for young children at-risk for learning disabilities*. Chapel Hill: The University of North Carolina at Chapel Hill, FPG Child Development Institute.

DEC/NAEYC. (2009). *Early childhood inclusion: A joint statement of the Division for Early Childhood (DEC) and the National Association for the Education of Young Children (NAEYC)*. Chapel Hill: The University of North Carolina at Chapel Hill, FPG Child Development Institute.

Division for Early Childhood Task Force on Recommended Practices. (1993). *DEC recommended practices: Indicators of quality in programs for infants and young children with special needs and their families*. Reston, VA: Council for Exceptional Children.

Division for Early Childhood (DEC). (1999). *Concept paper on the identification of and intervention with challenging behavior*. Reston, VA: Council for Exceptional Children.

Dunst, C.J., Johanson, C., Trivette, C., & Hamby, D. (1991). Family-oriented early intervention policies and practices: Family-centered or not? *Exceptional Children, 58*, 115–126.

Education for All Handicapped Children Act of 1975, PL 94-142, 20 U.S.C. §§ 1400 et seq.

Education of the Handicapped Act Amendments of 1986, PL 99-457, 20 U.S.C. §§ 1400 et seq.

Fox, L., Carta, J., Strain, P., Dunlap, G., & Hemmeter, M.L. (2009). *Response to intervention and the pyramid model*. Tampa, FL: University of South Florida, Technical Assistance Center on Social Emotional Intervention for Young Children.

Fox, L., Dunlap, G., Hemmeter, M.L., Joseph, G.E., and Strain, P. (2003). The teaching pyramid: A model for supporting social competence and preventing challenging behavior in young children. *Young Children, 58*(4), 48–52.

French, J.E. (2000). Itard, Jean-Marc-Gaspard. In A.E. Kazdin (Ed.), *Encyclopedia of psychology*. Oxford, UK: Oxford University Press.

Goldfarb, W. (1945). Psychological deprivation in infancy and subsequent adjustment. *American Journal of Orthopsychiatry, 15*, 247–255.

Goldfarb, W. (1949). Rorschach test differences between family-reared, institution-reared, and schizophrenic children. *American Journal of Orthopsychiatry, 19*, 624–633.

Goldfarb, W. (1955). Emotional and intellectual consequences of psychological deprivation in infancy: A re-evaluation. In P.H. Hoch & J. Zubin (Eds.), *Psychopathology of childhood* (pp. 29–44). New York, NY: Grune & Stratton.

Goodenough, F., & Maurer, K. (1961). The relative potency of the nursery school and the statistical laboratory in boosting I.Q. In J. Jenkins & D. Paterson (Eds.), *Studies in individual differences.* New York, NY: Appleton-Century-Crofts.

Hamm, E.M., Mistrett, S.G., & Ruffino, A.G. (2006). Play outcomes and satisfaction with toys and technology of young children with special needs. *Journal of Special Education Technology, 21*(1), 29–35.

Handicapped Children's Early Education Assistance Act, PL 90-538, 82 Stat. 901, 20 U.S.C. 621 §§ *et seq.*

Hanson, M.J., Gutierrez, S., Morgan, M., Brennan, E.L., & Zercher, C. (1997). Language, culture, and disability: Interacting influences in preschool inclusion. *Topics in Early Childhood Special Education, 17,* 307–331.

Hanson, M.J., Wolfberg, P., Zercher, C., Morgan, M., Gutierrez, S., Barnwell, D., & Beckman, P.J. (1998). The culture of inclusion: Recognizing diversity at multiple levels. *Early Childhood Research Quarterly, 13,* 185–209.

Hawkings, S., & Schuster, J. (2007). Using a mand-model procedure to teach preschool children initial speech sounds. *Journal of Developmental and Physical Disabilities, 19,* 65–80.

Hemmeter, M.L., Fox, L., Jack, S., & Broyles, L. (2007). A program-wide model of positive behavior support in early childhood settings. *Journal of Early Intervention, 29*(4), 337–355.

Hunt, J.M. (1961). *Intelligence and experience.* New York, NY: Ronald Press.

Improving Head Start for School Readiness Act of 2007, PL 110-134, 42 U.S.C. §§ 9801 *et seq.*

Individuals with Disabilities Education Improvement Act (IDEA) of 2004, PL 108-446, 20 U.S.C. §§ 1400 *et seq.*

Individuals with Disabilities Education Act (IDEA) of 1990, PL 101-476, 20 U.S.C. §§ 1400 *et seq.*

Individuals with Disabilities Education Act (IDEA) of 1991, PL 102-119, 20 U.S.C. §§ 1400 *et seq.*

Individuals with Disabilities Education Act (IDEA) Amendments of 1997, PL 105-17, 20 U.S.C. §§ 1400 *et seq.*

Itard, J.M.G. (1962). *The wild boy of Aveyron* (G. Humphrey & M. Humphrey, Trans.). New York, NY: Appleton-Century-Crofts.

Kaiser, A.P. (1993). Parent-implemented language intervention. In A.P. Kaiser & D.B. Gray (Eds.), *Enhancing children's communication: Vol. 2. Research foundations for intervention* (pp. 63–84). Baltimore, MD: Paul H. Brookes Publishing Co.

Kaiser, A.P. (2000). Teaching functional communication skills. In M.E. Snell & F. Brown (Eds.), *Instruction of students with severe disabilities* (5th ed., pp. 453–491). Columbus, OH: Merrill.

Kanner, L. (1967). Autistic disturbances of affective contact. *Nervous Child, 2,* 217–250.

Kirk, S. (1958). *Early education of the mentally retarded.* Urbana: University of Illinois Press.

Losardo, A., & Bricker, D. (1994). Activity-based intervention and direct instruction: A comparison study. *American Journal of Mental Retardation, 98,* 744–765.

McCormick, L., (2003). Policies and practices. In L. McCormick, D.F. Loeb, & R.L. Schiefelbusch (Eds.), *Supporting children with communication difficulties in inclusive settings: School-based language intervention* (2nd ed., pp. 155–188). Boston, MA: Allyn & Bacon.

McWilliam, R.A. (1996). *Rethinking pull-out services in early intervention: A professional resource.* Baltimore, MD: Paul H. Brookes Publishing Co.

National Center on Universal Design for Learning. (n.d.). UDL guidelines. Version 2.0. http://www.udlcenter.org/aboutudl/udlguidelines

Park, J., Turnbull, A.P., & Park, H. (2001). Quality of partnerships in service provision for Korean American parents of children with disabilities: A qualitative inquiry. *Journal of the Association for Persons with Severe Handicaps, 26,* 158–170.

Repp, A., & Horner, R.H. (Eds.) (1999). *Functional analysis of problem behavior: From effective assessment to effective support.* Belmont, CA: Wadsworth.

Sadao, K.C., & Robinson, N.B. (2010). *Assistive technology for young children.* Baltimore, MD: Paul H. Brookes Publishing Co.

Sameroff, A.J., & Chandler, M.J. (1975). Reproductive risk and the continuum of caretaking causality. In F.D. Horowitz, M. Hetherington, S. Scarr-Salapatek, & G. Siegal (Eds.), *Review of child development research* (Vol. 4, pp. 187–244). Chicago: University of Chicago Press.

Sandall, S.R., & Schwartz, I.S. (2008). *Building blocks for teaching preschoolers with special Needs.* (2nd ed.). Baltimore, MD: Paul H. Brookes Publishing Co.

Santos, R.M. (2001). Using what children know to teach them something new: Applying high-probability procedures in the classroom and at home. In M. Ostrosky & S.R. Sandall (Eds.), *Teaching strategies: What to do to support young children's development.* (Young Exceptional Children Monograph Series No. 3, pp. 71–80). Denver, CO: DEC/CEC.

Shonkoff, J.P., & Phillips, D.A. (Eds.). (2000). *From neurons to neighborhoods: The science of early childhood development.* Washington, DC: National Academy Press.

Skeels, M.H., & Dye, H. (1939). A study of the effects of differential stimulation on mentally retarded children. *Proceedings and Addresses of the American Association on Mental Deficiency, 44,* 114–136.

Spitz, R.A. (1945). Hospitalism: An inquiry into the genesis of psychiatric conditions in early childhood. *Psychoanalytic Study of the Child* (Vol. 1, pp. 53–74). New York, NY: International Universities Press.

Strain, P.S., McGee, G.G., & Kohler, G.W. (2001). Inclusion of children with autism in early intervention environments. In M.J. Guralnick (Ed.), *Early childhood inclusion* (pp. 337–363). Baltimore, MD: Paul H. Brookes Publishing Co.

Sugai, G. (2007). *Responsiveness-to-intervention: Lessons learned and to be learned.* Keynote presentation at and paper for the RTI Summit. Washington, DC: U.S. Department of Education. December.

Sugai, G., Horner, R.H., & Sprague, J. (1999). Functional assessment-based behavior support planning: Research-to-practice-to-research. *Behavioral Disorders, 24,* 223–227.

Thompson, R.A. (2001). Development in the first years of life. *The Future of Children, 11*(1), 21–33.

Thousand, J.S., & Villa, R.A. (2000). Collaborative teaming: A powerful tool in school restructuring. In R.A. Villla & J.S. Thousand (Eds.), *Restructuring for caring and effective education: Piecing the puzzle* (pp. 254–292). Baltimore, MD: Paul H. Brookes Publishing Co.

Turbiville, V.P., Turnbull, A.P., Garland, C.W., & Lee, I.M. (1996). Development and implementation of IFSPs and IEPs: Opportunities for employment. In S.L. Odom & M.E. McLean (Eds.), *Early intervention/early childhood special education: Recommended practices* (pp. 77–100). Austin, TX: PRO-ED.

Turnbull, A.P., Summers, J.A., & Brotherson, M.J. (1983). *Working with families with disabled members: A family systems approach.* Lawrence: University of Kansas Press.

Wolery, M. (2001). Embedding constant time delay procedures in classroom activities. In M. Ostrosky & S.R. Sandall (Eds.), *Teaching strategies: What to do to support young children's development.* (Young Exceptional Children Monograph Series No. 3, pp. 81–90). Denver, CO: DEC/CEC.

2

Culture, Teaming, and Partnerships

Linda McCormick

••••••••••••••••• **FOCUS OF THIS CHAPTER** •••••••••••••••••

- Definition and practices inherent in cross-cultural competence
- Cultural values in parenting
- Cultural values of professional fields
- Culturally appropriate intervention practices
- Partnerships with parents and other family members
- Partnerships with other professionals
- Teaming as both a process and an outcome

As the United States has become more heterogeneous, cross-cultural effectiveness has become an essential skill for all persons who work with infants, young children, and families: neonatal intensive care nurses, social workers, physicians, child care providers, educators, psychologists, physical therapists, occupational therapists, speech-language pathologists, and aides (Lynch & Hanson, 2004). Cross-cultural competence—learning to think, feel, and act in ways that acknowledge, respect, and incorporate ethnic, cultural, and linguistic diversity—is a goal that requires a commitment to personal openness and self-reflection. It entails a willingness to set aside held beliefs in favor of alternative perspectives.

CROSS-CULTURAL COMPETENCE

At the broadest level, culture is a framework that guides and provides boundaries for life practices. It includes differences in economic status, sexual orientation, gender, and lifestyle as well as ethnic, racial, and linguistic differences. The beliefs, values, and attitudes that are learned by young children through socialization are the core of culture. These vary depending upon sociocultural factors such as child-rearing practices, family traditions, sociolinguistic patterns, familial economic status, a family's immigration status and experience, and the length of a family's presence in the United States. Membership in a particular cultural group does not determine behavior, but it does make some types of behavior more probable than others, because members of a common culture typically have similar responses to behaviors and tend to interpret events in similar ways.

Cultural values and personal beliefs are more than just the background for one's relationships with others—they are the central operating system. Acknowledging this is critical, because these values and beliefs have the potential to overshadow efforts to alter our behavior or influence our practices (Harry, 1998). Not only do cultural beliefs, values, and attitudes impact all aspects of our daily behavior, they become yardsticks against which the behaviors and attitudes of others are judged.

Cultural diversity in the United States grows each year. By 2030, the non-Hispanic white population will be in the minority of the U.S. population under the age of 18 (U.S. Department of Education, 1999). There was a time when the United States was considered to be a melting pot, where people from different cultures and countries could forge a new and homogeneous society. More recently—at least since the 1980s—the melting pot metaphor has been replaced by a pluralistic view that recognizes and values the differences and contributions of every cultural group.

Cultural and ethnic diversity is nowhere more apparent than with the children and families served in early intervention (EI) services, early childhood special education (ECSE) settings, and other community programs. Unfortunately, in most states that diversity is not reflected among the professionals working in these programs or in the associated student populations. Challenges surrounding cultural diversity compound the potential for relationship difficulties and conflicts. The only way to address this issue is for both preservice students and personnel to work toward cross-cultural competence. Cross-cultural competence is thinking, feeling, and acting in ways that acknowledge, respect, and build on ethnic, cultural, and linguistic diversity. Achieving cross-cultural competence is not an endpoint so much as it is a process.

The first stage in the process is understanding and acknowledging the significance of culture and membership in a cultural group, the beliefs and practices of different cultures, and the difficulties inherent in immigration and acculturation (Lynch & Hanson, 2004). Cultures can be grouped generally as either individualistic or collectivist, and the difference is often reflected in the communication style of its members. Individualistic cultures have a low-context communication style while collectivist cultures have high-context styles. Low-context cultures such as Northern European and Anglo-American cultures focus on direct and precise communication, leading them to include as much verbal information as possible when they communicate. In contrast, high-context cultures such as Asian, Native American, Arab, Latino, and African American cultures rely more heavily on the context of the interaction (nonverbal cues) to convey meaning.

The second stage in the course of achieving cross-cultural competence, after acknowledging the significance of culture, is learning to 1) relate and communicate effectively with individuals who do not share one's ethnicity, culture, language, or other salient variables (Hanson, 2004), and 2) respect each family's values, traditions, and beliefs regarding child rearing and development, communication and decision-making styles, and views on receiving assistance from people outside the family. Once one acknowledges the fact that ethnic, cultural, and/or linguistic diversity are an asset, the challenge is to translate this respect and understanding into actions that create and maintain a supportive and sensitive environment. Understanding the differences in communication style noted above is one example of an especially important knowledge base that helps professionals relate to and build rapport with families.

Recommended practices of the Division for Early Childhood (DEC) of the Council for Exceptional Children (CEC) emphasize the importance of preparing professionals to work effectively with diverse families in both didactic program content and through field-based experiences. Primary goals of preservice and in-service cross-cultural curricula are to bring EI and ECSE service providers to the point of 1) feeling comfortable and effective in their interactions and relationships with families whose cultures and life experiences differ from their own, 2) knowing how to interact in ways that enable families from different cultures and life experiences to feel positive about the interactions and the interventionists, and 3) being able to develop and accomplish goals in partnership with the family they serve. These require a broad conceptual framework that goes beyond the needs of specific cultural groups.

A broad conceptual framework focuses on helping people avoid stereotyping and deal with the infinite range of differences both within and among cultural groups. The three essential components of preparation for cross-cultural competence are 1) self-examination and values clarification; 2) general knowledge of the values, beliefs, and behaviors that may be encountered in cross-cultural interactions; and 3) ability to apply principles of effective cross-cultural communication, both verbal and nonverbal, at interpersonal and systems levels (Lynch, 2011).

Cultural Values in Parenting

Parents bring their heritage, experiences, personalities, talents, skills, values, and beliefs to all interactions in EI/ECSE environments. Beliefs about parenting are culturally embedded. Family-centered practices support the ability of parents to facilitate their child's learning and development within the parameters of the family's cultural, religious, and familial traditions. The defining characteristics of family-centered practices are cultural and socioeconomic sensitivity, individualization in accord with family priorities and concerns, transparency in decision making, assistance in accessing community resources, and empowerment (Dunst, 1997).

How should (or how can) professionals respond when families' perspectives and visions of their children's social pathways differ from the state of the art in the field of special education? This was the key question that a 4-year study by Harry (1998) sought to answer. She examined the role of culture and social class on the social pathways established by seven culturally diverse families for their children with disabilities. At the beginning of the study, when parents noted that what they wanted for their children was a normal life, Harry assumed that what they wanted for their children essentially paralleled the values espoused by the field of special education. She thought that the families were saying that they wanted their children to have "lives that mirrored those of typically developing children, including concepts such as choice, friendship, independence, and equality of opportunity" (Harry, 1998, p. 58).

Over the 4 years of the study, Harry became convinced that she had been mistaken. In fact she noted major discrepancies between the parents' visions of a normal life for their children and the values espoused by the field of special education. The parents' visions for their children (those with and those without disabilities) had to be understood through their cultural background, their acculturation to new contexts, and their socioeconomic status. Parents viewed the friendships of their children as evolving more within the family than with peers outside the family circle (the typical Anglo-American vision). Personal choice did not rank highly as a value for any family member, and it was even less high for the child with a disability. Sometimes parents' visions for their children with disabilities were based on different assumptions than those held for their other children. Parents valued equality of opportunity for their children without disabilities, but generally they valued it less for their child with a disability. Independence did not mean a life apart from the family—for their typically developing children and, especially, for the child with a disability.

The children in Harry's study ranged in age from 8 to 18. The families were Indian (from Central America), Caucasian (from Palestine), African Caribbean (from Trinidad), African American, and American Chinese/Caucasian. It is interesting to compare her findings with those of Denney et al. (2001), who considered the beliefs and goals of Mexican families whose infants were in the neonatal intensive care units of two hospitals. Denney et al. were especially interested in the families' views about caregiving and development for their infants with prematurity, low birth weight, and/or intensive health care needs. What they learned was that the Mexican families were extremely frustrated by the practices of the hospitals. They complained that hospital practices were inappropriate and that they did not get enough information about how to care for their infants. The source of the latter problem was readily identified: information was not available because the physicians and nurses were not bilingual and access to translators was limited. The hospital caregiving procedures that concerned the Mexican families were 1) leaving infants fully exposed and unswaddled in their cribs (the reason for this was that physicians and nurses need to have quick access to intravenous catheters, ventilators, and monitoring equipment), and 2) giving mothers cold liquids and foods after birth. Based on their family beliefs and traditions in Mexico, parents believed that newborn babies should be dressed warmly, wrapped, and covered with blankets and that leaving babies unswaddled placed them at risk for illness. They believed that cold foods and liquids decreased the mother's ability to produce breast milk. These findings highlight the impact of communication difficulties. Limited access to translators contributed to lack of information, which in turn led to concerns about the appropriateness of the hospital procedures.

One can also learn several important facets about cross-cultural competency from this study. First is the importance of ensuring that parents have regular access to information (in their language) about the ongoing medical status and caregiving needs of their children. Second is the importance of professionals learning as much as possible about the cultural values and socialization practices of the ethnically and linguistically diverse families they serve. Whenever possible, caregiving practices that differ from those of the family should be modified, or, if modifications are not possible, families should be given a thorough explanation of the reasons for the practices. Finally, families must have an opportunity to say whom they want included in making treatment decisions and what they need in terms of training for the infant's homecare (Hanson, 2004).

Trusting relationships will develop if service providers embrace diversity and are open to and accepting of different opinions and beliefs. Family preferences must guide the course of relationships with professionals (e.g., Denney et al., 2001; Harry, 1998). Each family system is unique. Some families will have an extended base of support while others will include only the immediate family and depend on external support networks, such as neighbors.

Cultural Values of Professional Fields

Culture can be envisioned as a multitiered structure with macro- and microlevels (Banks 1997a, 1997b). The national culture of the United States is an overarching framework at the macro level. At the microlevel there are many ethnic cultures, subsocieties, and institutions. Microcultural groups participate to varying degrees in the macroculture, while retaining varying amounts of their separate cultural traditions. All individuals have characteristics of various different cultures: their macroculture (their country), their original or primary microculture (their family), as well as the other microcultural groups to which they belong. Thus, in addition to factors such as race, ethnicity, nationality, language, social class, and geographical location, each person's identity incorporates the beliefs and values of his or her professional or personal interest groups (Harry, 2002). This is something that people often fail to recognize. They readily recognize and cite their macroculture and their primary microcultural affiliations (the race, ethnicity, nationality, language, social status, and geographical location with which they identify), but they do not think of the variety of professional and interest groups to which they belong (parents, musicians, golfers, teachers, nurses, and so forth) as cultures. Some professional and interest groups have specific and well-defined beliefs and practices; others have only implicit beliefs and values.

As a professional microculture, special education has a profound impact on its members' cultural identity and, in turn, the interactions that they have with others (Kalyanpur & Harry, 2012). It is essential for professionals to recognize and understand professional acculturation, how it occurs, and its potential influences on the ability to appreciate and be open to the values of others (other professionals as well as families).

Personnel preparation programs (in all disciplines) explicitly teach the policies and practices of their field in much the same way as families teach their culture to their children (Skrtic, 1991, 1995). Professional acculturation is, of course, more formal and structured than child enculturation. For example, when students in the field of special education demonstrate that they have internalized the policies and practices of the discipline, they are certified as competent by their program and their institute of higher education and licensed to teach.

During the professional preparation period, the beliefs and values underlying the policies and practices of the field are not made explicit. However, they are embedded in assigned readings and class lectures or discussions. Over the course of professional preparation, these beliefs or core values become inculcated in or taken for granted by students to the extent that they are experienced as "the natural order of things" (Bowers, 1984, p. 36). Instead of being critically examined and reflected on throughout this period and continuously thereafter, they come to be accepted as the way things are intended to be.

The core values of the cultural foundation of special education policy and professional knowledge are *individualism*, *choice*, and *equity* (Kalyanpur & Harry, 2012). These core values are not difficult to identify as they are reflected in the six basic principles of the Individuals with Disabilities Education Act (IDEA) of 1990 (PL 101-476): zero rejection, nondiscriminatory assessment, free appropriate public education, least restrictive environment (LRE), due process, and parent participation.

The next consideration is the beliefs underlying the core values, and finally, what effect these values have on working with families. The belief underlying individualism is that all children have the right to a meaningful education that is appropriate to their abilities. The assumption is that an education will maximize each child's potential to get a job and become an independent, productive adult. This assumption is most apparent in the due process requirement of IDEA, which states that children with disabilities have the right to protection under the law. Parents of children with disabilities must be told their rights specific to their child's education. The belief underlying the core value of choice is that everyone has the right to the pursuit of happiness and to choose how they want to attain it. In IDEA, the right to choice is most evident in the principles of LRE and parent participation. The belief underlying the core value of equity is reflected in three of the basic principles of IDEA: zero rejection, nondiscriminatory assessment, and parent participation.

Beliefs determine core values and, in turn, values affect legislation and practice. As noted above, the core values are rarely stated explicitly, but they are inculcated in the course of the professional preparation program. Over time they come to be taken for granted as the natural order of things and are assumed to be universal values. When families and professionals share the same values, problems are minimized. When there is a common frame of reference, relationships have a high probability of being harmonious with minimal dissonance and generally straightforward communication. What many do not realize, however, is that these core values—individualism, choice, and equity—are not universal values. Some cultures in our multicultural society (and thus in our classrooms and early intervention programs) have very different concepts of self, choice, equity, and status.

It is useful to consider some examples of the disparity between the core values and defining features of special education and the values of other cultures (Kalyanpur & Harry, 2012). For example, the concept of individualism, which means that the individual (not society) comes first, is antithetical to the beliefs of most Asian American families. Of course, there is considerable diversity across the 28 different Asian groups in the United States (Asian American Heritage, 1995), but even taking that considerable diversity into consideration, most members of Asian American communities share a subset of common values. They are often troubled and confused by the belief in individual rights that underlies many Western cultures and, more specifically, special education policy and practices. It is contrary to their beliefs in 1) group orientation, 2) strong family ties, 3) emphasis on education, and 4) respect for authority and the elderly. Traditional Asian families place more value on the family unit than on the individual. Individual needs are considered to be subservient to those of the family and the community. Many Asian families consider harmonious interpersonal relationships, interdependence, and mutual obligations or loyalty essential for peaceful coexistence with family and others.

Where the Asian community is concerned, people have duties and responsibilities, not rights. Thus, it is easy to understand why Asian families, particularly those who have immigrated to the United States, may have difficulty with the concept of individualism and, hence, with claiming their child's right to an appropriate education. Even when made aware of their rights, they may not choose to be assertive in claiming them or accept the importance of protest when their child's rights are violated (Dentler & Hafner, 1997).

The concept of choice is also perplexing to many Asians. This value is baffling because some societies do not believe in allowing individuals freedom of choice in all matters. For example, some cultural groups do not believe that their adolescent children should choose their own friends, their occupations, or their marriage partners. Families from these cultures are mystified by the array of special education programs and service options for their children with disabilities.

Equity, the third core value of special education policy and practices, is as ingrained in the American collective conscience as individualism and choice. Here again, difficult as it is for many to accept and understand, equity is not a universal value. Some cultures believe that human beings are inherently unequal by reason of birth, caste, skin pigmentation, and economic and social status (Miles & Miles, 1993). They accept that some people should dominate others because of their backgrounds and status (e.g., education, age). There are traditions and expectations in these cultures to prevent the abuse of power in hierarchical structures. Those in more privileged positions are expected to fulfill certain obligations toward those who are less privileged. Families in these cultures expect professionals to protect, assist, and support their clients or students because the professionals have higher status. They find it difficult if not impossible to view themselves as equals and partners with professionals in making educational decisions (Kalyanpur & Harry, 2012).

Other families (e.g., African American parents) have different reasons for not feeling comfortable participating in decision making with professionals. Their own negative experiences in educational settings lead them to view the power dynamics between themselves and educational professionals as inherently unequal. The silence of these parents should not be taken as consent. Silence could have any number of meanings: for example, that the parents 1) do not expect their contributions to be respected, 2) view compliance and deferring to authority as the only way to get along, and/or 3) do not agree with what is occurring.

Cross-cultural competence begins with awareness and with questioning the influence that the assumptions of our field have on our beliefs and our practices. If not acknowledged and well understood, the values that underlie special education policies and practices and professional knowledge can contribute to difficulties in interactions with families. Cross-cultural competence is a lifelong goal that one only begins working toward during professional preparation. It is a basic skill set essential for partnerships with other teachers (co-teaching and itinerant consultation) and with parents.

Culturally Appropriate Intervention Practices

Cross-cultural competence is important in every phase of the intervention process: beginning with a family-professional exchange of information and planning for assessment. The following discussion and guidelines for conducting this process in a culturally sensitive manner draw from the fourth edition of a comprehensive reference and definitive resource on this subject—*Developing Cross-Cultural Competence* (2011), edited by Lynch and Hanson. The volume's authors provide the following guidelines for making this first step culturally appropriate in the process—establishing family-professional collaboration and assessment planning:

- Learn as much as possible about the ethnic and cultural groups represented in the community (e.g., languages and cultural values associated with child-rearing practices, health and healing, disability); the roles of community leaders and/or spiritual leaders in advising and counseling families; and the extent of cultural identification within the community at large. Keep in mind that the amount of exposure families have to different cultural groups may lead to mixing cultural practices.

- Learn some words and greetings in the families' language if families are English-language learners and ensure that trained interpreters are present for all assessments and meetings.

- Allow adequate time with interpreters to build rapport and determine families' concerns, priorities, and resources. Recognize that initially some families may not be comfortable with the amount of involvement expected in intervention programs in the United States.

- Minimize the use of written forms with families who are English-language learners or non-English speaking. Forms (in the family's language) should not be presented until the family signals readiness to participate in completing them.

- Recognize that many families experience power differentials between themselves and agency representatives and the effect of a perception of differential power on participation and decision making.

The second step in the intervention process, data gathering and assessment, presents the greatest challenge in terms of avoiding cultural bias. The vast majority of available assessment instruments are designed for English-speaking children and families who belong to the dominant culture in the United States. Children and families with other life experiences may not have been exposed to certain concepts reflected on these tests or had the opportunity to practice the required behaviors. Thus tests with mainstream U.S. norms may not give a true picture of the child's performance and potential. Lynch and Hanson (1993) cite the example of a young child whose family had recently moved to California from Samoa. During the initial assessment session in the EI program the child was clumsy and seemed delayed in motor development. However, when observed in his home, which was furnished with mats and low furniture like a traditional Samoan home, the child moved freely and functionally. It was obvious that the child had never moved around in a setting with the types of objects found in most homes and in the EI setting.

The interview process may be inappropriate for some families, even with a trained interpreter. Even professionals with the best of intentions in terms of sensitivity may find that family members are uncomfortable with the manner in which the interview is conducted as well as with the questions (e.g., about marital relationships). In another example, Lynch and Hanson (1993) describe a mother who told the interpreter that she was very uncomfortable and embarrassed when asked questions about her child's disability and service needs. She said that it reflected badly on her to have a child with a disability and she could not talk about service needs because that is the job of the professionals. The following guidelines can make data gathering and assessment more responsive and sensitive for families from diverse cultures:

- Select assessment instruments appropriate for the language and culture of the child and family.

- Work with a trained interpreter who can interpret cultural cues as well as language.

- Arrange assessment at a time when all the people important to the family can be present and conduct it in a setting where the family will be comfortable.

- Limit the number of assessors and the numbers of forms, questionnaires, and other types of paperwork.

- Explain every step in the process and its purpose as many times and in as many different ways as possible.

The third step in the intervention process is planning. The intervention will be effective only to the extent to which the people involved actually buy in at the planning stage. Participation and statement of the family's point of view may be very different for families from other cultures or families from sociocultural groups other than the mainstream. Some families may consider following the teacher's suggestions and making no demands to be active participants. In contrast, active participation for other families may include conducting research on recommended practices, asking questions, and constantly advocating for their child's needs. Incorporating the following guidelines will make planning more culturally responsive:

- Prepare the family by describing how the meeting will be conducted, its purpose, and who will be present.
- Limit the number of professionals present but encourage families to bring the people who are important to them (relatives, spiritual leaders, friends, and so forth).
- Make the meeting as comfortable as possible for the family by including practices that they consider culturally appropriate for meetings—serving tea, taking time to get socialized before beginning, and conducting the meeting in a formal manner.
- Encourage family input but be very careful not to embarrass the family by pressing them for perspectives.
- Confirm that the goals, objectives, and desired outcomes in the plan reflect the family's values and beliefs as well as their concerns and priorities for their child.

The fourth step is to put the plan into action. The likelihood of successful implementation of the intervention plan is maximized if professionals have used cultural- and family-specific information and worked closely with cultural guides and other care providers who are important to the family. The following guidelines should be kept in mind when implementing the intervention program:

- Ensure that the proposed goals and outcomes are the family's priorities.
- Clarify the family's definition of involvement and then make every effort to involve family members to the extent that they want to be involved in all aspects of the program.
- Provide continuous information to family members about the program and the child's progress.
- Invite the participation and advice of the cultural communities' leaders through advisory boards, roundtables, and councils.

The last step in the process is evaluation conducted to determine whether 1) the intervention objectives have been accomplished, 2) family members are satisfied with the outcomes, and 3) all services have been culturally appropriate, sensitive, and cost-effective. Broad guidelines to keep in mind include the following:

- Examine timelines and conditions associated with the child's progress to identify practices that need revision as well as those that are effective.
- Use interviews, short questionnaires in the families' language, and parent-led focus groups to get a clear idea of what the families and members of involved community agencies think of the program.
- Maintain logs of staff-development activities and new initiatives and revisit and assess program and/or agency progress on at least an annual basis.

As noted, this discussion of culturally appropriate intervention practices has drawn heavily from Lynch and Hanson (2011). They caution that skills and information are only the beginning of the path toward cultural competence. However, they are a good beginning. The impact of cultural diversity on services for young children and their families (whether or not the children have disabilities) has been well established. The more professionals learn about their own attitudes, values, and beliefs and how to provide culturally responsive practices, the better their ability to ensure a positive impact.

PARTNERSHIPS

Partnership is a vehicle through which people can relate to each other. Professional and parental partners may differ in some aspects of their relationship, but their core objectives are the same, and there is agreement that desired outcomes cannot be achieved by working alone. The essential features of a partnership are trust, transparency, and mutual accountability. The values and beliefs inherent in cross-cultural competence are enormously important in partnerships. Cross-cultural competence is requisite to true partnerships and collaboration, which in turn affect the success of all aspects of EI and ECSE. Service providers must be as committed to establishing and maintaining partnerships as to acquiring the knowledge and skills for child assessment, intervention, instruction, and program evaluation.

Partnerships with Parents and Other Family Members

The adults who know the child best are his or her parents and other family members. Services and supports for infants and young children differ from those for older children in several ways, most notably the emphasis on active involvement of family members. A key element of a family-centered approach and the collaborative team model (described in the following pages) is forming partnerships with families and working collaboratively with them to mobilize needed resources and supports and guide development and implementation of an individualized educational program. A review of the research literature on family-centered help-giving practices identified the following key elements in effective partnerships: 1) treating parents with dignity and respect, 2) sharing information to support informed decision making, and 3) providing choices to parents regarding their roles and desired services (Dunst, Trivette, & Hamby, 2007). The positive outcomes of these practices included improvements in parenting skills and in parents' sense of well-being, overall satisfaction with services and supports, feelings of competence, and judgments of their child's behaviors.

Research on parent-professional partnerships has studied the perspectives of both the parents and the service providers (e.g., Dinnebeil, Hale, & Rule, 1996; Park, Turnbull, & Park, 2001). High-quality partnerships are characterized by 1) good communication skills, 2) facilitative interpersonal factors, 3) professional expertise, and 4) practice of certain values and attitudes. The survey that generated this information asked 1,400 parents and service coordinators to describe the variables that the other person in the partnership brings to the relationship that either enhance or interfere with collaboration. The same communication and group-process skills that apply to collaborative team interactions apply to partnerships with parents. Most notably, these include good listening skills, openness to suggestions, and responsiveness. In successful partnerships, the two sides communicate openly and honestly about where they stand and how they feel. They listen to understand, not just to hear. Ideas and feelings are shared in an atmosphere of nonjudgmental acceptance. Facilitative interpersonal factors, the second characteristic of high-quality partnerships, are defined as honesty, tact, and the ability to establish a positive atmosphere. Interpersonal courtesies such as keeping appointments, being on time, being organized and prepared, and following through were also highly valued (Dinnebeil et al., 1996).

Respondents referred to professional expertise as "expert power." It is the extent to which a person is perceived as having the specialized knowledge necessary to perform a task or achieve a goal. A study by Park, Turnbull, and Park (2001) of partnerships between professionals and Korean American parents reported a similar finding. Parents appreciated professionals with good teaching skills, knowledge about planning for their children's future, and resourcefulness. They wanted professionals to encourage their children's potential and not emphasize what their children could not do. Most highly valued were professionals who were skilled at teaching academics and at decreasing challenging behaviors and who could teach parents how to help their children catch up academically. Thus, although a professional may be caring, committed, and enthusiastic, he or she is not viewed as an effective collaborator unless parents perceive the individual to be knowledgeable and competent in his or her field. Where values and beliefs are concerned, parents considered it essential for service providers to hold *and practice* a belief in family-centered practices. Professionals must be willing to carry through on commitments as well as to provide assistance with regard to family-centered practices.

Partnerships with Other Professionals

Partnerships are important because of the complex needs of infants and young children with disabilities and their families. No one person (infant specialist, ECSE teacher, early childhood education [ECE] teacher, parent, therapist, or physician) and no one discipline has an adequate knowledge base and a sufficient skill set to meet all of these needs singlehandedly. Inclusive programs that do not survive over time are marked by partnership difficulties—what Peck, Furman, and Helmstetter (1993, p.105) described as "acrimonious professional relationships" and "struggles over control of time, activities, and programs for individual children" (p. 197).

Partnership problems occur when professionals have significant philosophical differences with others and lack skills for effective negotiation and collaboration. Differences in philosophical perspectives (theoretical beliefs and practices) were once thought to be the sole source of conflicts between ECE teachers and ECSE professionals. Their major conflicts were thought to arise from basic differences in the philosophical underpinnings and, hence, the practices of the two fields. Most ECE teachers believe that children *discover* principles and *construct* knowledge and meaning from their own experiences in their environments (Bredekamp & Copple, 1997). They view their role as facilitating and guiding children through the discovery and construction processes. In contrast, ECSE teachers have traditionally focused on arranging the environment and providing direct instruction to ensure that children learn and then practice newly acquired skills.

Two studies contributed to a reexamination of ideas about observed conflicts between ECE and ECSE teachers. Apparently, the conflicts did not arise from either philosophical differences or disagreements about practices and procedures (Kilgo et al., 1999). Teachers in inclusive situations who were surveyed by Minke, Bear, Deemer, and Griffin (1996) minimized the importance of similar philosophies and practices. They attributed daily conflicts and dissatisfaction to lack of a "shared work ethic." They viewed mutual respect, affection, trust, and cooperation as the most important requirements for successful partnerships. The difficulties that plague relationships between ECE teachers and ECSE teachers are also evident in interactions with other professionals (e.g., audiologists, nurses, nutritionists, physicians, occupational therapists, family therapists, physical therapists, psychologists, social workers, speech-language pathologists). Interactions sometimes become tense, antagonistic, and even explosive. Differing philosophical perspectives undoubtedly play some role in these relationship difficulties. Professionals trained in a traditional medical perspective tend to focus on providing individual therapy with an emphasis on remediation of identified deficits. Their goal is to diagnose a child's difficulties, prescribe a remedy, and then work to fix the problem. In contrast, ECSE teachers have been acculturated in an educational model. Their goals derive from family preferences and the functional needs and desires of the children (Sandall, Hemmeter, Smith, & McLean, 2005). The focus is on maximizing opportunities for optimum growth and development and maintaining extant skills and abilities because many of the problems of infants and young children with disabilities cannot be "fixed."

Co-teaching is a service-delivery option in which two professionals, such as a special educator and a general educator, jointly provide instruction to a diverse, blended group of children in a shared classroom. The strength of the teachers' relationship is key to meeting the diverse social and instructional needs of all students. There is a growing knowledge base supporting this approach as a way to increase the participation of children with disabilities in general education classrooms (Friend & Hurley-Chamberlain, 2008; Kloo & Zigmond, 2008). Collaboration plays a more central role in co-teaching than in consultation and teaming, because the teachers' relationship is pervasive and intense. Co-teachers work together to plan the curriculum, teach the lessons, manage the classroom, and evaluate children's progress and the effectiveness of instruction. In these classrooms one hears not the terms "your children" or "my children" but rather "our children."

Co-teaching may take many different forms in a single day. Friend and Cook (2007) described five possible formats: 1) one teaching, one supporting; 2) station teaching; 3) parallel teaching; 4) alternative teaching; and 5) team teaching. In the *one teaching, one supporting* approach, one teacher has primary responsibility for designing and delivering the lesson to the whole class. The second teacher supports the lead teacher by observing designated children or moving around the room and providing assistance to those children who need it. In the *station teaching* approach, there is a clear division of instructional responsibilities. The teachers plan together. Each is then responsible for delivering part of the lesson to the whole class. The teachers also plan together in the *parallel teaching* approach. The class is divided into two heterogeneous groups, and each teacher delivers instruction to one of the groups. In the *alternative teaching* approach, one teacher provides extra practice or reteaches a specific skill or concept to a small group of children while the other teacher instructs a larger group of children in some concepts or activities that the small group can afford to miss. One advantage of this approach is that it gives all children opportunities to interact with a teacher in a small group. Group composition is varied on a regular basis to avoid the stigma of children with disabilities always being in the small group. Finally, in *team teaching* the teachers plan and jointly teach all of the children. They do not divide the lesson between them or separate the children into groups.

The itinerant teacher model is similar to the co-teaching model in that it relies heavily on collaboration. In the itinerant model, early childhood special educators function in many capacities, providing direct and indirect services to young children with disabilities in a variety of early childhood settings, traveling from site to site. Direct service entails working with one or more children to address specific individualized education program (IEP) objectives and help them join in classroom routines. Consultation involves collaborating with ECE classroom staff to plan and use strategies that address children's IEP objectives in the context of classroom routines and activities and help to make whatever environmental adaptations are necessary for children's access to and participation in the curriculum. The itinerant teacher also models specific teaching strategies and collaborates to facilitate development in the areas of social and communication skills. The roles of the itinerant consultant in community child care settings are similar to those in preschool classrooms. ECSE teachers are coaches, assessors, team members, and service coordinators.

TEAMING

Infants and young children with disabilities, particularly those with multiple disabilities, need the services of a diverse group of individuals with expertise in varying disciplines. There is no way that one or two service providers and/or disciplines can possibly meet their varied physical, medical, educational, and social-emotional challenges. Collaboration is therefore essential, and it is both a process and an outcome. At the most basic level, collaboration is sharing 1) information, knowledge, and skills; 2) classroom and/or center space; 3) ideas and creativity; 4) resources (e.g., time, materials, equipment); and, most important, 5) responsibilities. Learning to collaborate and function as a team takes a great deal of work, skill, commitment, and perseverance. An integrated team approach provides a context for collaboration. Teaming is a way to use the collective knowledge and expertise and improve the efficiency of a diverse group of individuals with different perspectives and different skill sets. It is essentially a mindset in which people truly believe that sharing and cooperating with one another enriches their decision-making potential and maximizes their effectiveness.

Part C of IDEA reinforces the importance of moving away from isolated, discipline-specific interventions to collaboration as part of an integrated team-based approach. The legislation explicitly states that service providers are to 1) consult with parents, others service providers, and representatives of appropriate community agencies regarding provision of services; 2) train parents and others regarding provision of services; and 3) participate in assessment and development of integrated goals and objectives for an individualized family service plan (IFSP).

How team members will coordinate, communicate, and make decisions is a function of the team model or framework they adopt. Traditionally, the three team models most often employed in early intervention and special education settings were the *multidisciplinary model*, the *interdisciplinary model*, and the *transdisciplinary model* (McCormick & Goldman, 1979). A fourth model, the *collaborative team model* (sometimes called the cooperative team model), combines the best features of the other three.

The multidisciplinary model is most often seen in medical settings. Professionals of different disciplines implement their respective discipline functions with minimal—if any—coordination, collaboration, or communication with one another. Professionals assess and attempt to remediate those aspects of the child's needs that fall within their disciplines' unique province (occupational therapy, physical therapy, speech–language pathology, and so on). This model has individual accountability but little, if any, sharing of information, joint planning, or team accountability.

The interdisciplinary model evolved in response to dissatisfaction with the lack of communication and the fragmented services in teams functioning with the multidisciplinary model. With the interdisciplinary model, communication occurs across disciplines: Professionals usually develop joint intervention goals and a unified intervention plan. A problem with this model lies in implementing the intervention recommendations. The recommendations are given to the person responsible for providing direct services, but they do not include a feedback loop. Information flows one way; there is no provision for monitoring and, if necessary, modifying the intervention recommendations if they do not prove to be practical and effective.

The transdisciplinary model came to be preferred over the interdisciplinary model because it provides a framework for professionals to share information and skills with one another and with the family (McWilliam, 2000; Sandall et al., 2005). The important characteristics of this model are joint functioning, continual staff development, and role release (Lyon & Lyon, 1980). *Joint functioning* means that whenever possible, team members perform required services together. Arena assessment is an example of joint functioning (Wolery & Dyk, 1984). In arena assessment, one person designated as assessment facilitator engages the child in specific activities while other team members observe and record their assessment of the child's performance. *Continuous staff development* means that team members help one another learn new skills. This emphasis on continual opportunities for skill development is particularly important: It means that team members are always learning new skills. *Role release* occurs when professionals on the team assist the direct service provider in performing a function that is typically part of the assisting team member's role. For instance, a speech therapist might help a teacher practice several of the children's therapy goals (e.g., asking and answering "wh" questions, using three-word sentences) at sharing time in morning circle.

The collaborative team model incorporates the best features of the transdisciplinary model (Thousand & Villa, 2000). Collaborative teams in EI/ECSE settings include service providers, family members, and members of relevant community agencies. Similar to the transdisciplinary model, there is joint functioning, continuous staff development, and role release, which means that in the course of working, team members acquire a shared understanding and knowledge of each other's expertise. Rather than each discipline specialist addressing his or her specific developmental domain (e.g., language, motor), the team works to design an integrated intervention. Rather than episodic and time-limited interventions (e.g., therapy in therapy rooms) this approach pools and integrates the expertise of team members. It acknowledges the integration of development across domains and maximizes the contributions of the discipline representatives who have expertise in the separate domains. The designated service provider relies on the other team members for consultation and support in implementing the plan.

The most critical competency for the collaborative team process is communication skills (Thousand & Villa, 2000). The two types of communication skills are 1) task-oriented skills and 2) relationship-oriented skills. Task-oriented skills include the ability to

- Clearly identify and define the problem at hand
- Determine potential strengths in the situation
- Keep an open mind to alternative solutions
- Develop appropriate goals and objectives
- Search for and analyze relevant information from different sources
- Interpret and clarify planning and implementation issues
- Combine and summarize related constructs and ideas
- Elicit input and consensus from others

Task-oriented communication skills facilitate problem solving and decision making. They are focused on clarifying problems and generating solutions. In contrast, relationship-oriented skills involve interpersonal communication competencies. They assist cooperation and collaboration. Relationship-oriented skills include the ability to

- Stimulate the participation of others
- Reconcile opposing positions in a positive manner
- Compromise for the sake of productive discussion

- View differences as negotiable
- Solicit and make use of feedback
- Clarify perceptions and feelings
- Communicate understanding and acceptance of the opinions of others
- Translate technical concepts into understandable terms
- Communicate accessibility, responsiveness, and honest concern
- Establish an atmosphere of trust, respect, and acceptance

There are many barriers to effective communication. Perhaps the greatest is talking too much rather than listening. Other barriers include not paying attention, giving advice too emphatically, making abrupt topic shifts, and asking unrelated questions. Positive communication is facilitated by facing the speaker with arms open and relaxed, mirroring the speaker's affect and movements, and smiling and nodding to acknowledge what is being said.

The barriers to effective collaboration at the interagency level are essentially the same as at the program level. They include 1) competitiveness, 2) parochial interests, 3) lack of communication skills, 4) resistance to change, 5) concerns about confidentiality, 6) inadequate knowledge about other agencies and programs, 7) negative attitudes, and 8) political naiveté.

Doing things "the way we've always done them" is always easier than trying new solutions, but the price an agency or a program-level team pays for this attitude may be high in terms of collaboration.

SUMMARY

This chapter has provided an introduction to three areas that embrace fundamental beliefs and values in the field of EI/ECSE: 1) cross-cultural competence; 2) partnerships with parents and other professionals, and 3) teaming. These concepts and practices are at the very core of recommended practices in the field and are essential to the delivery of high-quality services to infants and young children and their families. Cultural diversity and cross-cultural competence were considered from the perspective of working with families. Cultural diversity is incorporated in the other chapters of this text from the perspective of the child, with emphasis on environmental arrangements and instructional approaches for children from culturally and linguistically diverse backgrounds. Certainly, collaboration and teamwork are often challenging, but the skills that promote effective communication and build interpersonal connections can be learned.

•••••••••••••••••••• **STUDY QUESTIONS** ••••••••••••••••••••

1. Discuss the elements of culture, including how it is learned and how it affects behavior.

2. What are some ways to address the differences in background, race, and ethnicity between professionals and the families they serve?

3. What can professionals learn from the findings of Harry's (1998) study, which examined differences between parents' visions for their children and the values espoused by the field of special education?

4. Discuss the cultural underpinnings of the field of special education and the potential effect of these core values on interactions with families.

5. What characteristics would we expect to see in a teacher or other service provider who has cross-cultural competence?

6. Describe strategies to make data gathering, assessment, planning, and intervention more responsive and sensitive to families from diverse cultures.

7. What are some characteristics of effective parent–professional partnerships?

8. Enumerate and discuss difficulties that have the potential to disrupt professional relationships in EI and ECSE and how they can be addressed.

9. Describe and contrast key characteristics of the co-teaching model and the itinerant teacher model.

10. Describe and contrast the four team models with particular attention to the *collaborative team model*.

REFERENCES

Asian-American heritage: A resource guide for teachers, grades k–12. (1995). New York, NY: New York City Board of Education, Brooklyn, Office of Multicultural Education.

Banks, J.A. (1997a). Multicultural education: Characteristics and goals. In J.A. Banks & C.A. McGee Banks (Eds.), *Multicultural education: Issues and perspectives* (3rd ed., pp. 3–31). Needham Heights, MA: Allyn & Bacon.

Banks, J.A. (1997b). *Teaching strategies for ethnic studies* (6th ed.). Needham Heights, MA: Allyn & Bacon.

Bowers, C.A. (1984). *The promise of theory: Education and the politics of cultural change.* New York, NY: Longman.

Bredekamp, S., & Copple, C. (Eds.). (1997). *Developmentally appropriate practice in early childhood programs* (Rev. ed.). Washington, DC: National Association for the Education of Young Children.

Denney, M.K., Singer, G.H.S., Singer, J., Brenner, M.E., Okamoto, Y., & Fredeen, R.M. (2001). Mexican immigrant families' beliefs and goals for their infants in the neonatal intensive care unit. *JASH, 26*, 148–157.

Dentler, R.A., & Hafner, A.L. (1997). *Hosting newcomers: Structuring educational opportunities for immigrant children.* New York, NY: Teachers College Press.

Dinnebeil, L.A., Hale, L.M., & Rule, S. (1996). A qualitative analysis of parents' and service coordinators' descriptions of variables that influence collaborative relationships. *Topics in Early Childhood Special Education, 16*, 322–347.

Dunst, C.J. (1997). Conceptual and empirical foundation of family-centered practice. In R. Illback, C. Cobb, & J.H. Joseph (Eds.), *Integrated services for children and families: Opportunities for psychological practice* (pp. 75–91). Washington, DC: American Psychological Association.

Dunst, C.J., Trivette, C.M., & Hamby, D.W. (2007). *Research synthesis and meta-analysis of studies of family-centered practices.* Asheville, NC: Winterberry Press.

Friend, M., & Cook, L. (2007). *Interactions: Collaboration skills for school professionals* (5th ed.). Boston: Allyn and Bacon.

Friend, M., & Hurley-Chamberlain, D. (2007, January). Is co-teaching effective? *CEC Today.* http://oldsite.cec.sped.org/AM/Template.cfm?Section=Support_for_Teachers&template=/CM/ContentDisplay.cfm&ContentID=7504

Hanson, M.J. (2011). Diversity in service settings. In E.W. Lynch & M.J. Hanson (Eds.), *Developing cross-cultural competence: A guide for working with children and their families* (4th ed., pp. 2–19). Baltimore, MD: Paul H. Brookes Publishing Co.

Harry, B. (1998). Parental visions of "una vida normal/a normal life": Cultural variations on a theme. In L.H. Meyer, H.-S. Park, M. Grenot-Scheyer, I.S. Schwartz, & B. Harry (Eds.), *Making friends: The influences of culture and development* (pp. 47–62). Baltimore, MD: Paul H. Brookes Publishing Co.

Harry, B. (2002). Trends and issues in serving culturally diverse families of children with disabilities. *Journal of Special Education, 36*(3), 131–138.

Individuals with Disabilities Education Act (IDEA) of 1990, PL 101-476, 20 U.S.C. §§ 1400 *et seq.*

Kalyanpur, M., & Harry, B. (2012). *Cultural reciprocity in special education: Building family-professional relationships.* Baltimore, MD: Paul H. Brookes Publishing Co.

Kilgo, J.L., Johnson, L., LaMontagne, M., Stayton, V., Cook, M., & Cooper, C. (1999). Importance of practices: A national study of general and special early childhood educators. *Journal of Early Intervention, 22*, 294–305.

Kloo, A., & Zigmomd, N. (2008). Co-teaching revisited: Redrawing the blueprint. *Preventing School Failure, 52*, 12–20.

Lynch, E.W. (2011). Developing cross-cultural competence. In E.W. Lynch & M.J. Hanson (Eds.), *Developing cross-cultural competence: A guide for working with children and families* (4th ed., pp. 41–75). Baltimore, MD: Paul H. Brookes Publishing Co.

Lynch, E.W., & Hanson, M.J. (2004). Changing demographics: Implications for training in early intervention. *Infants and Young Children, 6*(1), 50–55.

Lynch, E.W., & Hanson, M.J. (Eds.) (2011). *Developing cross-cultural competence: A guide for working with children and their families* (4th ed.). Baltimore: Paul H. Brookes Publishing Co.

Lyon, S., & Lyon, G. (1980). Team functioning and staff development: A role release approach to providing integrated educational services for severely handicapped students. *Journal of the Association for the Severely Handicapped, 5*(3), 250–263.

McCormick, L., & Goldman, R. (1979). The transdisciplinary model: Implications for service delivery and personnel preparation for the severely and profoundly handicapped. *AAESPH Review, 4*, 152–161.

McWilliam, R.A. (2000). Recommended practices in interdisciplinary models. In S. Sandall, M.E. McLean, & B.J. Smith (Eds.), *DEC recommended practices in early intervention/early childhood special education* (pp. 47–52). Denver, CO: Division of Early Childhood (DEC) of the Council for Exceptional Children (CEC).

Miles, M., & Miles, C. (1993). Education and disability in cross-cultural perspective: Pakistan. In S.J. Peters (Ed.), *Education and disability in cross-cultural perspective* (pp. 167–235). New York, NY: Garland.

Minke, K.M., Bear, G.G., Deemer, S.A., & Griffin, S.M. (1996). Teachers' experiences with inclusive classrooms: Implications for special education reform. *The Journal of Special Education, 30,* 152–186.

Park, J., Turnbull, A.P., & Park, H. (2001). Quality of partnerships in service provision for Korean American parents of children with disabilities: A qualitative inquiry. *JASH, 26,* 158–170.

Peck, C.A., Furman, G.C., & Helmstetter, E. (1993). Integrated early childhood programs: Research on implementation of change in organizational contexts. In C.A. Peck, S.L. Odom, & D.D. Bricker (Eds.), *Integrating young children with disabilities in community programs: Ecological perspectives on research and implementation* (pp. 187–205). Baltimore, MD: Paul H. Brookes Publishing Co.

Sandall, S., Hemmeter, M.L., Smith, B.J., & McLean, M.E. (2005). *DEC recommended practices: A comprehensive guide for practical application in early intervention/early childhood special education.* Longmont, CO: Sopris West.

Skrtic, T.M. (1991). *Behind special education: A critical analysis of professional culture and school organization.* Denver, CO: Love.

Skrtic, T.M. (1995). Deconstructing/reconstructing the professions. In T.M. Skrtic (Ed.), *Disability and democracy: Reconstructing (special) education for postmodernity* (pp. 3–62). New York, NY: Teachers College Press.

Thousand, J.S., & Villa, R.A. (2000). Collaborative teaming: A powerful tool in school restructuring. In R.A. Villa & J.S. Thousand (Eds.), *Restructuring for caring and effective education: Piecing the puzzle together* (2nd ed., pp. 254–292). Baltimore, MD: Paul H. Brookes Publishing Co.

U.S. Department of Education, National Center for Education Statistics. (1999). *Teacher quality: A report on the preparation and qualifications of public school teachers* (NCES 1999–080). Washington, DC: NCES.

Wolery, M.R., & Dyk, L. (1984). Arena assessment: Description and preliminary social validation data. *JASH, 9,* 231–235.

3

Assessment and Planning

The Individualized Family Service Plan and Individualized Education Program

Linda McCormick

FOCUS OF THIS CHAPTER

Assessment
- Purposes of assessment
- Assessment approaches

Planning
- Planning the Individualized Family Service Plan
- Service coordinator responsibilities
- Planning the Individualized Education Program
- Writing high-quality goals and objectives

As discussed in Chapter 1, there are two sections of the Individuals with Disabilities Education Act (IDEA) of 1990 (PL 101-476) that provide specific mandates for early childhood intervention: Part C addresses services for children from birth to age 3 and their families, and Section 619 of Part B addresses services for children ages 3 through 5. This chapter is concerned with two key requirements of IDEA: assessment and planning. The plan for infants (birth to 3) is the individualized family service plan (IFSP). For school-age children (ages 3 and above), the plan is the individualized education program (IEP). The specifics of planning are described in Chapter 5.

The major changes in IDEA 2004 (PL 108-446) that relate to infants and young children with disabilities are so important that they bear repeating. These are the requirements that 1) the family's Part C service coordinator (or other representative of the early intervention program) must be invited to participate in the IEP meeting, 2) the information in the IFSP must be considered when developing the IEP, 3) parents must be given the option of continuing early intervention services until their child enters kindergarten, 4) parents and teachers may agree to make minor changes in a child's IEP during the school year without reconvening the IEP team, and 5) parents must receive quarterly reports on their child's progress toward meeting IEP goals and objectives.

Other requirements in Part C were strengthened and clarified. The meaning of "natural environments" was clarified. They are settings that are natural or typical for same-age peers who have no disabilities. There is a stipulation that early intervention services for infants and toddlers must be delivered in these settings. If this is not possible, when services will be provided in other than natural environments, then the IFSP must include a clear justification in writing for that decision.

IDEA strongly advocates for the involvement of parents throughout the assessment, planning, and intervention processes. The definition of *parent* was amended to give adoptive parents the same status as birth parents, and the role of foster parents was clarified. Foster parents may act as parents if 1) the birth parents' parental rights have been terminated under state law, 2) the foster parents have an ongoing, long-term parental relationship with the child, 3) the foster parents are willing to make the decisions required of parents under IDEA, and 4) the foster parents have no interests that would conflict with the child's interests.

Alignment with the state's early learning standards is a consideration in the assessment and planning process. Early learning standards (also known as learning guidelines, principles, or expectations) specify what preschool-age children should know and be able to do. All states have identified early learning standards for preschool programs and most have identified early learning standards for early intervention (EI) programs (National Research Council, 2008). They come in a variety of formats but they have a common purpose: to outline expectations for growth and development—specifically what should be taught and what children should learn prior to entering kindergarten.

ASSESSMENT

IDEA guarantees all students with disabilities the right to an unbiased evaluation to determine whether there is a disability, whether special education and related services are needed (because of the disability), and, if they are, what kind of services the student will receive. Children from cultures and communities where English is not the primary language must be assessed by someone skilled in the child's primary language. If this is not possible, assessment must include a specialist or mediator who is bicultural and speaks the language of the home. This person keeps the family informed of all aspects of the assessment process.

The role of families as equal and contributing partners is emphasized. As both decision makers and advocates, parents and other family members play a central role from the very beginning of the assessment process. Because they know the child best, they are the most reliable sources of social-emotional, developmental, and behavioral information.

Involvement of family members begins at the assessment and planning stage. For many families, this is their first introduction to the system. They may have questions as to why assessment is needed, what information is necessary, what the procedures are, who will be involved, and how the information will help the child. In addition to answering these questions, the assessment team encourages the family members to talk about the child's strengths and preferences (e.g., activities, toys, people, settings) and their concerns regarding both the upcoming assessment and intervention activities. Whether families choose to be actively involved from the beginning of the assessment and planning process or choose only limited participation, the main concern is encouraging and honoring their contributions.

Assessment Purposes

The major categories of assessment are *screening, diagnosis* and/or *eligibility determination, intervention planning,* and *monitoring and evaluation.* Each type of assessment uses different tools and procedures and each asks different questions.

Screening asks the question: Is there a possibility that this child has a problem? Screening programs typically utilize brief, inexpensive measures that can be administered in a short time with relatively little effort. The purpose is to identify children who should receive more comprehensive assessment and, possibly, intervention. IDEA requires screening activities called Child Find to identify children who should participate in a more thorough formal screening process.

Diagnosis asks two questions: Is there a significant problem? What is the nature and extent of the problem? Comprehensive diagnostic assessment of infants and toddlers considers medical issues and sensory and motor functioning as well as cognitive, motor, communication, social/play, and self-care/adaptive development. Methods for answering these questions include observations, interviews, case history, informal tests, and norm-referenced tests (described below).

Eligibility determination assessment asks the questions: Is the child eligible for services under IDEA? If yes, to what disability category will the child be assigned? A child age birth to 3 is eligible for services as "at risk" if it is judged that he or she will experience substantial developmental delay if early intervention services are not provided. States have the option of expanding the definition of "at risk" to include an infant or toddler who could experience developmental delays because of identified biological or environmental factors. Some examples of diagnosed physical or mental conditions that have a high probability of resulting in developmental delays are chromosomal abnormalities, genetic or congenital disorders, sensory impairments, inborn errors of metabolism, congenital infections, and disorders reflecting disturbance of central nervous system development. The child might also or alternatively be identified as developmentally delayed. When developing an application for a Part C grant, each state develops its own definition of developmental delay, which it uses to identify infants and toddlers with disabilities who are in need of services.

Preschoolers with disabilities may be eligible for services under any of the categories of disabilities specified in Part B for school-age children (Table 3.1). In addition, preschool and young children (ages 3–9) may be eligible under the more general designation of developmental delay (or a similar term selected by the state). Assessment by a multidisciplinary team determines if a child meets the eligibility guidelines for receiving special services in one of the categories.

Intervention planning asks "what" and "how" questions. What do we need to teach this child? What are appropriate instructional goals and objectives? What are the child's strengths relative to the demands or expectations in his or her natural environments? How will we teach this child? How should we arrange the environment to facilitate learning? There are many sources of information for intervention planning: observations of the child in his or her natural environments, interviews with the family and other caregivers, and information from other professionals who know the child. This assessment should be closely linked to the actual curriculum and daily activities and routines in the child's preschool program. The results are the basis for developing goals and objectives, planning instruction, arranging the learning environment, and adapting materials.

Monitoring asks very different questions: Is the child making progress in an instructional program? Is the programming effective? This process begins with 1) determining what behavior to measure, 2) defining the behavior in observable terms, and 3) selecting an appropriate system for recording and summarizing the data. *Evaluation* may be summative or formative. Summative evaluation takes place after the service has been provided to determine whether the goals and objectives have been achieved. Formative evaluation takes place before and during instruction and intervention to determine if the services are being provided as planned and whether they are effective. The purpose of formative evaluation is to identify strengths and weaknesses in the intervention/instructional process. The information generated by formative evaluation is used to make decisions about whether programming should continue as it is now being provided or whether there is a need to modify or completely change the intervention/instructional process.

Assessment Approaches

The two broad categories of assessment approaches are traditional and authentic assessment. The two approaches supplement and complement each other. Each has a role in the assessment process.

Table 3.1. IDEA eligibility categories

Specific learning disabilities: A disorder in one or more of the basic psychological processes involved in understanding or using language (spoken or written) that manifests itself in the inability to listen, think, speak, read, write, spell, or do mathematical calculations; included are such conditions as perceptual disabilities, brain injury, minimal brain dysfunction, dyslexia, and developmental aphasia; does not include learning problems that are primarily the result of visual, hearing, or motor disabilities, mental retardation, emotional disturbance, or environmental, cultural, or economic disadvantage

Speech or language impairments: A communication disorder such as stuttering, impaired articulation, language impairment, or voice impairment that adversely affects the child's educational performance

Intellectual disability: Significantly subaverage general intellectual functioning that exists concurrently with deficits in adaptive behavior and is manifested during the development period and adversely affects the child's educational performance

Emotional disturbance: A condition exhibiting one or more of the following characteristics over a long period of time and to such a degree that educational performance is adversely affected: 1) inability to learn that cannot be explained by intellectual, sensory, or health factors; 2) inability to build or maintain satisfactory relationships with peers and teachers; 3) inappropriate types of behavior or feelings under normal circumstances; 4) general pervasive mood of unhappiness or depression; and 5) tendency to develop physical symptoms or fears associated with personal or school problems

Multiple disabilities: Concomitant impairments such as intellectual disability-blindness, intellectual disability-orthopedic impairment, and so forth, which combined cause such severe educational needs that they cannot be accommodated in a special education program solely for one of the impairments

Hearing impairments: An impairment in hearing (permanent or fluctuating) that adversely affects the child's educational performance (but is not included under the definition of "deafness")

Orthopedic impairments: Includes impairments caused by congenital anomaly, impairments caused by disease such as poliomyelitis, bone tuberculosis, and other causes (e.g., cerebral palsy, amputations, fractures or burns that cause contractures) that adversely affect educational performance

Other health impairments: Limited strength, vitality, or alertness, including heightened alertness to environmental stimuli, that results in limited alertness with respect to the educational environment and is due to chronic or acute health problems such as asthma, attention deficit disorder or attention hyperactivity disorder, diabetes, epilepsy, a heart condition, hemophilia, lead poisoning, leukemia, nephritis, rheumatic fever, sickle cell anemia, and Tourette syndrome and adversely affects the child's educational performance

Visual impairments (including blindness): Impairment in vision that, even with correction, adversely affects the child's educational performance; includes partial sight and blindness

Autism: A developmental disability which significantly affects social interaction and verbal and nonverbal communication; generally evident before age 3 and adversely affecting educational performance; other characteristics include stereotyped movements, repetitive activities, resistance to change, and unusual responses to sensory experiences

Deafblindness: Concomitant hearing and visual impairments causing severe communication difficulties and developmental and educational needs so severe that they cannot be accommodated in special education programs solely for children with deafness or children with blindness

Deafness: Hearing impairment so severe that the child cannot process linguistic information through hearing, with or without amplification, thus adversely affecting educational performance

Traumatic brain injury: An acquired injury to the brain caused by an external physical force and resulting in total or partial functional disability or psychosocial impairment (or both) which adversely affects educational performance; includes open or closed head injuries resulting in impairments in one or more areas (language, cognition, memory, attention, reasoning, abstract thinking, judgment, problem solving, perceptual and motor abilities, psychosocial behavior, physical functions, information processing speech); does not apply to brain injuries that are congenital or degenerative, or induced by birth trauma

Developmental delay: A delay in one or more of the following areas: physical development, cognitive development, communication, social or emotional development, or adaptive development; applies to children birth to age 3 (IDEA Part C) and children from 3 through 9 (Part B) as defined by each state

Source: IDEA (2004).

Traditional Assessment Standardized, norm-referenced assessments compare the child's achievements with those of same-age peers. These tests are used primarily for making diagnostic, eligibility, and placement decisions. They do not consider what children can or cannot do in real-life situations, so they contribute very little information that is useful for planning decisions.

The basis for the selection of items to include in norm-referenced tests is the percentage of children who master a particular skill at a certain age and whether an item correlates well with the total test. For the results of these tests to be comparable across children, they must be administered under standardized procedures. *Standardized procedures* means that all children taking the test must have an identical experience, with exactly the same amount of assistance and the same directions, materials, and scoring criteria. Norm-referenced instruments provide very little information that is useful for making decisions about instruction and most do not include infants and young children with disabilities in the standardization population.

Professionals who administer norm-referenced tests recognize the importance of strict adherence to standardized procedures and the limitations of these tests where children with disabilities are concerned. Children with intensive special needs often display atypical responses to sound, sight, touch, and other stimuli. They also have sensory, cognitive, communication, motor, social-emotional, and health care issues that affect their ability to respond to questions and instructions. Consequently whatever ratings and scores they receive on these tests are not valid. It is difficult to imagine trying to assess the cognition functioning of a child with hearing impairment or fine motor limitations by asking him or her to point to a picture or stack blocks to match those of a model. Another problem that affects test scores for very young children with disabilities (and even infants and preschoolers without disabilities) is that they are very easily distracted and reluctant to follow directions. A final limitation of norm-referenced tests is that they do not consider the effects of environmental variables or instructional strategies. Standardized testing procedures and norm-referenced tests can be useful in determining eligibility for special services, but it is important to understand their limitations.

Authentic Assessment The National Association for the Education of Young Children (NAEYC/NASCE, 2003) and the Division for Early Childhood (DEC, 2003) have provided clear, consistent guidelines for authentic assessment—an approach that integrates individualized assessment, curriculum, and progress evaluation. Authentic assessments are criterion-referenced measures that provide highly specific information regarding a child's level of performance relative to the test's criterion (often referred to as "yardstick"). Appropriate criteria are those developmental skills or hierarchies of functional skills deemed important to school performance or daily living. Examples include the ability to establish and maintain play with peers, the ability to take action to meet needs such as feeding, dressing, self care, and early literacy and math skills, and the ability to communicate with other children and adults to share observations and ask questions. Curriculum-referenced tests are a type of criterion-referenced test where the child's performance is compared to a predetermined sequence of curriculum objectives. (The curriculum may be commercially available or designed by the teachers—either way it will be based on the state's common core standards. See Chapter 5 for a discussion of preschool standards.) These tests provide information as to what curriculum objectives the child has mastered, what needs to be mastered, and how well the child is benefiting from the instruction (so that adjustments can be made). Criterion-referenced instruments and curriculum-based measurements are useful for developing IEP and IFSP goals and objectives as well as for guiding the selection of instructional methods.

Criterion-referenced assessments based on developmental milestones do have some limitations where young children with severe disabilities are concerned. Wolery (2004) summarizes the limitations of these tests for assessing young children with severe disabilities with these points: 1) most were not intended to yield instructional goals, 2) just because items are adjacent does not mean that they are necessarily related to the same skill, 3) there is no evidence that the sequence of milestones is the best teaching sequence (especially for children with sensory and physical disabilities), and 4) many of the sequences have large gaps between items. The practice of targeting the first items that a child fails does not consider prerequisite skills for learning that item or achieving a milestone and the relationship of skills across developmental domains. The practice of targeting and teaching skills in the order in which they occur (or are thought to occur) in typical development may be appropriate for children with only minimal delay but it is not the best approach for children with more severe and pervasive delays. It is based on two misleading assumptions: 1) that the development of young children with disabilities is essentially the same as that of children without disabilities and 2) that children with disabilities are simply functioning at an earlier stage of development. There is no empirical support for either of these assumptions.

The process of developing intervention goals is clearly more complex than teaching the first items that a child fails on a supposedly developmentally sequential test. Developmental information is useful but it should not be the sole source of data for developing goals and objectives. Valuable intervention time (the child's and the service provider's) may be wasted trying to teach developmental skills when the nature of the child's disabilities may make them not only unattainable but also unnecessary. So much time and effort may go to trying to teach the skills observed in younger, typically developing children that the child with disabilities has little time to socialize and participate with peers in developmentally appropriate learning opportunities.

Authentic assessment is a process of documenting the learning and development of children during real-life activities and routines by familiar and knowledgeable adults in the child's life (Macy & Bagnato, 2010). The criterion or yardstick is the requirement for participating in these activities and routines. Authentic assessment provides realistic and practical information about the child's strengths. It identifies not only targets but also strategies for instruction: how the child learns best. Some approaches that come under the heading of authentic assessment are naturalistic assessment, curriculum-based assessment, play-based assessment, and ecological assessment. They use a variety of informal assessment techniques that involve 1) ongoing observation of the child engaged in meaningful tasks (with different persons, using different materials, and in multiple naturalistic environments); 2) systematic recording of the changes brought about through instruction; and 3) team decision making. Ecological assessment and portfolio assessment (also a type of authentic assessment) are described in Chapter 5.

Whichever authentic assessment approach is used to identify intervention goals and objectives, *functionality* is a critical concern for children with severe disabilities. Functionality is judged by the extent to which skills facilitate a child's participation and independence in family, school, and community activities. Assessment is organized around basic skills such as achieving mobility, feeding oneself, toileting, dressing, imitating peers, responding to directions, making choices, playing with toys, and taking turns. The idea is to identify age-appropriate goals that can have immediate usefulness and benefits for the child. Age-appropriate behaviors are based on skills and enable their same-age peers to participate in natural environments. Engaging with materials, toys, or activities that are not age appropriate is stigmatizing. An example of a violation of the precept of age appropriateness would be asking a preschooler with disabilities to play with infant toys (e.g., stacking rings) or to play Pat-a-cake. Wolery's (2004) guidelines for selecting appropriate intervention goals from criterion- and curriculum-referenced test results are presented in Table 3.2.

Child-centered planning begins with authentic assessment. Also called *MAPS* (McGill Action Planning System) (Vandercook, York, & Forest, 1989), *person-centered planning* (Mount, 1992), or *personal-futures planning*, child-centered planning is more than a procedure for gathering information, and it involves not just family members but all the people who have an interest in the child. Two premises guide this process: 1) that planning for a child's future should be in the hands of the people who love the child and 2) that a child who needs services should be thoroughly understood by the people who will provide those services. The outcome of the process is a positive and realistic picture of the child that appreciates his or her unique characteristics and creates a shared vision for the future. In addition to facilitating the child's participation in his or her natural environments, the goals and ideas generated by the child-centered planning process provide a measure of social validity that expands and supplements more objective measures of behavior.

The concept of social validity, first introduced by Wolf (1978), refers to whether the goals and focus of intervention are in line with the values and desires of the consumers and participants. Child-centered planning ensures social validity because it elicits the contributions and views of the consumers: 1) the immediate and extended family, 2) the child's peers (when appropriate), 3) friends and neighbors of the family, and 4) service providers (therapists, preschool staff, EI staff, and special education personnel). The vision that comes out of the child-centered planning process is a template against which to measure the validity of the goals and objectives, the intervention procedures, and the outcomes of intervention.

In summary, the shift in assessment practices beginning in the 1990s reflects what we have learned about the complex and holistic nature of development and the role of context and culture in learning. The assessment process involves multiple observations and other information-gathering activities. It addresses the limitations of assessment based on developmental milestones alone, the unnatural separation of development domains, the view that behavior is relatively stable over time, and the limited scope of test items. Behavior is assessed in the context of daily experiences. Authentic assessment produces

Table 3.2. Questions to consider when developing intervention goals from criterion- and curriculum-referenced test results

1. What were the items that the child failed designed to measure?
2. Are the items that the child failed important constructs or skills that the child needs to acquire?
3. Do separate items that the child failed represent classes of important behaviors?
4. What do the failed items say about the child's overall competence in the across-skill areas?
5. Why are these skills important to this infant or child?
6. Is this skill essential for the infant or child to function in present and future environments?
7. What are the prerequisites for this skill, and does the child have these prerequisite abilities?
8. How does performance of the skill relate to other skills in this domain or other developmental domains?
9. Is this skill an important prerequisite to other skills?
10. Should the focus of instruction for this skill be on acquisition, fluency, maintenance, or generalization?

Source: Wolery (2004).

an accurate and full description of the settings, tasks, and activities in which the child is likely to learn best and the important behaviors that will enable the child to participate successfully in these settings, tasks, and activities.

PLANNING

Once assessment is completed, family members assist the team in interpreting the results. If the assessment process has been conducted in a collaborative and respectful manner, there will be a positive and productive planning process. As noted, IDEA provides for two types of individualized plans: the IFSP and the IEP. Which plan is developed depends on the age of the child. Part B of IDEA states that eligible children up to age 6 may have an IFSP (if the state, the family, and the local service program want one), but most states provide an IFSP only for eligible children under age 3 and their families. When children transition to preschool at age 3, they are reevaluated and an IEP is developed. Table 3.3 provides a comparison of the federal requirements for the IFSP and the IEP. The remainder of this chapter describes the requirements for these plans as set forth in IDEA, and the major activity of the IFSP or IEP meeting, which is the development of meaningful and functional goals and objectives.

Planning the Individualized Family Service Plan

The IFSP is not a product so much as a process. Development of the IFSP is the first step in establishing and maintaining a productive and supportive professional–family relationship. The IFSP process continues throughout intervention to ensure effective EI in accordance with the law. There is continuous gathering, sharing, exchanging, and expanding of information as the family makes decisions about the EI they want and need for their child and themselves. The IFSP specifies desired outcomes for the child based on the child's development, and, if the family desires, it may also include outcomes for the family. Families may identify their resources, priorities, and concerns related to enhancing their child's development, but this is optional. Other ways that the IFSP differs from the IEP include the focus on natural environments, inclusion of the services of multiple community agencies, and the assignment of a service coordinator for every family. (The service coordinator's responsibilities

Table 3.3. Comparison of the IDEA requirements for the IFSP and the IEP

An IFSP must include	An IEP must include
A statement of the child's present level of development in these areas: physical (including vision, hearing, and health status); cognitive; communication; psychosocial; and adaptive behavior	A statement of the child's present levels of educational performance; for preschool children, a description of how the disability affects the child's participation in age-appropriate activities
A statement of family strengths, resources, concerns, and priorities related to the child's development	A statement of annual goals and short-term objectives detailing what the child is expected to learn over a specific time with criteria to determine if the goals/objectives have been achieved
A statement of the major outcomes expected to be achieved for the child and family	A statement of the special education and related services to be provided to help the child reach the goals and objectives
A statement of the frequency, intensity, and method of delivering the early intervention services necessary to produce desired outcomes for the child and family	The extent of time to which the child will participate with nondisabled peers in the general education setting, including district and state assessments and an explanation of the time the student will not participate with nondisabled peers
A statement of the natural environments where services will be provided or a statement explaining why services will not be provided in natural environments	
Projected dates for the initiation of services and anticipated duration of services	Projected dates that the special education program and other services will begin and anticipated duration of services
The name of a service coordinator responsible for implementation of the IFSP and coordination with other agencies/professionals	

are described below.) The appearance and organization of the form used for the IFSP are not important: it differs across states and programs. What matters is that it includes all of the information as specified by IDEA (shown in the first column of Table 3.3).

The transition requirement was strengthened in the 1997 IDEA (PL 105-17) reauthorization by the addition of specific directions for transition from the EI program. The IFSP must include a plan with the steps to be taken to support the transition of the child to preschool services under Part B is discussed at length in Chapter 14.

Developing the IFSP The goal of the IFSP process is to enable families to make informed choices about the services they want and need for their children and for themselves. To make informed choices and feel empowered to act on them, the family must have a trusting relationship and clear communication with EI service providers. Ultimately, the IFSP is as good only as the information from which it is constructed. The family members and the support network are the primary sources of this information. Family information gathering is most effective when EI providers understand and respect the impact of cultural, environmental, and social factors (e.g., background, socioeconomic status, education) on the families' views and beliefs about disability, parenting, child-rearing practices, and early intervention services. From the first contact (by phone or in person), the EI professionals begin building a trusting relationship.

Following the initial evaluation and assessment process, a meeting is scheduled. This meeting includes the family, the service coordinator, at least one member of the evaluation team, and any others that the family or service providers want to invite. The purpose of the meeting is to identify family strengths and needs in order to make decisions about what services are needed. It is important to emphasize that the term *strengths and needs* in this context refers to what the family identifies as issues related to supporting the child's development. Examples might be respite care, child care, specialized equipment, and other supports.

Service Coordinator Responsibilities

Minimum qualifications for service coordination include knowledge and understanding of 1) infants and toddlers with special needs and their families, 2) early intervention legislation, and 3) the nature and scope of services available under the state's early intervention program. The selection of a service coordinator is central to the IFSP process because this person is intended to serve as the single point of contact to help parents assess services. It is the obligation of the service coordinator to see that the family understands and receives the rights, procedural safeguards, and services that are authorized under the state's early intervention program. Table 3.4 shows early intervention services that are authorized by Part C. If there is a need for services that are not authorized by Part C, those services are described on the IFSP, but separate funding sources must be sought. If the family will be charged for some services (which is allowable under the law), this is discussed and noted on the IFSP.

While not always the case, the service coordinator is usually the professional whose background is most relevant to the needs of the child and the family. In addition to helping the family access and coordinate services and assistance among agencies, the service coordinator's activities include the following:

- Coordinating and monitoring evaluations and assessments
- Ensuring that parents receive the early intervention services described in their IFSP in a timely manner
- Coordinating and monitoring the provision of needed services so that there are no gaps or unnecessary overlaps
- Helping the family locate appropriate services and service providers as the child's needs change
- Facilitating and participating in the development, review, and evaluation of the IFSP
- Informing families of the availability of advocacy services
- Facilitating the development and continuous review of a transition plan

Part C is very specific about the service coordinator's responsibilities, but because the law permits some discretion in developing service coordination

Table 3.4. Part C early intervention services

Early intervention services may include any one or some combination of the following services:
- Assessments to identify...
   (a) The child's strengths and developmental needs
   (b) The family's concerns, priorities, and resources
- Assistive technology, including specially designed or altered adaptive assistive devices
- Audiology testing and referral
- Family training and counseling, as requested
- Health services to enable the child to benefit from other early intervention services
- Medical services for the purpose of diagnosis or evaluation—provided by a licensed physician to determine developmental status and the need for early intervention services
- Nursing services as necessary to enable a child to benefit from early intervention services
- Nutrition assessment and development and monitoring of a plan to address the child's nutritional needs
- Occupational therapy services to help the child learn skills for play and daily living and design and provide assistive devices
- Physical therapy to identify and help prevent or reduce movement problems
- Psychological assessment and counseling for the child, parents, and family regarding child development, child behavior, parent training, and educational services
- Service coordination to provide information and assist in obtaining needed services and resources in the community
- Social work assessment in the home and family environment and individual and family group counseling and other activities to build social skills
- Special instruction to assist the child in learning new skills
- Speech-language pathology that includes identification, referral, and provision of services to assist development of language and communication
- Transportation services as necessary to enable the child and family to receive early intervention services
- Vision assessment and referral for medical or other professional services necessary for habilitation or rehabilitation

systems, there is a great deal of variation across states. In some states, service coordinators have no responsibilities other than service coordination. In other states, service coordination responsibilities may be shared by all of the professionals on the early intervention team. Usually this depends on the needs of the child and the wishes of the family.

Expected Outcomes   The team develops a list of expected outcomes. The purpose of the expected outcomes is twofold: 1) to increase the family's capacity to support the child and 2) to increase the child's participation in valued activities in natural environments. Outcomes for the child are based on the child's development and behavior: outcomes for the family (if they want to include these outcomes) depend on what family members identify as their resources, priorities, and concerns related to enhancing their child's development.

Outcome statements should not be confused with traditional assessment-driven therapeutic goal statements. Outcome statements reflect the team's shared vision for the child and how that vision will be achieved. They should be written in the family's own words. Most statements will be altered or expanded numerous times in response to changes in the child's physical and developmental status and the family's preferences, resources, and challenges. Thus, they should be viewed as tentative.

The format for outcome statements is straightforward. It begins with a statement of what the child will do (as a result of the intervention) followed by the rationale (why this is important for the family and for the child's development). For example, Jace, a 3-year-old with Down syndrome, will sit in his highchair and feed himself finger foods (e.g., dry cereal, pieces of fruit) so that the family can enjoy breakfast together and Jace can become more independent.

In addition to methods for achieving the desired outcomes, the implementation plan lists what various people will do and when and where intervention will take place. In the case of Jace, teaching will occur at breakfast (and conceivably at other meals in the kitchen), and the people responsible will be the family members who are present at mealtimes. Family members will be taught how to physically shape Jace's fingers around a food particle and guide it to his mouth. Over and above the outcomes that focus on the child in daily activities, there may be other types of outcomes focused on activities that family members identify as important to the family's functioning. These might include finding out how to get help with financial planning or locating possible community supports. Other outcomes might focus on improving the family's health, safety, and quality of life (e.g., securing and moving to affordable housing, earning a GED). Finally, there may also be outcomes that specify agency or administrative activities: for example, identifying needs for additional assessment, equipment and materials (both acquisition and training for their use), transportation, and training and technical assistance.

Finally, the team decides for each outcome how to determine when the outcome has been achieved. The plan for evaluation should be appropriate to the setting and phrased in a meaningful way. Using the example of Jace at breakfast, data collection might be as simple as jotting notes on a pad or calendar kept on the kitchen table. The parent may estimate the percentage of his breakfast that Jace is feeding himself independently or count the number of bites that he eats on his own.

The culmination of the initial planning process is a draft IFSP with outcomes that reflect the family's long-term aims for their child and that can realistically be accomplished as part of the family's daily routines. (As noted above, the IFSP is an ongoing process, so it may undergo many revisions in the course of the family's tenure in the EI program.) The IFSP is reviewed at least every 6 months, or more frequently, to be sure that it continues to meet the needs of the child and family. There is a meeting at least once a year at which parents review their child's outcomes and the early intervention services to decide whether changes are needed. Table 3.5, based on Bruder (2000), provides a summary of the guidelines for IFSP development discussed in this section.

Planning the Individualized Education Program

The purpose of the IEP is to ensure that eligible students ages 3 through 21 receive an appropriate and individualized special education and related services. At the most basic level, the IEP is an agreement between the parents and the school specifying what the child's needs are and what the school system will do to address those needs. A student's IEP team (sometimes called the IEP committee) may include professionals (e.g., teachers, administrators, language interventionists, nurses, school psychologists, physical therapists,

Table 3.5. Guidelines for IFSP development

Focus on the family
Emphasize two points at the beginning of the relationship: 1) that the intervention team and the family are a partnership and 2) that the family's concerns, priorities, and resources will guide the IFSP process.

Identify the family's environments
Ask about the family's environments and the people, activities, and routines in those environments. Analyze the teaching/learning possibilities of family activities and routines. (Ecological assessment is described at length in Chapter 5.)

Engage in functional assessment
Try to get an accurate picture of the child's strengths, preferences, interests, and needs. Plan to observe the child in his or her natural environments to verify and complete the picture.

Review and respond to family questions
Review all the available information and respond to each family member's concerns about the child. Plan for assembling additional information if needed.

Decide expected outcomes
Collaborate to develop statements of activities that will increase the family's capacity to support the child and the child's participation in valued activities in natural environments.

Assign people and strategies to address the outcomes
The team (including the family) should decide upon and assign members the responsibilities for intervention services to accomplish the mutually agreed upon outcomes. Team members' responsibilities should depend on the needs of the situation, not the traditional functions associated with a specific discipline.

Decide on an implementation plan
Collaborate to decide on specific interventions and strategies to bring about the desired outcomes. Select interventions that will promote generalization of outcomes, target several skills during one activity, promote independence, and resemble typical interactions. (These interventions are described in Chapters 7-13.)

Plan ongoing and periodic evaluations
Evaluations should consider the rate and the quality of progress toward expected outcomes. Most important is whether the intervention strategies are resulting in developmental gains and increased participation in natural environments.

Source: Bruder (2000).

and/or occupational therapists), community members (e.g., child care providers, social workers), and family members (e.g., parents, grandparents, siblings, aunts, uncles). IDEA's Part B regulations specify that the IEP must include a number of statements.

- A statement of the child's present levels of academic achievement and functional performance, including (for preschool children) how the disability affects his or her participation in general education curriculum

For preschoolers, this statement, based on all of the information and data collected during the assessment process (e.g., observations, interviews, checklists) describes how the child's disability affects participation in appropriate preschool activities. The "present levels" statement for preschool children with significant disabilities should provide a picture (written in positive language) of the child's learning and performance in relation to the state's early learning/preschool standards, preschool curriculum expectations, and basic skills needed to participate in preschool activities. It should also provide information about how the child learns: specifics about what seems to facilitate and/or interfere with his or her learning.

- A statement of measurable annual goals, including short-term objectives/benchmarks (for children with significant disabilities)

Annual goals are measurable statements identifying the desired outcome of intervention or instruction. Goals and objectives should reflect specific performance expectations. They are the basis for a detailed, individualized instructional program aligned with the curriculum and/or the state's early learning standards. Each goal identifies the learner, the behavior that the child can reasonably accomplish in a 12-month period, the criteria to judge whether what has been taught has in fact been learned, and the time when the skill will be achieved.

Objectives or benchmarks are more specific. They are the small steps toward achievement of each annual goal. They include 1) the clearly defined behavior, 2) the conditions under which the behavior will be taught, and 3) the criterion for judging when the behavior has been learned. Thus, an objective/benchmark states the behavior the child needs to learn, the activity or activities during which the child will learn and demonstrate the behavior, and the standard for achievement of the desired learning. (Suggestions for expanding and judging goals and objectives are discussed below.)

One of the changes made by the 2004 IDEA Amendments was that benchmarks or short-term objectives are no longer required for all children. They are required only for children who will receive assessments aligned to alternative achievement standards (described below)—usually children with moderate to severe disabilities. Some states have opted to use benchmarks for all children. Benchmarks are particularly valuable for children with moderate to severe disabilities because they help the family monitor their child's progress toward meeting his or her annual goals.

- A statement of how the child's progress toward meeting the annual goals will be measured and when periodic reports on the child's progress will be provided

There must be a plan for continually, effectively, and efficiently monitoring and documenting progress toward achievement of the annual goals and periodic reporting of progress to the team (including the parents). This plan should be very specific. In addition to evaluation criteria stated in objective, measurable terms, it should describe the techniques that will be used to collect the data, the data-collection schedule, and how data will be analyzed, summarized, and used in modifying instruction when modifications are necessary. It should also include a statement of how and when program modifications will be undertaken.

- A statement of the special education and related services and supplementary aids and services to be provided to the child, or on behalf of the child, and program modifications (how the curriculum will be adapted) and what supports will be provided for school personnel

This statement lists the types of special education services that will be provided, the professionals who will provide direct services, and supports (e.g., transportation, speech-language therapy) as well as support and training for staff who work with the child. The purpose of the supports is to enable the child to 1) advance appropriately toward attaining the annual goals, 2) be involved in and make progress in the curriculum, and 3) be educated and participate with peers both with and without disabilities. Examples of possible supports and modifications include material adaptations, activity simplification, environmental supports, peer support, and special materials and equipment. Supports and modifications are addressed at length in Chapter 13.

- An explanation of the extent, if any, to which the child will not participate with children without disabilities in regular education classes and in extracurricular activities

The provision to educate children with disabilities to the maximum extent appropriate with children who are not disabled is at the very heart of the IDEA. This part of IDEA operationalizes that mandate. Removal of children with disabilities from regular educational environments should occur only if the nature or severity of the child's disabilities is such that he or she cannot achieve satisfactorily even with the use of supplementary aids and services. If the child will not participate in the regular classroom full time, the extent of nonparticipation must be explained. This section then specifies the percentage of time that a child will participate in the general education curriculum (including extracurricular and nonacademic activities) with his or her peers.

- A statement of individual accommodations that are necessary to measure the achievement and functional performance of the child on state or district assessments

IDEA requires that students with disabilities take part in state and district assessments. When it is necessary to make accommodations or modifications in how the test is administered or how a given child takes the test, the IEP team has the responsibility for deciding and documenting how the child will participate. The four broad categories of assessment accommodations are not unlike adjustments and modifications made in classroom instruction: timing and scheduling accommodations, response accommodations, setting accommodations, and presentation accommodations.

If the IEP team decides that a test is not appropriate for the child (even with accommodations), the child is given an alternative assessment. The IEP must include an explanation of that decision and the alternative assessment. Alternative assessment for preschool-age children (typically those with moderate/severe and multiple disabilities) may be aligned to the state's early learning standards and/or curriculum expectations.

- The projected date for beginning services and program modifications and the anticipated frequency, location, and duration of special education and related services and supplementary aids and services

This section details the specific services that the child will receive. The IEP may provide this information in a chart format with a column for the following types of information: 1) starting and ending dates of services, 2) where services will be provided, 3) number of times a per day or week that the child will receive services, and 4) how long (number of minutes) each session will last. The team also determines if the child needs to receive services beyond the typical school year (extended school year services). This decision is based on state and local educational agency guidelines.

In addition to the required statements, there are some special factors that must be considered when the IEP is developed (Development, Review, and Revision of IEP, 2006):

- Positive behavioral interventions, strategies, and supports if a child's behavior impedes his or her learning or that of others
- The child's language needs as they relate to the IEP (when there is limited English proficiency)
- Instruction in the use of braille for a child who is blind or visually impaired (unless the team decides that braille is not appropriate for the child)
- The child's language and communication needs if the child is deaf or hard of hearing, including opportunities for direct instruction in the child's communication mode and communication with peers and professionals in that mode
- Determination of the need for assistive technology devices and services

The requirement that the IEP must be finalized prior to actual placement can be a problem where preschoolers are concerned. If the child is not yet in his or her placement, as is often the case with preschoolers, members of the IEP team do not yet know what the child's strengths and needs are relative to the expectations of the preschool setting. To increase the validity and appropriateness of the goals and objectives on a child's first IEP, it is critical to ensure that assessment provides information about the child's specific developmental, instructional, and support needs and that the goals and benchmarks or short-term objectives (if appropriate) are developed by persons familiar with the child's daily functioning in natural environments.

When necessary, a second IEP meeting can be called a few weeks after placement to revise and/or rewrite the goals. This meeting can include all the service providers in the child's preschool setting. A general outline of the information that must be included in the IEP as compared with the IFSP is shown in Table 3.3.

Each child's IEP should be functional and individualized for that child, and it should be possible to teach and evaluate the targeted skills in the context of developmentally appropriate activities and routines. It should be family-sensitive and discipline-free. "Family-sensitive" means that it is nonjudgmental, positive, and free of jargon. It should be easily understood so that it can be successfully implemented by any adult who is associated with the child (e.g., teacher, paraeducator, therapist, family member). "Discipline-free" means that intervention areas are not assigned exclusively by professional discipline. It is a mistake to think of speech, language, and communication as the exclusive province of speech-language pathologists, motor skills as the exclusive province of occupational or physical therapists, and social and cognitive skills as the exclusive province of teachers. Assigning responsibility in this way gives the impression that the different disciplines have totally separate and distinct knowledge bases. This is not true. There is enormous overlap in both research and practice across disciplines, and, in fact, development in any one area—social, emotional, physical, cognitive, and language—affects and interacts with development in the other areas. There should be pooling of expertise. Moreover, assigning developmental areas to specific disciplines can have unfortunate consequences in that the focus of professionals tends to be myopic rather than holistic. This makes it more difficult to reach consensus as to the child's intervention needs, and when there is a lack of progress the blame may be placed on a single professional rather than thoroughly examining all aspects of the problem.

In addition to other instructional and functional goals, the team formulates long-term health goals and objectives. Backup staff members (e.g., nurses) are identified to assist with required services for children with chronic health needs. Included under this heading are children with asthma, diabetes, and cystic fibrosis as well as those who require health-related procedures such as gastrostomy tube feedings, nebulizer treatments, administration of oxygen, and suctioning a tracheostomy. The IEP also describes the specific health-related needs of children who require ongoing support and technology for survival as well as needs regarding equipment and staff training. Any services that can be performed by an individual other than a physician (e.g., school nurse, any other qualified person)—thus enabling the child to attend school with peers—are to be available to the child within the school setting. If a school or personal nurse is not available to administer health-related procedures, then the ECSE teacher and assistant should be trained by professional health personnel to assume primary responsibility for this support.

Writing High-Quality Goals and Objectives

Recommended practices require identifying skills that are functional for the child and then teaching and evaluating those skills in the context of developmentally appropriate routines and activities (Wolery, 2000). This is a conditional statement. If the first condition is not met—if the identified skills are not *functional*—then teaching and evaluating those skills in the context of developmentally appropriate routines and activities is extremely difficult, if not impossible. This is why formulating appropriate goals and objectives is so important. When the first condition is violated—when goals and objectives target isolated nonfunctional skills—they must be taught in another room or in a corner of the classroom. Children should not be removed from their peers and from the routines and activities that are the context and the curriculum of early childhood education. Activities in a developmentally appropriate classroom are not planned with one skill in mind (e.g., identifying colors); they are designed to provide opportunities for a variety of learning outcomes.

Notari-Syverson and Shuster (1995) identified five indicators of high-quality goals and objectives: functionality, generality, ease of integration, hierarchical relationship between the goals and objectives, and measurability. The questions presented in Table 3.6 address the five indicators. Introducing and discussing these questions at the IEP meeting provide an opportunity for the service providers and parents to clarify the reasons for intervention and instruction and reformulate or rephrase the objectives that do not measure up.

Functionality refers to the usefulness of the skill(s) for coping with the challenges of daily living and participating in routine activities. Interaction with peers and objects comes under this heading. The question is: Will this

Table 3.6. Rating the quality of goals and objectives

Functionality
- Will the skill enhance the child's ability to participate independently in all or most of his or her natural environments?
- Will the skill increase the child's appropriate interactions with peers and objects in his or her natural environments?

Generality
- Can the skill be taught and thus generalized across a variety of people, activities, materials, and settings?

Ease of integration
- Do the child's peers without disabilities demonstrate the skill within a variety of daily activities and routines?
- Are there naturally occurring antecedents and logical consequences for the skill in the child's daily activities and routines?
- Can the skill be elicited easily in a variety of activities and settings?

Hierarchical relationship
- Is the objective necessary for achieving the goal?

Measurability
- Can the skill be seen and/or heard so that it can be counted?
- Can the product(s) of the skill be recorded?

Source: Notari-Syverson and Shuster (1995).

skill increase the child's ability to engage with people, activities, and objects in the daily environment? Priority skills are those skills that are performed across environments (e.g., requesting help, replacing objects or materials after an activity) and are essential for completion of daily routines. Examples of the types of narrowly defined skills to be avoided are saying numbers 1 to 10 or stacking blocks. These skills are clearly not as important or meaningful as skills needed to achieve independence and to get along with others.

Generality, the potential for carryover, is an extremely important consideration when selecting instructional targets. Skills that represent a general concept or class of responses and skills that can be practiced across people, activities, materials, and settings fit into this category. The skills cited above (requesting help, replacing objects/materials after an activity) meet the criteria of generality as well as functionality.

Ease of integration refers to the ease of teaching the skill in the context of daily routines in natural environments. Serving children with disabilities in inclusive settings requires planning. Planning accommodations and adaptations is expedited when the child's IEP goals and objectives reflect the philosophy and practices of the program. Instruction can take advantage of naturally occurring antecedents and logical consequences that occur throughout the day. For example, requesting help and replacing objects or materials after an activity can be taught in numerous activities and across most daily environments (e.g., preschool, family child care setting, home), because they are needed in numerous activities and across many environments. Thus, these skills meet the criteria of ease of integration as well as generality and functionality. IEP goals and objectives should help children be viewed as members of the classroom community.

Hierarchical relationship refers to the association between the goals and the objectives that enable their attainment. It should be possible to state with assurance that when the child attains all the objectives that accompany a goal, that goal has been achieved. For example, under the goal "Jace will participate in the morning circle routine" are two objectives that focus on the specific behaviors that Jace will learn in order to participate in this particular activity with his peers. These objectives are: "In morning circle, Jace will indicate 'I am here' when his name is called on 3 consecutive days," and "In morning circle, Jace will respond to at least one question about the story of the day on 3 consecutive days." Jace is already performing the other behaviors that the teacher expects during morning circle. When he has learned these two additional behaviors, it can be stated with assurance that the goal of "participation in the morning circle routine" has been achieved.

Measurability refers to decisions about what data will be recorded and how they will be collected. In many cases it is possible to measure the products of a skill; for example, it is relatively simple to know whether a child is successful at cutting with scissors, pasting, molding with clay, painting, and/or marking on a paper in response to a question or a direction. Best examples of the behavior can be saved in a portfolio to document performance and progress. The alternative to permanent products is observation and recording of the child's behavior while the child is engaged in the target skill. The limited number of dimensions on which behavior may be observed and measured include

- *Frequency or number*—how often the behavior occurs relative to the number of opportunities or during a constant time period
- *Rate*—how frequently the behavior occurs relative to a unit of time
- *Duration*—how long the behavior lasts
- *Latency*—how long it takes the child to begin the behavior once the direction or cue has been given
- *Topography*—the shape of the child's response (how the child performs the behavior)
- *Magnitude*—the intensity of the child's response

The dimension to be observed and measured depends on the target behavior and what aspect of that behavior will be taught or changed. *Frequency or number* is the most commonly used measure. Recording frequency or number is appropriate when the observation period is held constant from one session to another or when the child has the same number of opportunities to respond each session. If the child has three opportunities to respond every day in the morning circle routine, then the number of responses in 3 consecutive days (because it is held constant) could be used as a criterion (e.g., "Jace will respond to at least two directions/instructions in morning circle for 3 consecutive days"). In situations in which opportunities to respond are not directly controlled, frequency can be used only if the observation period is held constant each day. The objective for Joey, who always plays with the same toy for the entire 20 minute free-play period, is an example: "Joey will select and play with at least three *different* toys during free-play period."

Rate is a measure of both fluency and accuracy. It is especially useful when the length of observations varies. Rate is computed by dividing the number of behaviors by the unit of time. For example, the objective for Abby is to increase the number of spoonfuls of food eaten with her self-feeder. Rate would be the best measure because the length of snack time and lunch varies from one day to the next. The first measurement for Abby during baseline was eight bites in 20 minutes, or 0.4 per minute.

Duration is an appropriate criterion when the length of time that a behavior lasts is of concern. There are two types: total duration and duration per occurrence. If, for example, the objective is to increase play with a peer during morning free play and at recess, then a decision needs to be made as to whether to record the time for each social play episode or the total duration of social play in one or both of the designated periods. When the duration of each play episode is recorded, the frequency of play episodes is also recorded. These data make it possible to calculate the frequency of play episodes, as well as mean, median, and mode duration of the behavior (if desired).

Latency is the time between the prompt, question, or instruction and the time when the child begins to respond. An example would be the time between the teacher's question "Which container has the red paint you need?" and the child pointing to or taking the can of red paint to his or her easel or the time between the question "Which color tells us it is now safe to cross the street?" and the child pointing to the green circle. Latency is important because it can affect the usefulness of a skill. The child's response must be prompt as well as accurate.

Topography refers to the precision or appropriateness of the performance. Measurement of topography assumes a description of both correct and acceptable and incorrect examples of the behavior. Topography may be reported as frequency, rate, percentage, or duration of the response. For example, topography might be rated on a 1–5 scale. Then the number of opportunities in which correct topography is observed (ratings of 4 or 5) may be compared with the total number of opportunities. Topography is not often a concern. An example of when it might be used is in judging the correctness of letter formation, in which case there is a permanent product, so measurement is straightforward.

Magnitude is the strength, force, or intensity of a response. Precise measurement of intensity requires some type of automated apparatus. However, in some cases the magnitude of a behavior can be determined, albeit subjectively, by evaluating the effect of the response on the environment. The force of a response may be determined to be acceptable or unacceptable depending on a criterion included in the operational definition of the behavior. For example, acceptable speech might be operationally defined as speech that is audible from a distance of 5 feet.

Some skills are easier to measure than others (e.g., the number of questions the child responds to about a story), but ultimately any behavior is measurable. The following are not behaviors and thus are not measurable: feelings (e.g., "improved self-concept"), sensory experiences (e.g., "hear his name"), and broad concepts (e.g., "increased receptive language skills"). If restated as behaviors, feelings, sensory experiences, and broad concepts can, however, be measured. For example, Jace's improved self-concept may be evident in increased responses to and initiations of peer play requests during recess. These behaviors can be measured. Sensory experiences, "hearing," "seeing," "feeling," and "smelling," are not measurable in natural environments, but it is possible to record children's responses to these experiences. For example, we can note whether Jace turns toward the person who says his name or comes when called. Broad concepts should be stated as the specific skills that constitute evidence of the category. It is possible, for example, to state numerous observable behaviors that are evidence of receptive language (e.g., "follows one-step directions," "answers questions about the story").

Some writers recommend expanding objectives to include information about intervention/instruction. Grisham-Brown and Hemmeter (1998) suggested adding a list of activities from relevant environments that will serve as contexts for instruction and a list of possible adaptations and/or instructional strategies to the traditional objectives format. They provide the following example of an expanded objective statement:

> When involved in an activity (described following) and given choices between two objects, Kendall will indicate her preference by looking at the desired object for 5 seconds across three activities for 3 days.
>
> Example activities include the following:
>
> *Home:* Mealtime (choice between two snacks), bedtime (choice between two books)
> *School:* Center time (choice between centers), snack time (choice between crackers and bananas)
> *Community:* Playground (choice between two pieces of play equipment), feeding the ducks (choice between feeding the ducks bread or crackers) (Grisham-Brown & Hemmeter, 1998, pp. 6–7)

Possible adaptations are 1) providing multisensory cues (e.g., visual, verbal, tactile) prior to asking the child to make choices; 2) using concrete objects that clearly represent the activity; and 3) using things with high color contrast such as red objects on a black background.

The target skill in this example is "making choices." Including a variety of different choice-making activities across the child's environments (home, school, community) has two advantages: There are frequent opportunities for practice, and programming for generalization is embedded in the instructional process.

Measurability Issues Adding the following four questions to the measurability indicator of Notari-Syverson and Shuster's (1995) quality monitoring scheme helps to differentiate among objectives that can or cannot be taught *and measured* in the context of routine activities:

1. *Does the objective propose to measure an appropriate dimension of the target behavior?* Consider this example of an inappropriate criterion: "Jace will respond to three routine questions (roll call, weather, day of the week) in morning circle by pointing to the appropriate picture on his communication device (without a prompt) 80% of the time for a week." "Pointing" requires measurement of frequency. Saying "80% of the time" is ambiguous: "80%" suggests that the percentage of opportunities will be measured, and "of the time" suggests measurement of a temporal dimension of the behavior, which is duration. To be measurable, the objective should read: "Jace will respond to three routine questions every day for a week (roll call, weather, day of the week) in morning circle by pointing to the appropriate

picture on his communication device (without a prompt)." Using percentage as the dimension of measurement (e.g., "80% of the time") is usually not appropriate and it always complicates data-recording requirements. (See additional discussion of the use of percentages below.)

2. *Does the objective propose to measure a meaningful dimension of the behavior performance that the adults in the child's environment consider worthwhile and valuable?* Consider this example: "Sarah will walk (with her walker) from the round table to the restroom door and from the round table to the outside door to get in line on four of five consecutive days." The problem here is that the parents and the teachers were not concerned with the target behavior of walking: Sara has already learned to use her walker. What they really wanted her to learn was to move faster and to do so consistently because it took her far too long to move from one place to another. Her parents and the teachers think she should be able to walk the distance in less than 4 minutes and that she should do it every day. This is the modified objective: "Sara will walk (with her walker) from the round table to the restroom door and from the round table to the outside door to get in line in 4 minutes or less, five consecutive opportunities."

3. *Is it clear how to elicit the desired performance?* Consider this objective: "When shown any two letters or small pictures and asked to say 'same' or 'different,' Jessie will respond correctly in 9 of 10 trials." The stimulus conditions are not clear. When the teacher was preparing to assess and then teach this behavior, he did not know how much disparity there should be between the letters or pictures and whether to present 10 pairs of letters and 10 pairs of pictures or one set of each for 10 trials. Restated, this objective reads: "When shown 10 pairs of two-inch letters or small pictures with minimal differences and asked to say 'same' or 'different,' Jessie will respond correctly in 9 of 10 trials."

4. *Can performance of the behavior be measured in the context of daily routines and activities?* Even though the objective in the above example has been restated so that the stimulus conditions are clear, it is not a good objective. Jessie's performance cannot be measured in the context of daily routines and activities. The teacher will have to present 10–20 trials in a massed trial format in order to assess and teach this behavior. This shows that the way an objective is written can actually limit the potential for embedding instruction and assessment into existing classroom activities and routines. Theoretically, ease of measurement should not be a factor in deciding whether a particular skill should be targeted for instruction. However, it must be a consideration in natural environments, because there are not sufficient staff in preschools to assign one person to do nothing but observe and record behavior. Thus, it is highly desirable to target behaviors that can be measured while simultaneously carrying out daily activities and routines. Here is a way to rewrite the objective so that performance can be measured (and taught) in the context of daily routines and activities: "When shown small objects with minimal variation in color, shape, size, and function (three to five a day in the context of ongoing activities) and asked to say 'same' or 'different,' Jessie will respond correctly in 9 out of 10 trials."

Problems related to measurability are among the five most common problems in IEP goals and objectives. Bateman and Linden (1998, p. 70) are particularly concerned with the use of percentages, noting that "percentages seem to be worshiped unduly"—people seem to think that by simply attaching a number (usually a percentage) to an objective they make it measurable. This is one of their examples of what they call a "not-so-wonderful goal": "Karen will improve her handwriting by 80%." The problem with this goal is readily apparent: If only 80% of the words in an essay were legible, then one of five words would not be legible. Performance of this behavior at the stated criterion level (80%) would not be acceptable.

The misuse of percentages where social behavior is concerned is even more worrisome. Consider, for example, this goal: "Levi will have acceptable behavior 80% of the time." Imagine what it would be like to be around a child whose behavior was unacceptable 20% of the time. Acceptable social behavior has not been learned if it is exhibited on only 8 of 10 occasions. How could "80% of the time" be a goal? Again, performance of the behavior at the stated criterion level would not be acceptable.

Finally, the following goal statement provides another example of the misuse of percentages: "Given a short paragraph, James will be able to identify the main idea with 95% accuracy." This is an example of the third measurability question discussed above. It is not clear what constitutes acceptable performance of the behavior, because the stimulus conditions are not clear. Should James be given 100 short paragraphs, from which he will need to identify the main idea in 95 of them? Or should he be given one paragraph in which he would be expected to *almost accurately* identify the main idea?

The examples of objectives provided by Bateman and Linden (1998) are obviously for school-age children. However, many goals and objectives developed for preschoolers are not-so-wonderful goals and they have other problems. Michnowicz, McConnell, Peterson, and Odom (1995) analyzed the goals and objectives in the IEPs of 163 preschoolers. Nearly 50% had no social goals or objectives whatsoever. When there were social goals and objectives, 68% of the social objectives lacked criteria and 45% were rated as unmeasurable as written.

When writing objectives, one needs to remember that "percentage" refers to the number of times a behavior occurs per total number of opportunities, multiplied by 100. Saying "80% *of* the time" is meaningless, because the total number of opportunities for the behavior to occur is not specified. Percent is a useful measure when accuracy is a primary concern and when a permanent product is generated, as is the case with a spelling test or a page of addition problems (not preschool activities). Percent data are also used to summarize the responses recorded in interval recording systems, which, as noted above, are not common in most classrooms because recording requires the observer's undivided attention. Teachers rarely have the time to collect this type of data. Moreover, percentages should not be used when the total number of opportunities to respond is less than 20, in which case one change in the numerator will produce greater than a 50% change.

The purpose of the criterion component of the objective is to tell the teachers what measurement system to develop so that they can judge whether what they have taught has in fact been learned. As noted above, the criterion component should include or at least imply the measurement procedures (the *how*), the schedule (*when* and *how often* measurement will occur), and an indication of *how well* the student is expected to perform for the behavior to be considered satisfactory. Unless the criterion component includes or implies a feasible and appropriate measurement system, the teacher cannot assess whether the child can perform the behavior. This leads to instruction of behaviors that are already in the child's repertoire.

SUMMARY

IDEA provides precise guidelines for assessment and planning for infants and young children with disabilities and their families. Assessment has a number of distinct purposes—screening, diagnosis, eligibility determination, intervention planning, monitoring, and evaluation. The purpose of assessment dictates selection of appropriate assessment strategies and/or instruments. Assessment results should inform the development of IFSP and IEP goals and objectives. The two broad categories of assessment approaches are traditional assessment and authentic assessment. Planning (IFSP and IEP development) requires information about the child's performance in natural environments; thus, it usually relies on authentic assessment approaches. Traditional assessment provides information about the child's present levels of performance and areas of need, but it offers little information to guide development of outcome statements or objectives. Parent priorities and needs related to participating in natural environments always have a significant influence on the development of goals and objectives. Finally, when writing behavioral objectives, it is critical that targeted skills are functional and measurable in the context of developmentally appropriate routines and activities.

STUDY QUESTIONS

1. Describe the IDEA requirements related to assessment.
2. Describe the major reasons and purposes for assessment and the questions that each type of assessment addresses.
3. Compare and contrast traditional and *authentic assessment approaches*.
4. Discuss the limitations of norm-referenced tests where children with intensive special needs are concerned.
5. Discuss the advantages and disadvantages of *criterion-referenced assessments*.
6. Define *functionality* as it applies to assessment and planning for young children with disabilities.
7. Describe the procedures and goals of the *child-centered planning* process.
8. Compare and contrast IDEA requirements for the IFSP and the IEP.
9. Describe the process through which the IFSP is developed and evaluated.
10. Describe the responsibilities of the service coordinator.
11. Compare and contrast IEP goals and objectives or benchmarks.
12. Describe indicators of high-quality goals and objectives.
13. List the dimensions on which behavior may be observed and measured and the measurement procedures suitable for each dimension.
14. Discuss reasons why it is so important to develop objectives that can be taught and measured in the context of routine activities.

REFERENCES

Bateman, B.D., & Linden, M.A. (1998). *Better IEPs: How to develop legally correct and educationally useful programs* (3rd ed.). Longmont, CO: Sopris West.

Bruder, M.B. (2000). Family-centered early intervention: Clarifying our values for the millennium. *Topics in Early Childhood Special Education, 20*, 105–115.

Development, Review, and Revision of IEP, 34 C.F.R. § 300.324 (2006). Retrieved from http://idea.ed.gov/explore/view/p/,root,regs,300,D,300%252E324

Division for Early Childhood (DEC). (2007). *Promoting positive outcomes for children with disabilities: Recommendations for curriculum, assessment, and program evaluation.* Missoula, MT: Author.

Grisham-Brown, J., & Hemmeter, M.L. (1998). Writing IEP goals and objectives: Reflecting an activity-based approach to instruction for young children with disabilities. *Young Exceptional Children, 3*(1), 2–10.

Individuals with Disabilities Education Act (IDEA) of 1990, PL 101-476, 20 U.S.C. §§ 1400 *et seq.*

Individuals with Disabilities Education Act (IDEA) Amendments of 1997, PL 105-17, 20 U.S.C. §§ 1400 *et seq.*

Individuals with Disabilities Education Improvement Act (IDEA) of 2004, PL 108-446, 20 U.S.C. §§ 1400 *et seq.*

Macy, M., & Bagnato, S.J. (2010). Authentic alternatives for psychological assessment in early childhood intervention. In C. Reynolds (Ed.), *Oxford handbook of psychological assessment.* New York, NY: Oxford University Press.

Michnowicz, L.L., McConnell, S.R., Peterson, C.A., & Odom, S.L. (1995). Social goals and objectives of preschool IEPs: A content analysis. *Journal of Early Intervention, 19,* 273–282.

Mount, B. (1992). *Person centered planning: Promises and precautions.* New York, NY: Graphic Futures.

National Association for the Education of Young Children (NAEYC/NASCE). (2003). *Early childhood curriculum, assessment, and program evaluation: Building an effective, accountable system in programs for children birth through age 8.* Washington, DC: NAEYC.

National Research Council. (2008). *Early childhood assessment: Why, what, and how.* Washington, DC: The National Academies Press,

Notari-Syverson, A.R., & Shuster, S.L. (1995). Putting real-life skills into IEP/IFSPs for infants and young children. *Teaching Exceptional Children, 27*(2), 29–32.

Vandercook, T., York, J., & Forest, M. (1989). The McGill Action Planning System (MAPS): A strategy for building the vision. *Journal of the Association for Persons with Severe Handicaps, 14,* 205–215.

Wolery, M. (2000). Recommended practices in child-focused interventions. In S. Sandall, M.E. McLean, & B.J. Smith (Eds.), *DEC recommended practices in early intervention/early childhood special education* (pp. 29–37). Denver, CO: Division of Early Childhood of the Council for Exceptional Children.

Wolery, M. (2004). Using assessment information to plan intervention programs. In M. McLean, M. Wolery, & D.B. Bailey (Eds.), *Assessing infants and preschoolers with special needs* (3rd ed.). Columbus, OH: Pearson.

Wolf, M.M. (1978). Social validity: The case for subjective measurement, or how applied analysis is finding its heart. *Journal of Applied Behavior Analysis, 11,* 203–214.

4

Naturalistic Curriculum Model

Mary Jo Noonan

••••••••••••••• **FOCUS OF THIS CHAPTER** •••••••••••••••

- Curriculum models in early intervention and preschool special education
- Naturalistic approaches in early intervention curricula
- Age appropriateness and developmentally appropriate practice
- Implementing the naturalistic curriculum model

Curriculum is often defined as an organized and sequenced set of content to be taught: It is the "what to teach" (Bailey, Jens, & Johnson, 1983). Another, broader definition includes instructional techniques, or "how to teach," so that curriculum is defined as content and teaching techniques ("what and how to teach"). And sometimes content is not specified; instead, curriculum is defined by a process for deriving content and planning instruction, rather than specific content and procedures. In this chapter, curriculum includes all three approaches: content, techniques, and a process for deriving content and planning instruction.

A number of factors influence the general curriculum of early childhood programs. Some programs adopt published curricula, typically covering a range of themes that are of interest to young children. Suggested activities may be included to assist teachers in addressing the various topics associated with each theme. A common theme of a general early childhood curriculum, for example, is "community," and topics addressing the community theme might include places, people, and activities in the local community. Examples of published general early childhood curricula include The Creative Curriculum (Dodge, Colker, Heroman, & Bickart, 2002) and Meaningful Curriculum for Young Children (Moravcik, Nolte, & Feeney, 2013). Other early childhood programs follow a curriculum linked to a program philosophy and approach to early childhood education, such as Montessori (Gutek, 2004) or Reggio Emilia (Edwards, 1998). These early childhood curricula define the content and sequence of instruction, the teaching approach, and related program variables such as instructional materials, classroom arrangement, parent involvement, and scheduling.

In addition to published curricula and program approaches, educational standards influence the content of general early childhood curricula. States throughout the United States are defining early learning standards for early childhood education, usually addressing birth through age 5 or ages 3 to 5 (Neuman & Roskos, 2005). All 50 states have adopted common core standards for kindergarten through grade 12 (Carmichael, Martino, Porter-Magee, & Wilson, 2010). The standards identify benchmarks or goals that all children are expected to achieve in language arts and mathematics. While the standards are not a curriculum, they do affect instructional priorities in early childhood programs and will shape the content of instruction in the inclusive classroom.

CURRICULUM MODELS IN EARLY INTERVENTION AND PRESCHOOL SPECIAL EDUCATION

Three types of models have characterized early intervention curricula for infants and young children with special needs: 1) developmental, 2) developmental-cognitive, and 3) behavioral (Bailey et al., 1983; Hanson & Lynch, 1989). These models are continually being modified so that they are more immediately relevant to the needs of young children and their families. The most recent modifications focus on children interacting with the social and physical environment—naturalistic considerations. This chapter briefly reviews traditional curriculum models and their current naturalistic modifications. The naturalistic components of the models are then synthesized and presented as a naturalistic curriculum model for early childhood education.

Finally, this chapter provides a series of steps for implementing the naturalistic curriculum model.

Developmental Model

The developmental curriculum model was perhaps the initial approach to early intervention for infants and young children with disabilities. It was borrowed from the compensatory programs for children living in poverty in the 1960s (e.g., Head Start; see Chapter 1). It is sometimes referred to as an enrichment model because compensatory early childhood programs attempted to enhance or enrich the experiences of children living in poverty by providing them with experiences similar to those of their age peers living in more economically privileged circumstances.

The goal of the developmental model is to guide infants and young children through the typical sequences (or milestones) of child development. It is primarily a content model. The content includes the skills of physical development (gross motor and fine motor), adaptive development (self-help and daily living skills), social development, and communication development. Instructional strategies simulate activities engaged in by infants, toddlers, and preschoolers who do not have disabilities. The activities provide opportunities for demonstrating or encouraging the targeted milestones. Current approaches to developmental curricula such as activity-based instruction recommend that developmental skills be embedded and taught during naturally occurring activities and routines (Macy & Bricker, 2007).

Current applications of the developmental curriculum model also include an emphasis on infant/child and caregiver interaction (Ammaniti et al., 2006). Both partners in the interaction are considered the appropriate unit of focus for assessment and instruction because interaction is a cyclical process: The behavior of each member of the dyad affects the behavior of the other member. The shift in the developmental model to include this more naturalistic perspective (child and caregiver interaction) is compatible with the philosophy of early intervention as family centered rather than being focused solely on the child (Dunst, Trivette, & Hamby, 2007).

Developmental-Cognitive Model

The developmental-cognitive model is a theory-driven model based on the work of Jean Piaget (1952, 1954). Piaget posited that cognitive development occurs as a result of physiological growth and the child's interaction with the environment. This curriculum model is considered an interactionist approach defined by content and instructional techniques. The content is similar to the developmental model and emphasizes skill sequences of the sensorimotor period of intellectual development (birth through age 2). Cognitive skill sequences typically address five areas of intellectual development: object permanence (understanding that objects exist even when not in sight), means for obtaining environmental ends (using objects as tools to accomplish a goal), causality (using people or mechanical objects to make things happen), imitation (copying verbal and gestural behavior), and schemes (interacting with objects appropriate to the nature of the objects). Some curricula also include skills from the preoperational period of intellectual development (ages 2–7 years).

The instructional approach of the developmental-cognitive model reflects Piaget's interactionist theory: Tasks that are challenging are presented to the child to create a state of cognitive "disequilibrium." As the child attempts to solve the challenge of the task, he or she must intellectually organize the new information and adapt previously learned information in light of the new. The cognitive processes of organization and adaptation are referred to as "equilibration." In the 1970s, this model was applied to early intervention in the constructive interaction adaptation model (Bricker, Bricker, Iacino, & Dennison, 1976) and also in a compensatory education curriculum model (Weikart, Rogers, Adcock, & McClelland, 1971).

As the developmental-cognitive model was applied to early intervention, some researchers added a social development component (Toth, Munson, Meltzoff, & Dawson, 2006). This naturalistic perspective is based largely on the work of Jerome Bruner, a psycholinguist (Bruner, 1975, 1977). Bruner described early social skills as social-cognitive behaviors that serve an early communication (or prelinguistic) purpose. Such skills include following an adult's visual line of regard (the infant's gaze shifts to look where the adult is looking), joint attention (adult and infant demonstrate concurrent and sustained attention to the same object/activity), and turn taking.

In addition, the developmental-cognitive model includes a naturalistic component of environmental control (Dunst, Trivette, Raab, & Masiello, 2008). Infants and children learn environmental control when their behavior has a predictable effect on their social and physical environments. Environmental control is significant because it decreases children's dependence on adults to identify and meet their needs. Teaching environmental control skills involves attending to the child's subtle ways of responding to environmental stimuli and reinforcing behaviors that could be communicative. For example, if an infant winces when a spoon of food is presented, the parent withdraws the food, saying, "Oh, you don't want any more of that right now," and gives the child some milk instead. Responding to the infant's wince as communication may eventually teach the child environmental control (in this case, how much or when he or she is fed) using specific facial expressions.

Behavioral Model

The behavioral curriculum model is an instructional techniques model based on the principles of behavioral psychology. Behaviorists such as B.F. Skinner (Skinner, 1953), Sidney Bijou, and Donald Baer (Bijou & Baer, 1961, 1965) described human development and learning as resulting from environmental interactions in which individuals experience relationships among stimuli, actions, and the consequences of actions (reinforcement or punishment). As a curricular approach, interventionists or teachers alter stimuli to be more noticeable or meaningful to a child (e.g., pointing to a stimulus), help a child make a correct response so the consequence can be experienced, or provide more individualized or powerful reinforcement to strengthen the consequence. These techniques are termed *direct instruction* and include strategies such as prompting, shaping, and reinforcing. Direct instruction is implemented in a precise and consistent fashion. Learning is monitored through frequent data collection, and instruction is modified based on data evaluation.

In the behavioral model, naturalistic components include goal selection and instructional techniques. Goal selection is referenced to environmental needs or expectations. One method to determine environmental needs is to ask parents, caregivers, and other family members to describe their routines, the child's participation in the routines, and what they would like the child to learn associated with the routines (McWilliam, Casey, & Sims, 2009; Wolery, 1996).

Instructional techniques in the behavioral model have shifted from teacher-focused direct instruction techniques to more naturalistic procedures. For example, instead of teaching a preschooler to use two-word phrases by looking at picture cards and describing them ("big truck"), two-word phrases are taught throughout the day in free play, snack time, circle time, and storytime when the child initiates speech (Kaiser & Trent, 2007). Naturalistic techniques include teaching skills in sequence with other skills as they would typically occur, at the times when they are needed, using natural stimuli and consequences, and with strategies that promote independent, child-initiated behaviors. These techniques of enhanced milieu teaching (EMT) and activity-based interventions are described in detail in Chapter 7.

The naturalistic concern that newly acquired skills are generalized is addressed in the behavioral model by planning for generalization when skills are initially taught. Instructional procedures referred to as "general case" methods facilitate generalization by targeting a broad skill (e.g., grasping small objects) rather than a discrete skill (e.g., grasping a raisin) and providing instruction in several situations in which the skill is needed (Horner & McDonald, 1982). For example, the toddler who has difficulty with finger feeding because of poor fine motor skills has the objective to improve grasping (not just finger feeding) and is taught to grasp many small objects of various weights and shapes throughout the day.

The developmental, developmental-cognitive, and behavioral models have each incorporated naturalistic strategies and perspectives (see Table 4.1 for a summary of the models and their naturalistic components). The boundaries that once differentiated these models are becoming blurred as each emphasizes naturalistic considerations. The following assessment and intervention practices reflect the growing emphasis on naturalistic curriculum procedures (Sandall, Hemmeter, Smith, & McLean, 2005):

- Relying on assessment materials that capture the child's authentic behaviors in routine circumstances
- Assessing children in familiar contexts
- Assessing not only immediate mastery of a skill but also generalization
- Using a variety of appropriate settings and naturally occurring activities as teaching/learning contexts
- Providing services in natural learning environments as appropriate, such as home or community settings
- Fostering positive relationships, including peer–peer, parent/caregiver–child, and parent–caregiver relationships across environments
- Embedding and distributing specialized procedures (e.g., naturalistic strategies, prompt/prompt fading strategies) within and across activities

Table 4.1. Traditional curriculum models in early intervention and early childhood special education

Curriculum model	Curriculum type	Key features	Naturalistic components
Developmental	Content	Developmental skill sequences	Sequence of infant/child and caregiver interaction
Developmental cognitive	Content and teaching techniques	Developmental skill sequences	Sequences of social-cognitive development
		Sequences of cognitive skill development	Sequences of environmental control skills
Behavioral	Teaching techniques	Direct instruction	Skill sequencing
			Incidental and milieu teaching techniques
			Generalization strategies

Assessment is an integrated part of the naturalistic curriculum model. It is the process through which individualized curriculum goals are identified. Assessing the child in natural environments while participating in activities that are typical of same-age peers accomplishes three objectives: First, it ensures that intervention goals represent skills that are relevant to the child and family and have immediate usefulness. Second, it increases the likelihood that assessment results accurately reflect the child's abilities and needs (Farrell, 2009). Finally, it provides information as to where, when, and how services should be provided. Note that natural environments address social situations as well as physical situations.

NATURALISTIC APPROACHES IN EARLY INTERVENTION CURRICULA

The goal of the naturalistic curriculum model is to enhance the young child's environmental control, participation, and interaction in everyday experiences consistent with the cultural values and expectations of the family. The naturalistic model is a process model of curriculum: Content is derived through environmental assessment, and instruction uses naturalistic behavioral techniques. Natural environments are the "sources and contexts" of intervention (Dunst, Hamby, Trivette, Raab, & Bruder, 2000, p. 151). This model is appropriate for all infants and young children with disabilities, including those who have frequently been provided services in segregated environments (children with severe/multiple disabilities and those with autism). The sections below describe the major components of the naturalistic curriculum model: content, context, methods, cultural relevance, and evaluation. Note that contextual and cultural considerations are embedded throughout the model. The chapter emphasizes ways in which the what (content), where (context), and how (methods) of this model differ from traditional approaches and discusses additional concerns of cultural relevance and evaluation.

Content of Instruction

Content is the *what* of instruction—*what* to teach. In the naturalistic curriculum, goals for each child are developed on an individualized basis, reflecting the skill demands of natural, age-appropriate environments. The content "grows with the child" and is responsive to the requirements of the increasing number of environments that young children participate in as they get older. Chapter 5 describes the process of identifying these goals.

Age-Appropriate Skills *Age appropriate* means that the skills and activities are the same as those for infants and children who do not have disabilities. The naturalistic model encourages participation and interaction across the full range of family routines and activities. Family routines and activities and age-related expectations for infants and young children are influenced by the family's culture and values. For example, whether a caregiver immediately responds to an infant's crying is influenced by culture and child-rearing values. Similarly, expectations that toddlers help out with household chores (e.g., whether the child takes his or her dish to the sink) is heavily influenced by culture and family values. Therefore, the naturalistic curriculum model includes strategies to obtain family/caregiver information about family routines, activities, and expectations for their child's participation therein.

For young babies, the most important aspect of the environment is parent–infant interaction. Infants "control" their environment through behavior that affects the quality and quantity of incoming stimulation. This is one of the first ways infants learn to affect their environments.

The work of Brazelton has been particularly influential in understanding and designing interventions to promote infants' control of their environments (Als et al., 1979; Brazelton, 1982). According to Brazelton, the newborn engages in a neurological and physiological system of interaction, disorganization, reorganization, and then a return to interaction. As infants attend to and interact with the environment, they eventually become overstimulated. This overstimulation causes neuromotor and physiological disorganization. When disorganization occurs, the infant may fuss and withdraw from the environment by looking away or falling asleep. Withdrawing from the environment allows the infant to reorganize neurologically and physiologically and reestablish homeostasis (internal stability) and energy/drive for subsequent environmental input when desired.

Parents usually learn to recognize their infant's signals and determine when interactions are appropriate. They notice when the infant has received adequate stimulation and needs to rest. A successful parent–infant interaction is one in which there is mutual responsiveness, with the parent and infant each responding according to the signals of the other. For example, when the parent talks to the infant, the infant stops moving and stares at the parent. The parent pauses and talks again; the infant shows intent interest. The cycle is repeated several times. Finally the infant looks away. The parent recognizes this as a signal that the baby has tired and needs a rest from interaction, ceases the game, and rocks and cuddles the baby gently.

When an infant has a disability, however, his or her signals may not be easy to recognize or interpret. Infant specialists may observe the infant–caregiver dyad and provide feedback or reinforcement when the parent or caregiver shows sensitivity to the infant's behavior and effectively obtains, maintains, or terminates the infant's attention (Chen, Klein, & Haney, 2007). In this way, parents learn to become responsive to their infant, and the infant learns age-appropriate social-interaction skills. The distinctive feature of Brazelton's (1982) approach to enhancing infant–caregiver interaction is to provide feedback and reinforcement when the caregiver demonstrates appropriate sensitivity or responsiveness to the infant's behavior. The interventionists never take the infant from the caregivers to demonstrate interaction skills. Instead, the interventionists promote parent competence and self-confidence by observing and reinforcing instances of appropriate responsiveness (Dunst et al., 2010). Watching the caregiver's interaction style also allows interventionists to learn about cultural and interpersonal styles that are effective, albeit different from their own styles. Cripe and Venn (1997) extended this approach—building on effective strategies used by caregivers—to intervene with families who have toddlers and preschool-age children.

As the infant gets older, interaction with the physical environment increases. The social environment expands beyond parents to include siblings, relatives, and family friends. The naturalistic curriculum will include a wider range of behaviors to accomplish environmental interaction and control, particularly social, cognitive, and communication skills. For example, the infant may demonstrate environmental control by crying when a sibling takes a toy away, which results in the parent retrieving the toy for the infant.

During the first year of life, the infant learns the turn-taking and signaling skills that form the basis of later social and communication interactions. Like sensorimotor behaviors in Piaget's model, social-cognitive skills develop in a progression leading to mental representation (thinking) and symbolic thought; that is, the ability to use words to represent thoughts and actions (Seibert, Hogan, & Mundy, 1982, 1987). When parents respond to an infant's vocalizations as a request to repeat a playful episode, they are teaching the infant that the vocalization is a communication signal: "Do it again." For example, the parent's pause after a playful episode, the infant's communicative signal, and the repetition of the play is a turn-taking routine, much like the turn taking involved in conversation.

During the toddler years, the child's play expands in sophistication, and he or she shows an interest in the play of other children. Toddlers participate increasingly in the routines of other family members, sometimes as play (e.g., sweeping with a toy broom as the father sweeps the kitchen floor) and sometimes as a contributing member of the family (e.g., carrying a dish to the table, taking a turn playing ball with a sibling). Much of a toddler's participation in routines and activities in the home involves daily living activities such as dressing or bathing. Initially, participation may be in the form of cooperation: lying still while having a diaper changed or raising arms as a T-shirt is removed. Toddlers also begin to learn skills that will be useful in preschool, many of which are group participation skills (following simple directions, sharing, attending to a task or speaker). As in the case of social interaction routines, cultural and individual parent/caregiver preferences influence family daily living routines and expectations for child participation. And finally, during the preschool and kindergarten years, play, self-help, and school-related skills are expected and required. Note that play skills are legitimate content for early childhood curriculum, as well as an important context for addressing other intervention needs, such as communication or social skills (NAEYC, 2009; Wolery & Hemmeter, 2011).

The age-appropriate content of the naturalistic curriculum model includes the skills needed by the young child to participate in natural social and physical environments. Each family's social and physical environments are unique and influenced by culture, individual preferences, and interpersonal styles. Environments expand as the infant grows and develops, and the content of the naturalistic curriculum model expands accordingly to address the increasing range of behaviors needed for control, participation, and interaction. When a discrepancy exists between age-appropriate and readiness levels, a teacher should adapt the age-appropriate content to the child's abilities and needs.

A current emphasis in general early childhood curriculum is *developmentally appropriate practices* (DAP; Copple & Bredekamp, 2009). Two foundational concepts of DAP—age appropriateness and individualization—have important implications for the naturalistic curriculum model. Early childhood programs that ascribe to DAP emphasize a child-centered curriculum characterized by individual choice-making and play, rather than a teacher-directed, highly structured curriculum with a specific set of objectives identified for all children. The DAP model is based on the assumption that if children are allowed to explore their interests, their interests will guide them to choose and learn content that they are developmentally ready to learn.

Infants and children with severe disabilities, however, will not always be ready to learn the same activities as their age peers with mild or no disabilities. To support the inclusion of infants and young children with disabilities in early childhood programs, however, curricular activities should be age appropriate, even when the activities do not correspond to readiness levels. The activities of the general early childhood curriculum serve as a context for instruction. Specific objectives and the way in which children with disabilities participate in activities are individualized to address unique needs. For example, a preschool child with a disability selects a puzzle during morning free play and hands the pieces one at a time to a peer who puts the puzzle together. She has chosen an age-appropriate activity that is also of interest to her friend who does not have a disability. Although not able to assemble the puzzle, she is able to select puzzle pieces and to play cooperatively with a peer. Chapters 12 and 13 provide numerous strategies and examples for promoting peer interaction and independence in age-appropriate activities and inclusive settings.

Skills for Participating in Present and Future Environments The naturalistic curriculum model selects curricular content by identifying and analyzing the routines and activities of natural environments. There are a number of ways to approach the identification and analysis of routines and activities. One method is to interview parents or caregivers, asking them to describe their daily routines and activities and the infant's or child's present participation in these routines and activities. Potential goals and objectives are formulated as each routine and activity is discussed (McWilliam et al., 2009). The routines and activities identified in this ecological assessment will reflect the child's capabilities, interests, and temperament. For example, a child recovering from a hospital stay may play for short periods of time and only with one or two other children to avoid roughhousing. In contrast, another child may enjoy roughhousing and show the greatest amount of participation with large groups of children.

The uniqueness of each family is reflected in an ecological assessment of the home. Routines and activities will vary from one family to another depending on factors such as family members present in the home, work and/or school responsibilities, social/recreational interests and preferences, and interpersonal needs and strengths. Culture will be reflected in the family's lifestyle and will likewise influence the daily routines and activities from which curricular content is derived. For example, culture might guide family member roles (who does which chores), arrangements for mealtimes and sleeping, and the extent and nature of participation in social or religious activities.

Another ecological assessment strategy, focused on skills needed in future environments, is the survival skills model. Survival skills are behaviors that early childhood educators expect or require of children in childcare, preschool, or kindergarten settings (Noonan et al., 1992; Rous & Hallam, 2012; Vincent et al., 1980). Although many readiness assessments for preschool or kindergarten focus on preacademic skills, educators tend to expect young children entering early childhood programs to demonstrate social and communication skills (Wesley & Buysse, 2003). Survival skill assessments and related instructional approaches are discussed in Chapter 14.

The naturalistic model may include early intervention goals derived from the developmental and developmental-cognitive models. In these models, intervention goals are identified by comparing the child's skills to sequences describing typical development: Instruction begins with the skill that the child fails to demonstrate in the sequence of a developmental assessment. Developmental assessment usually includes social, communication, daily living, fine motor, gross motor, feeding, and cognitive skill sequences.

Developmental curricula and related assessments may be appropriate if they result in meaningful, age-appropriate instructional goals. These conditions would conceivably be met for children who are at risk or who have mild delays/disabilities—the majority of children served in most early intervention programs. Skill needs identified through developmental assessment for children with severe or multiple disabilities, however, would be far below the children's chronological ages, and thus ill-fitting with age-appropriate early childhood settings. Instead, skill adaptations may be more practical goals for achieving age-appropriate and functional skills for these children.

Context for Instruction

Context is the *where* of instruction. It is a characteristic of the naturalistic model that differentiates it from other early intervention curriculum models. The naturalistic model focuses on natural experiences (social and nonsocial) for determining the content of instruction, selecting and implementing the instructional methods, and evaluating child progress. Instruction is conducted as "situated learning," occurring in the context of family-guided routines (Dunst, Raab, Trivette, & Swanson, 2010). As an example of the importance of typical experiences in the naturalistic curriculum model, consider a 2-year-old named Missy who attends a community playgroup once a week. The playgroup usually consists of five 2- to 3-year-olds who participate together in a song time, a physical development activity, and a snack. Missy plays with the other children and follows the simple rules of the activities, such as passing toys and taking turns. Observations in the home and reports from the family, however, indicate that Missy is usually on the sidelines watching as her two sisters (ages 4 and 5) play. Missy's parents would like her to play with her sisters. Note that home experiences provide very different information than the playgroup regarding Missy's social and play skills. An instructional plan is designed to reflect the characteristics of the home environment. Given that the home environment includes Missy's 4- and 5-year-old siblings, the instructional plan is directed at the play behavior of the siblings as well as Missy. Missy's sisters are taught to invite Missy to play with them and are shown various ways that Missy can join in, even when she doesn't know how to play their games. Missy is taught to crawl close to her sisters when she wants to play with them. The success of instruction is evaluated in the home, during after-school hours, and on the weekends when the sisters typically play together. In all phases of this instruction—goal selection, instruction, and evaluation—the context has a significant influence.

For newborns, the most important environment is their home, the environment in which most of their social experiences occur. As the infant develops beyond the first few months of life, the social interaction context of the family expands and begins to include the extended family and friends. In addition, the infant increasingly attends to environmental stimuli, including objects. In the toddler and preschool years, the physical environment broadens to include settings outside the home, such as the neighborhood, playgrounds, parks, and shopping centers. Toddlers and preschoolers interact extensively with objects in their environment and are becoming more and more independent in their interactions. Their social spheres now include peers, as well as neighbors and family members.

At all ages, culture, individual lifestyles, and family preferences will influence the proportion and amount of time the child spends in various environments. For example, some families may have a large extended family that provides childcare as needed. They choose not to enroll the child in preschool. Weekend social activities are family gatherings and church activities. In contrast, other families may not live near their extended families and rely on community childcare programs and in-home babysitting services. They have smaller social networks comprised of a few friends and/or work colleagues. They regularly participate in their community's weekend family events, such as children's activities at the museum and recreation center sports.

The context for instruction in the naturalistic curriculum model is natural experiences. Natural experiences are the source of curricular content, as well as the instructional environments. The number and variety of natural experiences expand as infants and young children grow and at all times include an array of experiences that are unique to each family.

Instructional Methods

Methods are the *how* of instruction. The naturalistic curriculum model uses instructional methods that are minimally intrusive, that is, instruction that appears similar to naturally occurring events. In some cases, the instruction will be barely noticeable to an observer, as a teacher or parent interacts with a child in a very typical fashion. What the observer might now know, however, is that the interactions are planned in advance, including such strategies as creating opportunities to practice emerging skills, providing subtle prompts that assist a child or serve as a model for a new skill, or responding to a child's interest in an activity with encouragement to demonstrate an acquired skill at a more complex level.

Another criterion for instructional methods in the naturalistic curriculum model is "goodness of fit." This means that the methods must be suited to the child's temperament. *Temperament* refers to a personal behavioral style that includes the dimensions of activity level, intensity, mood, persistence, and reaction to new experiences. Its greatest influence is not on what a child does, but how he or she does it (Pelco & Reed-Victor, 2003). A concern for temperament means that teachers must pay close attention to a child's response to instructional methods. For example, if a child "resists" the instructional prompt of physical guidance, the teacher should try other types of prompts (e.g., a model) to be minimally intrusive from the perspective of the child.

Instructional Procedures for Newborns and Infants During the neonatal period, while curricular content focuses on parent–infant interaction, the primary instructional procedure is Brazelton's approach (described below) to observe parent–infant interaction and provide positive and descriptive feedback when the parent is responsive to the infant's signals (Als, Lester, & Brazelton, 1979; Brazelton, 1982). For infants beyond the first few months, a number of early interventionists suggest instructional techniques similar to Brazelton's, but focused on a larger repertoire of interactions, compatible with broadening social experiences (Dunst et al., 1987; McCollum & Stayton, 1985). For example, to assist the infant in gaining control over the environment and to teach parents to be more effective in promoting social interactions, Dunst et al. (1987) recommend the following interaction approaches:

- Being sensitive to the child's behavior
- Reading the child's behavior as intents to interact
- Responding to the child's initiations
- Encouraging ongoing initiations
- Supporting and encouraging competence

These interaction approaches can be implemented through guided learning, violations of expectations, introduction to novelty (Dunst, 1981), and enhanced milieu teaching (Kaiser & Trent, 2007). Note that families of some cultural backgrounds may not view parent-infant interaction as a priority (Chen & McCollum, 2001).

In *guided learning*, play or instructional situations are carefully arranged so that they attract the infant's attention, appear highly motivating, and are at a level of difficulty that is optimally challenging. An example of guided learning is to present a 10-month-old girl who explores objects (a cognitive skill) by banging them with a variety of other objects (e.g., wooden spoon, metal spoon, whisk broom) and a variety of surfaces for banging (e.g., an aluminum cookie sheet, wicker basket, magazine). The situation is enticing to the infant because she enjoys banging objects, and the availability of several objects and surfaces is challenging. The environmental arrangement of the task guides learning. It also reflects sensitivity to the infant's present level of performance, encourages her to participate in the activity without adult instruction, and supports and encourages competence.

The procedure of *violating expectations* requires that a predictable and repetitive play sequence be established. The sequence is then altered without warning. Violations of expectations surprise the infant, often increasing the infant's attention and curiosity (motivation) and stimulating a communicative response (a quizzical look at the adult, a vocalization, or a laugh), as if to say, "What happened?" An adult who covers and uncovers her smiling face repeatedly with a cloth in a game of peekaboo violates the infant's expectations if she uncovers her face and is suddenly not smiling or has her eyes closed. The infant will usually respond to such a violation with a communicative response, and the adult should respond to any communication by the infant as a request to reestablish the expected sequence.

Using novelty is a minimally intrusive technique that can motivate exploratory behavior. For example, rather than place all the infant's toys around her, a caregiver would give her only one or two toys a day. Changing the toys from day to day will encourage play because they seem more interesting. This technique encourages infant-initiated behaviors.

Enhanced milieu teaching (EMT) refers to a group of instructional techniques in which a predetermined child behavior is used to identify occasions for instruction (Kaiser & Trent, 2007). For example, when an infant reaches for a toy that is out of reach (the predetermined behavior), instruction is conducted to encourage more developmentally sophisticated behavior (the desired response is modeled or prompted, "Tell me what you want"). EMT is a strategy that responds to the infant's behavior as an intent to interact and thus may shape social interaction behaviors. EMT is discussed at length in Chapter 7.

Instructional Procedures for 2- through 6-Year-Olds EMT methods are important instructional procedures for 2- through 6-year-olds. They are highly effective for promoting independent and child-initiated behaviors. Systematic teaching procedures that involve more controlled and adult-directed instruction are also included in the naturalistic curriculum model but with specific techniques to facilitate generalization. For example, the general case instructional procedure (Horner & McDonald, 1982) is teacher-directed and more tightly structured than incidental teaching, but it is effective in promoting generalization.

General case instruction uses two strategies: objectives are described as generalized skills rather than discrete skills ("child will grasp raisins or small candies, T-shirt bottom, and cup" rather than "child will grasp raisins"), and generalized skills are taught across a number of situations with a variety of materials (e.g., at breakfast, when getting dressed in the morning, after recess). In selecting situations or materials, choose those that represent the range of characteristics of situations or materials to which the skill is intended to generalize. Both of these techniques are a part of general case instruction.

Instructional procedures within the naturalistic model emphasize instruction that is as subtle as possible while still being effective (minimally intrusive); that promotes generalization; and that fits into the natural settings, routines, and activities of the child and the family. The more naturalistic the instruction, the greater the likelihood that newly learned skills will be generalized and used in the natural situations in which they are needed.

Cultural Relevance

Research has shown that culture influences learning, largely through its effect on learning styles and interpersonal communication (Tharp & Dalton, 2007). In the naturalistic curriculum model, a number of psychocultural variables are embedded so that instruction is responsive to the child's learning and communication style. These variables include, but are not limited to,

- Instructional arrangements (individual work, group work, oral presentation, and so forth)
- Teaching procedures (connection to children's experiences, pace of instruction, and so forth)
- Communication style (eye contact, direct prompting, questioning, calling on children, and so forth)
- Reinforcement strategies (public acknowledgment, type of reward, and so forth)
- Performance expectations (remaining seated, oral response, voluntary response, and so forth)

Although these variables may have a profound impact on learning, individuals are not usually cognizant of them. Thus, a child's parents or caregivers probably cannot inform others of their child's learning style and communication preferences. The teacher will need to observe family interactions with the child who has a disability, as well as with other members of the family, for evidence of learning style and communication preferences. Once identified, these may be included in the instructional plan. For example, parents may wait for what seems to be an extended period of time for children to respond to a direct question. Lengthy wait time has been found to be characteristic of many Native Americans (Yamauchi & Tharp, 1995). Failure to incorporate long wait times in instructional plans may result in ineffective teaching. For young children, this may mean a slower pace for typical give-and-take games between parents and children. Chapter 7 describes strategies for addressing cultural relevance throughout instruction.

Evaluation Methods

The primary focus of evaluation in the naturalistic curriculum model is generalized outcomes in natural settings. Generalization is promoted through general case instruction (described in Chapter 6) and assessed in settings that are similar to the instructional settings but in which instruction has not occurred. For example, a 4-year-old is taught to ask for a turn at play rather than take objects from his sister and the children next door. Generalization is assessed in natural noninstructional settings, including the childcare program and the park on Saturdays. The assessment is conducted under naturalistic conditions in which the skill is expected, rather than in clinical or contrived settings typical of traditional assessments. Chapters 5 and 6 review strategies for evaluating children's instructional progress.

IMPLEMENTING THE NATURALISTIC CURRICULUM MODEL

The following steps are a guide to implementing a naturalistic curriculum. They include descriptions of how content and strategies from the traditional models and related services can be included at each step.

Step 1: Conduct Ecological Assessment

As described in Chapter 5, ecological assessment begins with listing the routines, activities, and expectations typical of the child's day. The child's participation in these routines and activities are assessed to determine his or her current skill levels and instructional needs.

Step 2: Develop Instructional Goals and Objectives

Recall that goals are broad statements, such as "Juanita will participate in mealtime." One or more objectives may then be written for each goal. Instructional objectives in the naturalistic model have the following characteristics:

- Instructional objectives support participation in naturally occurring routines and activities.
- The context(s) for instruction is specified.
- Instructional objectives address generalized skills.
- A functional criterion is included.

The following objective illustrates these four characteristics: Given a small spoon with a built-up handle at snack and lunch at preschool and dinner at home (naturally occurring routines, generalized across settings and adults), Juanita will grasp the spoon and scoop thick-pureed or sticky foods such as mashed potatoes, pureed vegetables, or pudding (generalized across food types) and raise the spoon to her mouth with half or more of the food remaining on the spoon, maintaining a grasp until she has the food in her mouth (functional criteria) for five of six scoops, for five consecutive meals. (A comprehensive discussion of developing instructional objectives for individualized family service plans and individualized education programs is included in Chapter 3.)

Step 3: Develop Instructional Plans

Individualized instructional plans are formulated for each objective. In addition to identifying information such as date, name of child, and objective, all instructional plans should include six components (see Figure 4.1):

1. *Contexts or occasions for instruction:* When and in what situations will the instructional plan be implemented? Who will provide the instruction?
2. *Physical positioning or materials arrangement:* Does the child require any special seating arrangements to demonstrate the skill objective? How or where are the materials presented? Are any specialized materials needed?

Figure 4.1. Instructional plan format.

General Case Intervention Plan			
Child: Fia Corrado	**Interventionist(s):** Lani Smith, Mom, Dad, and Kimo		**Date:** 2/4/13
Objective: When Fia wakes up in the morning or after a nap, she will vocalize any sound(s), such that the sounds are audible outside the room where she has been sleeping on 8 of 12 consecutive opportunities.			
Contexts/ occasions for intervention: When you notice that Fia is awake, in the morning, after a nap, at home, or preschool *Physical positioning and/or materials:* On her right side, with one pillow between her knees and one under her head; with her left knee and hip flexed *Intervention techniques:* 1. Approach Fia and talk to her until she vocalizes, or for 3 minutes (do for 5 days). 2. Enter the room so Fia can see you, wait 6 seconds before talking to her. After 6 anticipated correct responses (within the 6-second delay), move to Step 3. 3. Wait outside the room for 10 seconds.	*Child response:* Fia will vocalize any sounds, such that they are audible outside the room where she has been sleeping. *Task analysis (if applicable):* n/a		*Consequences for correct response:* Pick Fia up immediately and say, "Oh you are ready to get up now!" and carry her out of the room. *Consequences for incorrect or no response:* Approach Fia and say: "Are you ready to get up?" Wait 6 seconds. If she vocalizes, respond as you would for a correct response. If she doesn't, leave the room for 6 seconds. If she vocalizes within that time, enter the room and respond as you would for a correct response. If she doesn't vocalize, pick her up and try again next time.

3. *Instructional techniques:* What procedures will be used to teach the skill and increase the likelihood of the child demonstrating the skill correctly? What will be provided to motivate and assist the child to make the correct response?

4. *Child's response:* In precise and observable terms, what is the expected response? Will any approximations or variations of the skill be accepted as correct?

5. *Consequences for correct response:* How will the child be shown that he has made a correct response? Is the natural reinforcer obvious, or can it be made more obvious? Will any further instruction be provided when the child responds correctly?

6. *Corrections for incorrect response:* What instructional techniques will be implemented if the child does not respond or makes an incorrect response? If the child makes a correct response following the correction procedure, is reinforcement provided?

Because most instruction will be implemented across more than one situation, and because objectives are developed as general case objectives, instructional plans are written as general case plans (Horner, Sprague, & Wilcox, 1982). Chapter 6 focuses on the development of instructional plans and provides detailed descriptions of each of these instructional components.

It is also necessary to develop data collection systems in order to monitor the effectiveness of instruction. The type of data collected must correspond to the criterion level specified in the goal. For example, if the child's goal is to share materials at least three times during three consecutive play sessions, the number of times (or frequency) the child gives materials to a peer must be recorded. Data are graphed so that progress may be monitored. If progress does not occur, or occurs too slowly, the instructional plan must be modified. Chapter 5 provides a complete discussion of measurement, data collection, and evaluation methods.

Step 4: Prepare an Instructional Schedule

Once instructional objectives and plans have been developed, teaching opportunities must be identified and scheduled. A scheduling matrix (see Figure 4.2) is useful for creating an individualized schedule. The first step in constructing

Figure 4.2. Example of a scheduling matrix.

Child: Fia Corrado	Additional Objectives								Date: 2/4/13
Daily Schedule	Sitting	Reaching	Self-feeding	Dressing	Toy play	Take turns	Vocalize	Receptive labels	Point for choice or request
6:30–6:45 a.m.									
Wash up									
Diaper change									
Dressing									
6:45–7:15 a.m.									
Breakfast									
7:45–9:00 a.m.									
Playpen (Mom's chores)									
Diaper change									
9:00–9:30 a.m.									
Play with Mom									
9:30–11:00 a.m.									
Lunch									
Self-feeding									
11:30–noon									
In kitchen with Mom									
Noon–1:30 p.m.									
With Mom—errands, park, or walk									
1:30–2:00 p.m.									
Diaper change									
Clean up & relax									
2:00–3:00 p.m.									
Nap									
3:00–5:30 p.m.									
With sibling									
Take turns									

the matrix is to complete the left column by listing daily activities. If the child is enrolled in a center-based or home-based infant program that meets one or two hours per week, two matrices may be developed—one for the infant program and one for days when the infant does not receive services from the infant program. If the child attends childcare or preschool, the daily program schedule is listed as it occurs during the child's daily schedule.

The second step is to list the child's instructional goals across the top of the matrix. In the third step, the box under each instructional goal corresponding to its associated activity is checked to indicate that the goal will be taught during that time. The team reviews the entire daily schedule to determine if other activities might also be appropriate times for instruction. If so, the corresponding box is also checked. For example, if a toddler has a goal to share during playtime with neighborhood peers, the box under the *sharing* goal and next to the *playtime with neighborhood peers* activity is checked. The team also checks the box next to the *free-time* activity during morning preschool and *playtime with siblings* in the late afternoons.

If it is not possible to address all instructional goals as often as desired, the team (including the family) should establish priorities and decide which goals will receive the most attention. If there are not enough natural opportunities for addressing some of the instructional goals, it may be necessary to create naturalistic occasions. For example, a preschool child may receive instruction on changing her T-shirt after naptime if more instructional opportunities to work on her dressing goal are needed.

Given the current emphasis on teaching during natural learning opportunities, much of the child's instruction may occur at home. The implication of this is that early intervention teachers must shift their focus from teaching children to supporting families and caregivers in their efforts to enhance their children's learning (Bruder, 2010). The family and caregivers must decide when they are best able to implement instructional plans. A family may feel too rushed to work on a self-feeding plan in the morning while preparing for work and school, but may feel comfortable to do so at the evening meal and at lunchtime on weekends. If the child attends childcare or a preschool program, the instructional needs (and individual matrices) of the other children, as well as staffing ratios, must be considered in finalizing the schedule for the entire group of children.

Step 5: Implement Instruction

After the instructional plans have been developed and scheduled, teaching begins. Instructional plans are implemented as accurately as possible so that their effectiveness can be determined. Program staff and family members who implement the same instructional plans may observe one another periodically to be certain that they are implementing the plans in the same manner.

Step 6: Monitor Progress

Progress on instructional plans should be evaluated regularly. How frequently data are collected will vary. For some instructional plans, very precise data will be collected by the infant specialist when the baby attends the infant program once a week. The family may keep simple data (a checklist) indicating which days they were able to implement the instruction and whether the child performed the skill independently or with help. If the child attends a preschool program, data may be collected daily on high-priority instructional plans; lower priority goals may be monitored less frequently.

Because most instructional goals will be formulated as general case objectives, it is also necessary to assess whether generalization has occurred. Generalization is assessed by observing the infant or child in situations in which the skill has not been taught, but in which its use would be expected. For example, the skill of sharing was taught at preschool, with a sibling, and with neighborhood peers. Generalization is assessed by observing the child at a family picnic with cousins or with peers at a baby sitter's home. Generalized objectives are mastered only when generalization to new (noninstructional) situations is demonstrated.

The more frequently data are collected, the more accurately progress can be monitored. When enough data have been collected and graphed to create a fairly clear picture of performance (usually five or six data points), the data are reviewed and a decision is made whether to continue the plan as is or to change it. If progress is not as expected, only one part of the instructional plan is modified so that the effectiveness of the change can be evaluated (again, after five or six data points are collected). Frequent progress monitoring will result in a dynamic instructional plan that is responsive to child performance.

These six steps yield an individualized curriculum that is based on the unique ecology of an infant or child and family. It begins with the assessment process and continues through the development, implementation, and ongoing evaluation of instructional plans. As noted, Chapter 5 describes instructional planning in detail.

SUMMARY

The naturalistic curriculum model draws on the naturalistic trends emerging from the developmental, developmental-cognitive, and behavioral curricula models. It respects the unique culture, preferences, and lifestyle of each family by promoting increased participation and interaction in natural environments, including the home, neighborhood, childcare, and school environments. Goals are derived through ecological assessment procedures and address skill needs associated with age-appropriate activities as well as social interaction with parents, siblings, and other significant individuals. Once goals are established, instructional plans are developed using systematic teaching procedures. The child's progress is then monitored through frequent data collection to ensure program effectiveness. When progress is not as expected, instructional plans are modified accordingly.

This chapter has described the naturalistic curriculum model for infants and young children. The intent of the model is to develop individualized intervention plans that address the unique needs of children in their home, school, and community environments. Subsequent chapters provide more detail on conducting assessment and intervention procedures in naturalistic settings (Chapters 5 and 6, respectively) and specialized intervention procedures that address particular instructional needs, such as adaptations for physical disabilities, strategies for behavioral challenges, and approaches to promote independence and social interaction (Chapters 7–14).

STUDY QUESTIONS

1. Identify and describe the three traditional curriculum models associated with early intervention and early childhood special education.
2. Discuss the naturalistic trends associated with each traditional curriculum model.
3. What is the goal of the *naturalistic curriculum model*?
4. What is the content of the naturalistic curriculum model? Describe at least two strategies for developing goals in the naturalistic curriculum model.
5. Explain the following statement: *In the naturalistic curriculum model, age appropriate activities are the context for instruction.*
6. Describe *naturalistic environments* that a 1-year-old, 2-year-old, 3-year-old, and 5-year-old might experience. How might the experiences and needs of a child in naturalistic environments vary from age 1 to age 5?
7. Discuss what it means to use *minimally intrusive* teaching procedures.
8. Discuss the focus of a naturalistic curriculum for an infant from 1 month to 5 months of age.
9. Identify and briefly define two instructional approaches in the naturalistic curriculum model that are appropriate for 2- through 5-year-olds.
10. Discuss how teaching in natural settings promotes *generalization*.
11. List and briefly describe the six steps in implementing the naturalistic curriculum model.

REFERENCES

Als, H., Lester, B.M., & Brazelton, T.B. (1979). Dynamics of the behavioral organization of the premature infant. In T.M. Field, A.M. Sostek, S. Goldberg, & H.H. Shuman (Eds.), *Infants born at risk* (pp. 173–192). New York, NY: Spectrum.

Ammaniti, M., Speranza, A.M., Tambelli, R., Muscetta, S., Lucarelli, L., Vismara, L., Odorisio, F., & Cimino, S. (2006). A prevention and promotion intervention program in the field of mother–infant relationship. *Infant Mental Health Journal, 27*(1), 70–90.

Bailey, D.B., Jens, K.G., & Johnson, N. (1983). Curricula for handicapped infants. In S.G. Garwood & R.R. Fewell (Eds.), *Educating handicapped infants: Issues in development and intervention* (pp. 387–415). Rockville, MD: Aspen.

Bijou, S.W., & Baer, D.M. (1961). *Child development: Vol 1. A systematic and empirical theory.* New York, NY: Appleton-Century-Crofts.

Bijou, S.W., & Baer, D.M. (1965). *Child development: Vol. 2. Universal stage of infancy.* New York, NY: Appleton-Century-Crofts.

Brazelton, T.B. (1982). Early intervention: What does it mean? In H.E. Fitzgerald, B.M. Lester, & M.W. Yogman (Eds.), *Theory and research in behavioral pediatrics* (Vol. 1, pp. 1–34). New York, NY: Plenum.

Bricker, D., Bricker, W., Iacino, R., & Dennison, L. (1976). Intervention strategies for the severely and profoundly handicapped child. In N. Haring & L. Brown (Eds.), *Teaching the severely handicapped* (Vol. 1, pp. 277–299). New York, NY: Grune & Stratton.

Bruder, M.B. (2010). Early childhood intervention: A promise to children and families for their future. *Exceptional Children, 76*(3), 339–355.

Bruner, J. (1975). The ontogenesis of speech acts. *Journal of Child Language, 2,* 1–19.

Bruner, J. (1977). Early social interaction and language acquisition. In H. Schaffer (Ed.), *Studies in mother-infant interaction* (pp. 271–289). New York, NY: Academic Press.

Carmichael, S.B., Martino, G., Porter-Magee, K., & Wilson, W.S. (2010). *The state of state standards—and the common core in 2010.* Washington, DC: Thomas B. Fordham Institute.

Chen, D., Klein, M.D., & Haney, M. (2007). Promoting interactions with infants who have complex multiple disabilities: Development and field-testing of the PLAI curriculum. *Infants & Young Children, 20*(2), 149.

Chen, Y.J., & McCollum, J.A. (2001). Taiwanese mothers' perspectives of parent-infant interaction with children with Down Syndrome. *Journal of Early Intervention, 24,* 252–265.

Copple, C., & Bredekamp, S. (Eds.) (2009). *Developmentally appropriate practice in early childhood programs serving children from birth through age 8* (3rd ed.). Washington, DC: National Association for Education of Young Children.

Cripe, J.W., & Venn, M.L. (1997). Family-guided routines for early intervention services. *Young Exceptional Children, 1*(1), 18–26.

Dodge, D.T., Colker, L.J., Heroman, C., & Bickart, T.S. (2002). *The creative curriculum for preschool.* Washington, DC: Teaching Strategies.

Dunst, C.J. (1981). *Infant learning.* Allen, TX: DLM/Teaching Resources.

Dunst, C.J., Hamby, D., Trivette, C.M., Raab, M., & Bruder, M.B. (2000). Everyday family and community life and children's naturally occurring learning opportunities. *Journal of Early Intervention, 23,* 151–164.

Dunst, C.J., Lesko, J.J., Holbert, K.A., Wilson, L.L., Sharpe, K.L., & Liles, R.F. (1987). A systematic approach to infant intervention. *Topics in Early Childhood Special Education, 7*(2), 19–37.

Dunst, C.J., Raab, M., Trivette, C.M., & Swanson, J. (2010). Community-based everyday child learning opportunities. In K.R. Harris & S. Graham (Eds.), *Working with families of young children with special needs* (pp. 60–92). New York, NY: Guilford.

Dunst, C.J., Trivette, C.M., & Hamby, D.W. (2007). Meta-analysis of family-centered helpgiving practices research. *Mental Retardation and Developmental Disabilities Research Reviews, 13*(4), 370–378.

Dunst, C.J., Trivette, C.M., Raab, M., & Masiello, T.L. (2008). Early child contingency learning and detection: Research evidence and implications for practice. *Exceptionality, 16*(1), 4–17.

Edwards, C.P. (1998). *The hundred languages of children: The Reggio Emilia approach—advanced reflections.* Greenwich, CT: Ablex.

Farrell, A.F. (2009). Validating family-centeredness in early intervention evaluation reports. *Infants & Young Children, 22*(4), 238–252.

Gutek, G.L. (2004). *The Montessori method: The origins of an educational innovation: Including an abridged and annotated edition of Maria Montessori's the Montessori method.* Lanham, MD: Rowman & Littlefield.

Hanson, M.J., & Lynch, E.W. (1989). *Early intervention: Implementing child and family services for infants and toddlers who are at-risk or disabled.* Austin, TX: PRO-ED.

Horner, R.H., & McDonald, R.S. (1982). Comparison of single instance and general case instruction in teaching a generalized vocational skill. *Journal of the Association for the Severely Handicapped, 7*(3), 7–20.

Horner, R.H., Sprague, J., & Wilcox, B. (1982). General case programming for community activities. In B. Wilcox & G.T. Bellamy (Eds.), *Design of high school programs for severely handicapped students* (pp. 61–98). Baltimore, MD: Paul H. Brookes Publishing Co.

Kaiser, A.P., & Trent, J.A. (2007). Communication intervention for young children with disabilities: Naturalistic approaches to promoting development. In S.L. Odom, R.H. Horner, M.E. Snell, and J. Blacher (Eds.), *Handbook of developmental disabilities* (pp. 224–246). New York, NY: Guilford.

Macy, M.G., & Bricker, D.D. (2007). Embedding individualized social goals into routine activities in inclusive early childhood classrooms. *Early Childhood Development and Care, 177,* 107–120.

McCollum, J.A., & Stayton, V.D. (1985). Infant/parent interaction: Studies and intervention guidelines based on the SIAI Model. *Journal of the Division for Early Childhood, 9*(2), 125–135.

McWilliam, R.A., Casey, A.M., & Sims, J. (2009). The routines-based interview: A method for gathering information and assessing needs. *Infants & Young Children, 22*(3), 224–233.

Moravcik, E., Nolte, S., & Feeney, S. (2013). *Meaningful curriculum for young children.* Upper Saddle River, NJ: Prentice Hall.

National Association for the Education of Young Children (NAEYC). (2009). *Developmentally appropriate practice in early childhood programs serving children from birth through age 8: A position statement.* Washington, DC: NAEYC.

Neuman, S.B., & Roskos, K. (2005). The state of state pre-kindergarten standards. *Early Childhood Research Quarterly, 20*(2), 125–145.

Noonan, M.J., Ratokalau, N.B., Lauth-Torres, L., McCormick, L., Esaki, C.A., & Claybaugh, K.W. (1992). Validating critical skills for preschool success. *Infant-Toddler Intervention, 2*(3), 187–202.

Pelco, L.E., & Reed-Victor, E. (2003). Understanding and supporting differences in child temperament: Strategies for early childhood environments. *Young Exceptional Children, 3*(3), 2–11.

Piaget, J. (1952). *The origins of intelligence in children.* New York, NY: International Universities Press.

Piaget, J. (1954). *The construction of reality in the child.* New York, NY: Basic Books.

Rous, B.S., & Hallam, R.A. (2012). Transition services for young children with disabilities. *Topics in Early Childhood Special Education, 31*(4), 232–240.

Sandall, S., Hemmeter, M.L., Smith, B.J., & McLean, M.E. (2005). *DEC recommended practices: A comprehensive guide for practical application in early intervention/early childhood special education.* Longmont, CO: Sopris West.

Seibert, J.M., Hogan, A.P., & Mundy, P.C. (1982). Assessing interactional competencies: The early social-communication scales. *Infant Mental Health Journal, 3,* 244–258.

Seibert, J.M., Hogan, A.P., & Mundy, P.C. (1987). Assessing social and communication skills in infancy. *Topics in Early Childhood Special Education, 7*(2), 38–48.

Skinner, B.F. (1953). *Science and human behavior.* New York, NY: Free Press.

Tharp, R.G., & Dalton, S.S. (2007). Orthodoxy, cultural compatibility, and universals in education. *Comparative Education, 43*(1), 53–70.

Toth, K., Munson, J.N., Meltzoff, A., & Dawson, G. (2006). Early predictors of communication development in young children with autism spectrum disorder: Joint attention, imitation, and toy play. *Journal of Autism and Developmental Disorders, 36*(8), 993–1005.

Vincent, L.J., Salisbury, C., Walter, G., Brown, P., Gruenewald, L.J., & Powers, M. (1980). Program evaluation and curriculum development in early childhood special education: Criteria of the next environment. In W. Sailor, B. Wilcox, & L. Brown (Eds.), *Methods of instruction for severely handicapped students* (pp. 308–328). Baltimore, MD: Paul H. Brookes Publishing Co.

Weikart, D.P., Rogers, L., Adcock, C., & McClelland, D. (1971). *The cognitively oriented curriculum.* Washington, DC: National Association for the Education of Young Children.

Wesley, P.W., & Buysse, V. (2003). Making meaning of school readiness in schools and communities. *Early Childhood Research Quarterly, 18*(3), 351–375.

Wolery, M. (1996). Using assessment information to plan intervention programs. In M.E. McLean, D.B. Bailey, & M. Wolery (Eds.), *Assessing infants and preschoolers with special needs* (2nd ed., pp. 491–518). Englewood Cliffs, NJ: Prentice Hall.

Wolery, M., & Hemmeter, M.L. (2011). Classroom instruction. *Journal of Early Intervention, 33*(4), 371–380.

Yamauchi, L.A., & Tharp, R.G. (1995). Culturally compatible conversations in Native American classrooms. *Linguistics and Education, 7,* 349–367.

5

Planning and Monitoring

Linda McCormick

•••••••••••••••• **FOCUS OF THIS CHAPTER** ••••••••••••••••

- Purposes of assessment, planning, and monitoring
- Child-centered planning procedures
- Ecological theory and assessment procedures
- Planning and organizing portfolio assessment

As noted in Chapter 3, assessments used with young children should be used only for their intended purposes—screening, diagnosis and/or eligibility determination, intervention planning, and monitoring/evaluation.

PURPOSES OF ASSESSMENT, PLANNING, AND MONITORING

Assessment, planning, and monitoring are closely related and interdependent activities that address the following questions:

- *What* does this child need to learn? What the child needs to learn depends on the expectations of daily activities, curriculum objectives, and early learning standards. The focus is on identifying behaviors that will have developmental and functional usefulness and benefits for the child in present and future environments (e.g., kindergarten).

- *How* will we teach this child? Specialized instructional procedures include naturalistic approaches such as milieu teaching, activity-based intervention, embedded and distributed trials, and high-probability procedures. These procedures incorporate environmental arrangement, adaptations, and prompts and prompt-fading procedures. Specialized instruction may also involve assistive equipment or technology, peer-mediated strategies, and systematic instruction.

- *When* and *where* will instruction be provided? Naturalistic instructional approaches require presentation of brief instructional trials throughout the day in age-appropriate activities and routines. Decisions need to be made as to who will be responsible for implementing the special instruction at the specified points throughout the day.

- *How* will we track the child's progress? The only way to ensure that teaching has been effective is to monitor the child's behavior during and after instruction. Decisions need to be made as to precisely what type of data will be collected, when and by whom, and what data collection procedures to use.

At the broadest level the focus is twofold: teaching the child to participate in age-appropriate activities and routines in the setting (e.g., moving about the room, making choices about activities and materials, playing alone and with peers, responding to peer and adult initiations, participating in conversations) and helping the child accomplish the developmental skills identified in the individualized education program (IEP) (e.g., requesting desired objects, using plurals, producing three-word phrases, asking and answering questions, recognizing and naming shapes and colors). This requires direct, systematic, and individualized instruction embedded in activities throughout the day. Child-centered planning, ecological assessment/planning, and portfolio assessment assist in 1) identification of specific instruction and intervention targets, 2) determination of where and when individualized instruction will be provided, and 3) measurement of child progress. Procedures for implementing the specialized instructional procedures (*how* to teach) are described in detail in subsequent chapters.

CHILD-CENTERED PLANNING PROCEDURES

Child-centered planning is a way for people close to the child to share their understanding and visions for the child. It can generate information for Individualized Family Service Plans (IFSPs) or IEP development or it can be incorporated as part of the ecological assessment process. Child-centered planning is a variant of the McGill Action Planning System (MAPS) (Vandercook, York, & Forest, 1989), personal futures planning (Mount & Zwernick, 1988), and Choosing Options and Accommodations for Children (COACH) (Giangreco, Cloninger, & Iverson, 2011). MAPS was the first of these assessment strategies. Developed at McGill University for school-age individuals, it is most often undertaken when the student with disabilities has had experiences in integrated settings long enough to develop relationships with peers. The focus is on identifying the gifts, talents, skills, and opportunities of the person with disabilities and then formulating these as positive goals and potential job opportunities. The plan is intended to be dynamic, changing as changes occur in the individual's lifestyle and participation in the community. Similar to MAPS, COACH is most often used with school-age persons. It is multilayered in that the procedures go beyond identification of priority learning outcomes by family members and the student with disabilities. There are specific guidelines for converting the outcomes into IEP goals and objectives and then developing supports that will help the student achieve the objectives in inclusive educational settings.

Child-centered planning is for young children. The goals are 1) to learn things about the child that only those who love him or her and have an investment in the child's future can articulate (the immediate and extended family, peers of the child with disabilities when appropriate, friends and neighbors of the family, related services providers, community preschool staff, early intervention staff, and special education personnel) and 2) to generate information that can then be used to plan and evaluate intervention and instruction. Child-centered planning provides an opportunity for the family and others who have a deep commitment to the child to contribute to planning, in addition to participating in the more formal assessment process that uses traditional testing instruments. This information has social validity. Social validity refers to the degree to which the goals and objectives and the subsequent intervention that are the outcomes of the child-centered planning process are desired and valued by the family and other significant persons in the child's world (Wolf, 1978).

The first step is bringing these important people together to construct a coherent picture of the child's strengths and gifts and their dreams for his or her future. This planning session may last anywhere from 1 to 3 hours. (Sometimes an additional session is necessary.) There should be a flip chart on an easel, a chalkboard, or large sheets of chart paper mounted on the wall with a separate paper (or section of the chalkboard) for recording responses to each question. The facilitator (usually the teacher or another service provider) asks the following questions to draw out the participants' thoughts and feelings:

- What is (*child's name*)'s history?
- What are (*child's name*)'s strengths and gifts?
- What are (*child's name*)'s needs?

Table 5.1. Child-centered planning vision for Kaitlin

Kaitlin will:
- Continue to be happy and healthy
- Move on her own
- Play with toys and enjoy games with her brother
- Enjoy being read to
- Feed herself
- Express her wants and needs so that anyone can understand
- Walk with a walker
- Sit up without assistance
- Have friends
- Always be in class with peers who do not have disabilities

- What is your fondest dream for (*child's name*)'s future?
- In your opinion, what would an ideal day be like for (*child's name*)?
- What is your worst nightmare where (*child's name*) is concerned?

The meeting lasts until all of the participants have had a chance to express their thoughts and all responses have been recorded. After the meeting, the information from the chart paper or the chalkboard should be transferred to regular-size paper and distributed to the participants for their comments and additions. Finally, the edited and expanded responses are condensed as a vision that provides one source of information for goals and objectives (and for the child's portfolio, if the teacher uses portfolio assessment). Table 5.1 shows the shared vision for a 3-year-old with severe disabilities that was developed through the child-centered planning process. This is exactly as the statements were recorded in the planning session.

As noted, the shared vision for the child's future that comes out of the child-centered planning process contributes to planning for intervention and instruction. At the same time it provides a standard against which to judge the outcomes (social validity) of the goal and objectives and the intervention procedures. The goals and objectives and the intervention procedures have social validity if they reflect the vision developed by the participants in the child-centered planning process.

ECOLOGICAL THEORY AND ASSESSMENT PROCEDURES

Ecological theory has roots in anthropology. When noted anthropologist Ruth Benedict (1934) published her ideas about the relationship between humans and their social-cultural environment in 1934, she used the term *cultural relativity* to describe the notion that human behavior cannot be properly understood unless it is interpreted within a larger cultural context. Simply stated, a behavior that is appropriate in one cultural context (e.g., separate sleeping arrangements for infants and young children) may be regarded as inappropriate in another. Ecology, now a branch of biology, studies the relationship between living organisms and their physical environment.

Many decades after Benedict's work, psychologists introduced ecological principles into the domain of psychology with studies of the effects of the physical environment on people's social behavior, and, vice versa, the effects of social behavior on the physical environment (Barker, 1968; Bronfenbrenner, 1979). These ecological psychologists insisted that the only way to get a valid picture of a child's functioning is by observing the child's behavior in the context of normally occurring routines in familiar settings.

Bronfenbrenner, probably the best known of the ecological psychologists, described the child as embedded in a series of interrelated systems that interact with one another and with the child to influence development. These nested systems both affect and are affected by the developing child. He labels the system closest to the child in the immediate environment the *microsystem* (the family, child care settings, school). The microsystem is embedded within three more distal systems: the *mesosystem*, the *exosystem*, and the *macrosystem*. The child does not participate directly in these distal systems, but events that occur in them can indirectly influence the child (e.g., the parent's worksite). The macrosystem, the furthest removed and most inclusive of the systems, is the social-cultural context (e.g., cultural beliefs, social structures).

Assessment based on ecological theory was first applied to developing goals and objectives for adolescents with severe and multiple disabilities by Brown and et al. (1979) in the late 1970s. It is now widely used with children of all ages and types of disabilities and in many environments, including inclusive preschools and family childcare. The information generated through the ecological assessment process is used for three purposes: 1) to develop instructional goals and objectives, 2) to plan for adaptations and supports, and 3) to select activities and routines for which special instruction is appropriate and necessary. The ecological assessment process is basically the same regardless of the setting. It may be implemented in a classroom setting, a home, a child care setting, or a community setting before or immediately after enrollment of the child with disabilities.

This chapter describes the implementation of ecological assessment in an inclusive early childhood program. Curriculum development typically draws from many sources, including recommended developmentally appropriate practices (Copple & Bredekamp, 2009). The focus is on mediating the understandings that children construct from their interactions with the environment in a way that advances their learning and development. The broad goals are for children 1) to actively initiate and engage in interactions with their social and the physical environments, 2) to learn to make choices, 3) to develop social relationships, and 4) to feel independent, safe, secure, competent, and accepted. Daily activities and routines are chosen to reflect what children are interested in and enjoy, and the curriculum is sensitive to children's cultural values, beliefs, and styles and the range of developmental levels represented in the class. They also reflect the state's preschool standards.

The preschool common core standards for 3- to 5-year-olds vary somewhat from state to state, and they may have different titles (e.g., guidelines, benchmarks). They are not a curriculum per se but they contribute to curriculum development. They are most appropriately viewed as expectations for learning and development, suggesting knowledge and skills that should be demonstrated by preschool children. Most importantly, all of the standards, including those for social-emotional development, language arts literacy, mathematics, science, and social studies can be addressed in the daily routines and activities that are characteristic of preschool classrooms.

Ecological assessment uses a matrix format similar to the matrices used for activity-based planning (Pretti-Frontczak & Bricker, 2004) and routines-based intervention (McWilliam, 2012) to identify behaviors that are necessary for participation in daily routines and activities. Figure 5.1 shows a completed ecological assessment form for Jace, a 3-year-old with Down syndrome. Jace is in his first week in preschool. (This example includes only the first two pages of a four-page completed form.) The following are the steps that the team followed in the assessment process (McCormick & Noonan, 2002).

Step 1: List Daily Activities and Routines in the Classroom and Other Naturalistic Settings

List these in the first column of the form in the order in which they typically occur. Because there are many teaching opportunities in every transition, some teachers like to list transitions as separate activities. For example, Transition from Arrival to Circle could be a separate routine and listed after Arrival. Transition from Circle to Art would be listed as another routine after Circle, and Transition from Art to Snacks would be a routine after Art in the first column.

Step 2: List Major Behavioral Expectations

Completing this step requires reflection and discussion. List broad expectations for each activity in the first column under the name of the activity or routine. Include those general expectations that differentiate the activity or routine from other activities and routines throughout the day. Every child in the class will not demonstrate every one of the behaviors every day. These are expectations for all of the children. Avoid being too specific. For example, it is better to say "answer questions about the story" than "answer *three* questions about the story."

Expectations should be positive and involve active engagement with the environment. "Sit quietly and don't bother peers" is an example of an expectation that violates this admonition. Keep in mind that children learn nothing that has functional or developmental value from "waiting in line" or "sitting quietly." For the brain and the body to grow, there must be active and positive engagement with the environment.

Developing the list of expectations for all activities in a typical day takes time, but once completed this list can be used for all children as long as the activities and routines remain the same. The one factor that will affect the expectations is the time of year. Expectations for children new to preschool in August will obviously be different from expectations at the midpoint and later in the school year. Many teachers have three or four different "expectations lists" that they use, depending on the time of year.

Step 3: Score "Can Do" or "Needs to Learn"

Discussion now shifts from activities, routines, and expectations for the class as a whole to the strengths and instructional needs of the child with disabilities.

Figure 5.1. Completed ecological assessment for Jace

Ecological assessment

Team members: Dayana, Melissa, Brandi, Yusong, Andreia

Child: Jace **Date:** 2/2/11

Activities/routines and expectations	Can do	Needs to learn	Comments	Objectives
Activity/routine: arrival/free play				
Say "Hi" and respond to "How are you?"		✓	No response—does not look at teacher, just goes inside.	Greet teacher (eye contact and verbalization) at the door.
Put belongings in cubby.	✓		Looks for his photo and pushes his backpack into his cubby.	
Select toy and play table or a center.		✓	Just wanders around the room.	Select a toy or activity center.
Play/share toys with peers.		✓	When led to a chair or center, he plays alone.	Play cooperatively with peers.
Put toys away when the signal sounds.		✓	Doesn't want to stop playing—refuses to help with cleanup.	Return toys to the shelf.
Activity/routine: circle				
Move to carpet area/sit in circle when music begins.	✓		Follows the other children and sits—needs help crossing his legs.	
Raise hand/say, "I am here" when photo is held up.		✓	Raises hand (when prompted) but does not vocalize.	Respond to roll call photo without prompting and vocalize.
Sing/do hand motions or rhythm instruments.		✓	Sometimes imitates motions but doesn't sing.	
Answer when asked questions about the story.		✓	No response.	Respond to questions about a story (by pointing to pictures or verbalizing).
Activity/routine: art				
Put on a smock.		✓	Needs physical assistance.	Independently put on a smock and close the Velcro tabs.
Get materials from the supply table as directed.		✓	Needs physical/verbal prompts.	Independently retrieve art materials from the supply table.
Use materials properly.		✓	Cannot cut or squeeze glue—does fine with crayons.	Demonstrate cutting and gluing skills.
Follow verbal/visual activity directions.		✓	Does not watch peers, so check the visual directions.	Follow verbal/visual directions for art activities.
Clean up/remove smock.		✓	Doesn't want to stop—ignores the cleanup signal.	Put materials away when an activity is over.
Activity/routine: snacks				
Wash and dry hands—throw away the paper towel.	✓		Can do, but wants to play in the water.	
Find a chair and sit.	✓		Follows peers.	
Pass plates and napkins.	✓		Manages with peer assistance.	
Eat and drink independently.	✓		Does fine with a cutout cup. Eats most of the food he is given.	
Throw trash in container.	✓		Imitates peers.	

Source: McCormick and Noonan (2002).

Rate whether the child can (and does) perform the expected behavior or needs to learn it. If team members feel that they know the child well enough, they can complete this rating without observations. They just go down the list one by one, reach consensus, and check whether the child can perform the behavior or not. Then they write comments as to what the child actually does when called upon to perform the identified behavior. If team members are not familiar enough with the child's behavior to reach consensus, then the child should be observed for a day or two to ascertain specific strengths and instructional needs related to the expectations.

Step 4: Formulate Goals and Objectives

As noted in Chapter 3, goals are short statements identifying the desired outcome of intervention or instruction. They describe behaviors that the child can reasonably be expected to accomplish in a 12-month period. For example, a goal could be "fully participate in the daily morning circle." Morning circle typically includes a variety of activities designed to foster language skills, turn-taking, and social-emotional development. Expectations include greeting one another, identifying one's own name in written form, listening to and responding to questions about stories, singing, identifying numbers and sounds of the alphabet, and much more. Morning circle behaviors that the child cannot yet perform would be stated as objectives.

Note that objectives for Jace are stated in the fifth column of the ecological assessment form (Figure 5.1). Goals and objectives for Jace for the first three activities of the day are restated as a list on Table 5.2. As instructional targets, these objectives meet the criteria for meaningfulness and functionality in that they promote his full participation in activities and routines that define the class environment.

Table 5.2. Goals and objectives for Jace

Goal: Jace will participate in the morning arrival and free play routines.
- Jace will use eye contact and a verbalization (a greeting or an approximation) to address the teacher every morning upon arrival.
- Jace will select a toy and take it to the play table or go to an activity center every morning upon entering the classroom.
- Jace will share toys and take turns with peers during free play every day.
- Jace will return his toys to the shelf when the signal sounds every day.

Goal: Jace will participate in morning circle.
- Jace will raise his hand (without prompting) and approximate "I'm here" or "here" when his photo is displayed at roll call every day.
- Jace will respond (by pointing and/or verbalizing) to at least one question about the story every day.

Goal: Jace will participate in art activities.
- Jace will put on his smock independently and close the Velcro tabs as directed for daily art activities.
- Jace will retrieve art materials from the supply table when the directions are given.
- Jace will cut paper (using adapted scissors) in daily art activities.
- Jace will squeeze the glue bottle and aim the glue as directed in daily art activities.
- Jace will follow the steps in the visual directions posted on the easel each day.
- Jace will participate in cleanup and return art materials to the supply table each day.

An important advantage of using ecological assessment to identify instructional goals and objectives is that targeted behaviors are already embedded into the daily activities and routines. This simplifies planning for provision of teacher trials in the various activities. Procedures for embedding objectives when they have come from an assessment procedure other than ecological assessment are described in Chapter 6.

Step 5: Plan Instruction

Figure 5.2, an instructional planning form, shows a portion of the planning form used in preparation for developing a more detailed lesson plan for Jace. The objectives briefly stated in the first column are from the last column of the ecological assessment form. The other four columns detail required skills to perform the objective (What to Teach), instructional procedures (How to Teach), Adaptations and Supports, and Persons Responsible.

The What to Teach column lists the specific skills to teach to Jace in order to accomplish the objective (to look at the teacher and to verbalize in response to the teacher's greeting). The third column, How to Teach, describes the specialized instructional procedures that will be used to teach the identified skills.

In many ways, the planning that goes into the third column is most critical. Children with disabilities need specialized instruction—individualized instruction that is specially planned and provided to teach specific skills. Specialized instruction is basic to providing services for young children with

Figure 5.2. Instructional planning form

Child: Jace				
Objectives (briefly)	What to teach	How to teach	Adaptations and supports	Persons responsible
Greet teacher: • Morning • Recess	Look at teacher. Verbalize in response to teacher greeting.	Position your face at Jace's eye level. When he attends, provide greeting. Use mand model (say "Hi") with progressive time delay.	Be sure to position your eyes at Jace's eye level.	Dayana, Brandi, or Yusong
Choose toy or activity	Move independently to toy shelf. Select toy. Sit (at table or on floor) and manipulate toy. or Move to a center and engage in center activity.	Physically guide Jace to toy shelf or activity center. Display a preferred and nonpreferred toy. Say, "What do you want?" Prompt Jace to select the preferred toy (progressive time delay). Same procedure for center. Say, "Where to you want to play?" Guide Jace to the center (physical prompt–progressive time delay).	Arrange Jace's favorite toy and a nonpreferred toy on a shelf at eye level.	Dayana, Brandi, or Yusong

disabilities. *Individualized instruction* in this context should not be defined to mean one-to-one instruction, although one-to-one instruction may occasionally occur in inclusive classrooms (with children without disabilities as well as those with disabilities). Specialized or individualized instruction provides environmental support, adult and peer assistance (encouragement, feedback, prompts), adaptations, and special equipment or technology to maximize the child's learning.

The belief that specialized instruction should not interfere with children's interactions and participation in the classroom has led to the development of instructional approaches that resemble the methods used with typically developing children in early childhood programs. These approaches, called naturalistic approaches, provide brief instructional trials interspersed throughout the day in age-appropriate activities and routines. They are as much about when instructional trials are provided as how they are provided. Planning is essential. Some examples of naturalistic approaches are 1) enhanced milieu therapy, 2) activity-based instruction, 3) embedded and distributed time delay trials, and 4) high-probability procedures. These approaches are described in Chapters 6 and 7.

Adaptations and supports are listed in the fourth column of Figure 5.2. They also require team collaboration and careful planning. The broad goal of independent functioning is foremost. Adaptations and supports are provided only when necessary and then just enough to facilitate participation. Table 5.3 provides examples of task adaptations and ways to provide supports during instruction. Finally, the team should discuss and decide who will be responsible for providing the instruction and supports for each objective and list these names in the last column of the instructional planning form.

Step 6: Plan Data Collection

The last step in the ecological assessment process is to develop a comprehensive monitoring and evaluation and plan. There should be a data collection form for each activity for which specialized instruction will be provided.

Table 5.3. Adaptations and supports

Provide scaffolding	Provide support, assistance, and encouragement until the child performs a new skill independently or gives evidence of understanding a new concept.
Provide practice	Give the child many opportunities and encouragement to repeat tasks and routines.
Change the task	Modify the task as necessary for the child to be successful, or provide a different task that accomplishes the same function.
Change the materials	Provide alternate materials (e.g., different size, texture) to accomplish the task.
Augment directions	Provide visuals depicting the sequence of steps in activities and routines, and cue the child to use these devices.
Change the response requirements	Require a less sophisticated response (e.g., a word approximation rather than a word) or a response in a different modality (pointing rather than verbalizing).
Assign a partner	Ask a peer to act as a model and/or helper for the task.
Provide adaptive equipment	Provide whatever devices (e.g., switches, environmental control units) are necessary for meaningful participation and task completion.

Figure 5.3. Data collection matrix

Name: Jace	Activity: arrival/free play		Week: 4/11 to 4/15			
Objective	Type of data	Monday	Tuesday	Wednesday	Thursday	Friday
Greet teacher	Frequency count Indicate type of prompt					
Select toy or activity Take to table or activity center	Frequency count Indicate type of prompt					
Share and take turns	Anecdotal notes Indicate peer(s)					
Return toys to shelf	Frequency count Indicate type of prompt					

The data collection matrix for Jace (for specialized instruction during "arrival/free play") is shown in Figure 5.3 This matrix form lists objectives (in the first column) and the types of data that will be collected (in the second column). It is on a plastic clipboard on a hook near the door to the classroom. There is a similar form for other activities. These are also on clipboards near where the activity takes place or on the corner of the teacher's desk. Data are recorded each day on this grid or on attached sheets.

The purpose of data collection is to determine whether instruction is accomplishing the desired outcomes. There are a number of decisions that need to be made. The first is whether to collect quantitative or qualitative data. Both quantitative and qualitative data collection procedures yield valuable and meaningful information about observable behavior that contributes to the evaluation process. Each has strengths as well as weaknesses. The decision which to use depends on the behavior that is being observed.

Quantitative Data As discussed in Chapter 3, quantitative data provide information about the frequency/number, rate, duration, latency, topography, or magnitude of a behavior. They answer questions about the effect of an intervention on particular observable behavioral outcomes. Specific questions that focus on highly discrete behaviors (the types of behaviors often defined on IEPs) generate objective quantitative data. Procedures for quantitative data collection, reporting, and analysis are discussed at length in Chapter 5.

Qualitative Data Qualitative data provide information about complex, broadly defined, quality-of-life outcomes such as communication, how children interact with others, and general comfort and well-being in the setting or activity. These questions require subjective, qualitative data with a focus on describing and to some extent, interpreting the nature of what is observed. A major difference between quantitative and qualitative data is that the latter does not require definition of the specific dimensions of the behavior prior to data collection. Examples of questions that require qualitative data are the following: "What types of activities does Jace engage in during free play?" "Which peers is Abby most attracted to?" "When and with whom does Anisa attempt communication?" "What does Anisa communicate about?" "In what activities and with whom does Jace initiate interactions?"

It is most important to record and analyze the data in a systematic and rigorous fashion—whether the lens is finely focused to collect quantitative data or focused widely on a broad spectrum of the child's behavior and the context in which the behaviors are embedded to yield qualitative data. Observers must remember to 1) match the data collection procedure to the question and 2) use multiple data sources whenever possible.

At the end of the week, the data from all of the activity matrices are graphed or otherwise summarized and analyzed to determine whether progress is satisfactory or whether there is a need to modify the program. Permanent product samples and anecdotal records are also collected every day and reviewed weekly, and selections are made for the portfolio.

PLANNING AND ORGANIZING PORTFOLIO ASSESSMENT

Portfolio assessment is formative assessment that relies on compilation of the child's work and other artifacts. A portfolio consists of a compilation of information that has been purposefully collected and assembled in an organized fashion. Portfolios provide a picture of the child's progress toward achievement of his or her goals and objectives over a specified period of time (typically a school year). An electronic or web-based portfolio can assemble basically the same products electronically, serving as a permanent record of the child's progress.

Well-developed portfolios provide a representative sample of a broad spectrum of behavior, using triangulation to document significant and meaningful behavior change in developmental, academic, and social arenas. Triangulation, a concept from qualitative research, refers to collecting material in as many different ways and from as many diverse sources as possible. Portfolios provide repeated examples of the child's behavior in different situations. The greater the variety of data provided, the better the overall picture. For example, a preschooler's portfolio might include audios documenting the child's improving oral language skills, teacher observation notes, photos of the child engaged in play with peers, parent reports of improved behavior at home, and a checklist showing improvements in independent toileting skills.

As an individualized assessment procedure, a portfolio does not compare one child with other children. This is especially important for culturally and linguistically diverse children. Portfolios can answer questions that cannot be answered by traditional assessment and data collection procedures. For example, they can answer such questions as "How well is Jace participating in art activities?" "How well is Jace following the snack routine?" "How well is Jace communicating with peers throughout the school day?" It is tempting to avoid qualitative questions such as these because data collection may be more difficult than simply tallying responses. Qualitative questions such as the above are challenging because the child's behavior is related to specific contextual variables.

As portfolios address qualitative questions concerning a child's progress, they may include work samples that illustrate the learning process rather than a product or outcome (e.g., showing the process of how the child learns to hold and use a utensil rather than noting the outcome of being able to eat independently). Electronic portfolios (or e-portfolios) provide an alternate presentation format that allows for digital work samples, such as photographs, video clips, and audio files. In addition to illustrating the child's learning process, e-portfolios are well suited to documenting longitudinal progress. The e-portfolio makes it possible to include many times more photographs than paper-based portfolios (Kristovich, Hertzog, & Klein, 2004). While there would not be space for 25 photographs showing a child's day-to-day progress in skill acquisition, 25 photographs is a relatively small amount of data in an e-portfolio. Other advantages of e-portfolios are the potential to use multiple forms of evidence and easy access and storage (Kankaanranta, 2001). A child's speech acquisition can be documented with 1) graphs portraying the acquisition of targeted communication skills, 2) photographs of the child interacting in increasingly larger groups of children as speech improves, and 3) recorded audio samples to accompany the photographs. Photographs of artwork can be included, allowing the child to take the original home to show his or her family. Digital storage and portfolio sharing may be conducted on the web, on CD/DVD, or both. One early childhood program that implemented a web-based communications project found that it fostered and increased communication among teachers, families, and children (Kristovich et al., 2004). Children enthusiastically explained their projects to their families when they viewed the photographs, videos, and work samples together on the web.

Portfolios, whether electronic or paper-based, provide information for monitoring and evaluating a child's progress and making informed decisions about future programming. Data collected through interviews (with the child or the child's significant others), observations (both descriptive and interpretive), photographs, audio- and/or videotapes, anecdotal records, and reflective journals show the child's progress in daily activities.

Planning and Construction

Selection and organization of materials and data for inclusion in the portfolio is guided by the child's IFSP or IEP goals and objectives and information collected with the ecological assessment. There should be a specific purpose for including each entry related to the child's developmental and instructional goals. Samples of the child's writing, painting, cutting, collage construction, drawing, and quotations taken early in the school year and then near the end of the year are included so that it is possible to see progress. Other possible entries include observational data, summaries of work samples, pre and post checklists, calendars, summaries of accomplishments, summaries of anecdotal records, graphs, rating scales, language samples, notes from interviews with the child about his or her favorite activities, photos, videos, and audio. Each entry should have a descriptive label that tells the date, the person who provided the entry, and a notation as to why it is important. Involve children as active partners in the development and selection of materials for their portfolios.

Photographs of group projects (e.g., cooking experiences, special school events, field trips) document the participants in action as well as the outcome of their efforts. Photos should be mounted in such a way that there is adequate space for text describing the activity, whatever comments are dictated by the child, and notations as to how the relevant skills and concepts are evident in the picture. Photographs are particularly beneficial for documenting the performance and products of children with severe disabilities. For example, the portfolio might include photos of the child building block structures, riding a tricycle at recess, interacting with peers, pouring juice at snacks, and stacking cups at the sand table.

Photos are also a way to show growth in confidence:

- A photo of the child purposefully moving his wheelchair in the direction of the activity center for free play
- A photo of the child in a wheelchair confidently leading her class down the hall and then down the sidewalk to the waiting bus

They can also show growth in social and communicative interactions:

- A photo of the child adding paper to a collage he is making with a peer
- A photo of the child giving a picture communication card to her peer in exchange for a toy
- A photo of the child responding to the request of a peer to share a toy

Photos such as these also show parents that their child is an active member of the class.

Teachers can document the child's progress in classroom routines and activities with anecdotal records that are brief, factual, and nonjudgmental. A special form specifically for anecdotal notes can be developed and made available for adults in the class, or anecdotes can simply be recorded on index cards. If an anecdotal record form is provided, there should be a place to note the child's name, date and time, activity context, and the name of the recorder, in addition to the specific child behavior (e.g., a skill related to an IEP goal).

Organization

There are a number of ways to organize and store the information in a paper-based portfolio. The portfolio may be an expandable folder, a cardboard or plastic box, a large loose-leaf notebook, or some other container. The only requirement is a way to divide the content into sections with marker tabs for easy filing and retrieval. Portfolios may be organized by content areas, time periods (months, quarters, semesters), IEP goals and objectives, activities, or thematic units. The first page of each section describes the contents of that section. The first section of the portfolio should provide a list of the child's IFSP or IEP goals and objectives, a description of the classroom with the program philosophy, curriculum objectives, a table of contents, and a copy of a letter to parents explaining the purpose of the portfolio and its organization.

Portfolios should be kept in a location that is easily accessible with portfolio supplies nearby (e.g., blank forms, a hole punch, plastic bags or clear envelopes for tapes and other three-dimensional objects, pencils, pens). Set aside time each day to select materials and place them in the appropriate sections. Photograph and print pictures of projects that are too large to fit in the portfolios. Teachers typically include no more than two or three entries within each section of the portfolio each week.

Remember, the portfolio has two purposes: 1) to document the child's learning and development and 2) to improve present instruction practices and future programming. As everyone on the team should assist in data collection, they should also be involved in regular portfolio review meetings to consider patterns of child behavior, whether the children are progressing at a desired rate, and areas of the program that need improvement. Because portfolio assessment provides information about the learning *process* as well as the *products* of learning, analysis of the portfolio information together with other data is invaluable when deciding whether instructional arrangements should be continued, modified, or expanded.

Perhaps the most challenging aspect of portfolio assessment is finding the necessary time to collect, select, review, and evaluate work samples. However, most teachers consider it worth the effort, because, in addition to providing instructionally relevant information about their students' growth and development, portfolio assessment shows respect for children, and it is far more meaningful to parents and administrators than the scores generated by traditional assessment procedures. Documenting functional behavior in natural contexts establishes a critical link between assessment and instruction. Parents gain an understanding of their children's interests as well as their development and accomplishments in the context of the daily routines and activities of the preschool program.

SUMMARY

This chapter has described three planning and evaluation/monitoring processes: 1) child-centered planning, 2) ecological assessment, and 3) portfolio assessment. Child-centered planning generates a vision for the child that can serve as a social validity standard for goals, objectives, and intervention procedures. Ecological assessment identifies the behaviors that, when learned, will enable the child to fully participate in activities with typically developing peers in inclusive settings (preschool classroom, child care setting, after-school care) and natural environments (home, extended family settings). Portfolio assessment is a way to collect data for purposes of planning and modifying instruction and to monitor progress. Portfolios, both electronic and paper-based, use numerous methods and sources of information across contexts and across people to formulate a picture of children's abilities in actual activities in natural environments. They differ from traditional assessment tools and procedures in that they are multidimensional.

•••••••••••••••••••• **STUDY QUESTIONS** ••••••••••••••••••••

1. What are the four questions that need to be addressed when planning instruction?
2. Discuss the role of *child-centered planning, ecological assessment and planning,* and *portfolio assessment* in the context of the four basic purposes of assessment.
3. Describe the child-centered planning meeting(s).
4. Describe the goal of the child-centered planning process.
5. Describe the roots of ecological theory and ecological assessment.
6. List the steps in the ecological assessment process.
7. Describe quantitative and qualitative data collection procedures to determine whether desired outcomes are accomplished.
8. Describe portfolio assessment procedures.
9. Describe the issues that need to be considered when preparing a portfolio.
10. Describe the materials and data that are typically included in a portfolio.

REFERENCES

Barker, R.G. (1968). *Ecological psychology.* Stanford, CA: Stanford University Press.
Benedict, R. (1934). *Patterns of culture.* Boston, MA: Houghton Mifflin.
Bronfenbrenner, U. (1979). *The ecology of human development: Experiments by nature and design.* Cambridge, MA: Harvard University Press.
Brown, L., Branston, M.B., Hamre-Nietupski, S., Pumpian, L., Certo, N., & Gruenwald, L. (1979). A strategy for developing chronological age-appropriate and functional curricular content for severely handicapped adolescents and young adults. *Journal of Special Education, 13,* 81–90.
Copple, D., & Bredekamp, S. (Eds.) (2009). *Developmentally appropriate practice in early childhood programs serving children from birth through age 8* (3rd ed.). Washington, DC: National Association for Education of Young Children.
Giangreco, M.F., Cloninger, C.J., & Iverson, V.S. (2011). *Choosing outcomes and accommodations for children (COACH): A guide to educational planning for students with disabilities* (3rd ed.). Baltimore, MD: Paul H. Brookes Publishing Co.
Kankaanranta, M. (2001). Constructing digital portfolios: Teachers evolving capabilities in use of information and communications technology. *Teacher Development, 5*(1), 259–275.
Kristovich, S., Hertzog, N.B., & Klein, M. (2004). Connecting families with innovative technology in an early childhood gifted program. *Journal of Early Intervention, 26,* 247–255.
McCormick, L., & Noonan, M.J. (2002). Ecological assessment and planning. *Young Exceptional Children Monograph #4* (pp. 47–60). Division for Early Childhood (DEC) of the Council for Exceptional Children. Longmont, CO: Sopris West.

McWilliam, R.A. (2012). *Routines-based early intervention: Supporting young children and their families.* Baltimore, MD: Paul H. Brookes Publishing Co.

Mount, B., & Zwernick, K. (1988). *It's never too early, It's never too late: A booklet about personal futures planning for persons with disabilities, their families, friends, case managers, service providers, and advocates* (Publication 42-88-109). St. Paul, MN: Governor's Planning Council on Developmental Disabilities.

Pretti-Frontczak, K., & Bricker, D. (2004). *An activity-based approach to early intervention* (3rd ed.). Baltimore, MD: Paul H. Brookes Publishing Co.

Vandercook, T., York, J., & Forest, M. (1989). The McGill Action Planning System (MAPS): A strategy for building the vision. *Journal of the Association for Persons with Severe Handicaps, 14,* 205–215.

Wolf, M.M. (1978). Social validity: The case for subjective measurement, or how applied analysis is finding its heart. *Journal of Applied Behavior Analysis, 11,* 203–214.

6
Instructional Procedures

Mary Jo Noonan

•••••••••••••••••• **FOCUS OF THIS CHAPTER** ••••••••••••••••••
- Systematic instruction in natural settings
- Effective assistance: prompting
- Effective motivation: encouragement
- Promoting generalization
- Implementation of systematic instruction
- Monitoring systematic instruction

Systematic instruction is the consistent application of teaching procedures that are individualized to address the child's personal, learning, and developmental characteristics. Aspects of systematic instruction include how materials are arranged, when and how reminders are provided, and how to provide physical guidance. Encouragement procedures provide motivation and are included in instruction to arouse interest and to reinforce desired responses. *Naturalistic* and *systematic* instruction are not incompatible constructs. Although the systematic emphasizes consistency, it does not require unnatural and mechanistic instruction. Furthermore, it does not require instructional plans to be so rigid that the teacher or infant specialist responds without regard for the interests or spontaneity expressed by the child. Furthermore, rather than being mechanistic and artificial, systematic instruction can and should be designed to utilize the natural supports to learning that are present in typical environments. Young children with disabilities need specialized instruction, but they also learn from typical *untouched* environments. The job of special educators is to tweak these environments by embedding systematic instruction in a way that is effective but not unnecessarily intrusive (McWilliam, 2012).

A systematic instructional approach provides for program integrity and accountability. Strategies are precisely formulated and are always conducted in a similar manner when teaching a specific skill, whether instruction is embedded or provided directly (Wolery & Hemmeter, 2011). Furthermore, when a teacher or infant specialist shares the education plan with other members of the intervention team, the plan on paper is an accurate representation of what is being implemented. The extent to which a systematic instructional plan is teacher-directed and structured corresponds with the needs of the child. When new skills pose difficult challenges, considerable teacher direction may be needed; conversely, when skills are nearly accomplished, less structure and teacher direction are required. Finally, consistent instruction allows for objective evaluation of program effectiveness. Evaluation is important so that the plan can be modified if progress is not as expected. It is also important to the field of early intervention that effective procedures be documented.

SYSTEMATIC INSTRUCTION IN NATURAL SETTINGS

As previously noted, the instructional situation is a key feature that distinguishes the naturalistic curriculum model from other models. Systematic instruction does not require exclusion; instead (and as discussed in Chapter 1) the quality of instruction is improved when it is linked to naturally occurring routines, activities, prompts, and reinforcement (Leach, 2012). The most fortuitous natural learning opportunities are those that promote development/learning through four qualities: interest, engagement, competence, and mastery (Dunst, Bruder, Trivette, Raab, & McLean, 2001). Learning opportunities that attract a child's interest and result in high levels of engagement are ones that the child will likely attempt and continue to pursue. In addition, learning opportunities that increase a child's competence and feeling of mastery will be highly reinforcing.

Teaching during naturally occurring routines and activities is vital to the success of the naturalistic curriculum model because naturally occurring prompts (assistance) are available, as are motivational variables (encouragement) that maintain new skills in the absence of instruction. Naturally occurring prompts and motivational variables should be identified during assessment or while planning instruction so that they may be highlighted (made more noticeable) or paired with instructional counterparts. These strategies are discussed in greater detail below.

Embedded Learning Opportunities

Providing instruction during naturally occurring routines and activities is known as conducting an *embedded learning opportunity*, or *ELO* (Grisham-Brown, Pretti-Frontczak, Hawkins, & Winchell, 2009). During ELOs, the child practices other skills between the embedded instruction, and instructional trials are dispersed throughout the day. This teaching arrangement provides a variety of natural stimuli, prompts, and corrections during instruction. For many infants and young children, this results in effective learning with the benefit of promoting generalization. For other children, however, it may be ineffective because the variety of stimuli may lead to confusion and an apparent nonsystematic approach to instruction. It may also be difficult to include an adequate amount of instruction during the day relying solely on ELOs. When ELOs are not sufficient or effective, more intensive instruction may be warranted (see discussion of the *response to intervention* service delivery model in Chapter 1). One intensive approach is direct instruction.

Direct Instruction

In direct instruction, also known as discrete trial instruction (McEachin, Smith, & Lovaas, 1993), a teaching trial (prompt, student's response, and correction or reinforcement) is presented and then repeated several times. For example, if a child is being taught to point to a photo on a communication board, a teacher sits down with the child and spends 5 or 10 minutes repeatedly guiding the child's hand within 2 inches of the picture, reinforcing her with a favorite toy if she points to the picture or, if she doesn't point to the picture, guides her hand to touch the picture as a correction. In direct instruction, as soon as the teaching sequence is completed, the toy (reinforcer) is taken back from the child, and the trial is repeated.

Although direct instruction seems incongruent with the naturalistic curriculum model, as an intense and explicit form of instruction, it may provide the necessary extra instruction required by a child with special learning needs in some situations (Buysse & Hollingsworth, 2009; Wolery & Hemmeter, 2011). Bambara and Warren (1993) suggested four situations when it may be appropriate. First, some skills occur repeatedly in natural situations, such as infant games (peekaboo) or self-feeding (scooping cereal). Second, if a child is having difficulty learning a particular step in a chain of skills, providing several warm-up practice trials of the difficult step may increase the child's success when practicing the chain. Third, warm-up sessions may help the child learn difficult or complex discriminations, such as the front and back of his clothing. Repeatedly asking the child to point to the discriminating features indicating the back of his shirt and pants could be practiced several times before changing his clothes. Similarly, functional academics (often involving complex discriminations) may be most efficiently taught in a direct instruction format initially (e.g., telling time). And fourth, some children may have difficulty learning certain skills in natural settings, possibly because of distracting stimuli. Using direct instruction may help them learn the skill initially, before being taught to use the skill in natural situations. Bambara and Warren (1993) caution, however, that direct instruction should be used only as an adjunct to naturalistic instruction: It should never be the sole means of instruction, because it mitigates against generalization. Furthermore, it is extremely important to include specific strategies that promote generalization (see section on general case instruction under "Promoting Generalization") within direct instruction (Strain, Wolery, & Izeman, 1998). Finally, teachers must be sensitive to the child's interest and responsiveness during direct instruction. If the child loses interest quickly or is not cooperative during direct instruction, this may suggest that naturalistic instructional situations would be more effective.

EFFECTIVE ASSISTANCE: PROMPTING

The assistance component of systematic instruction is implemented *before* a child is expected to demonstrate a response. Asking a child to respond without assistance is using a trial-and-error method, an instructional approach associated with errors (Bereiter & Englemann, 1966) and confusion. Instead, assistance is provided to increase the likelihood of correct responding and more efficient learning. Assistance strategies include prompting, cuing, shaping, and fading.

Assistance procedures can also be provided *after* the child attempts a target response. If the child does not respond, or does not respond as desired, assistance is a correction procedure. The correction procedure should be different from the assistance initially provided, because an ineffective procedure should not be repeated. Correction procedures should also have a high probability of resulting in the desired response so that a second error does not occur. Assistance can also be provided after the child demonstrates a correct response to highlight the desired response. For example, a child says, "Doll," and a parent says, "Doll—yes, that's your baby doll."

Prompts

Anything that helps a child make a desired response is a prompt. There are two kinds of prompts: natural and instructional. Natural prompts are environmental stimuli that "occasion a response" (Holland & Skinner, 1961). Prompts do not cause or elicit a response; instead, they signal a response. This happens when reinforcement regularly follows an appropriate response. A toddler, for example, quickly learns that when Dad says, "Let's watch cartoons!" (prompt) if she turns on the TV (response), Dad will watch cartoons and play with her (outcome). The predictability of the prompt-response-outcome relationship increases the likelihood that an appropriate response occurs when a natural prompt is present.

Instructional prompts are provided when natural prompts are inadequate or ineffective to teach a new skill. An instructional prompt can be as subtle as a glance or as intrusive as physical guidance. The amount of assistance provided by a prompt depends not only on its intensity but also on the child's ability to use it. If an infant does not understand speech, a verbal direction will not provide assistance. Likewise, if a child does not imitate, a model cannot serve as a prompt. For some infants and children, however, verbal directions and models are effective. Good prompts are ones that help a child make a response, rarely result in errors, and are as nonintrusive as possible while still being effective (Wolery & Hemmeter, 2011). Prompts that are associated with high levels of correct responding are also referred to as *controlling prompts*.

Prompts can be identified by the type of assistance they provide. Commonly used prompts include the following:

Indirect verbal: Asking a question or making a statement that implies what is needed. For example, "What do we need to do now that we're home from our walk?" (meaning "Go to your room for a nap") or "It's time for breakfast" (meaning "Raise your arms and I'll pick you up and take you into the kitchen").

Direct verbal: Making a specific statement to inform a child what needs to be done. "Say 'good morning'" or "Put your arm through the sleeve" are direct verbal prompts.

Gestural: Moving a hand or body part as a nonverbal prompt. It may be a conventional gesture that people are acquainted with, such as pointing, or an unconventional gesture known only to the child and/or her family, such as a sibling stamping his foot to prompt his sister to run to him.

Model: Demonstrating a desired response. The demonstration can be verbal or gestural. Verbal models might encourage a child to name things. Gestural models often prompt a child to engage in a variety of actions with objects (e.g., demonstrating how to roll, bounce, or shake a small ball).

Tactile: Touching the child. The tactile prompt is used to get the child's attention or as a reminder that a certain body part must be moved to make a response. Touching an infant's chin, for instance, may prompt the infant to open his mouth to eat.

Partial physical assistance: Guiding a child by touching or manipulating a body part. The prompt is partial because complete control is not provided; the child must do some of the response. Guiding a child's elbow, or supporting the weight of an object as an infant picks it up, are examples of partial physical assistance.

Full physical assistance: Providing complete control by touching or manipulating a body part. Guiding an infant's hand and helping her push a button with her finger is a full physical assistance prompt.

Spatial: Placing a stimulus in a location that increases the likelihood of a correct response. Positioning a preschooler's toothbrush in front of other toothbrushes on the counter is a spatial prompt.

Movement: Altering the location of a stimulus to attract attention. A parent may hold up two shirts and ask the child if he or she would like to wear the blue one or the red one, moving each shirt forward as she mentions it. The movement prompt assists the child to look at both shirts before choosing.

Visual/pictorial: Providing assistance through pictures (drawings or photographs), colors, or graphics. Placing a red mark on the back of an inside neckline, waistband, or clothing tag is an example of a visual/pictorial prompt to help a child put clothing on properly.

Auditory: Using sound (other than speech) to assist a child to make a desired response. Tapping an object is an auditory prompt.

When formulating systematic instruction, prompts are operationally defined, not simply identified by type. For example, in a plan to teach a toddler to point to and choose a toy, a partial physical assistance prompt is defined as "grasping her shoulders to maintain a forward and relaxed position." Clear definitions are necessary for consistent implementation.

Prompts can be used individually, simultaneously, or sequentially (Snell & Brown, 2011). When an individual prompt is used, the prompt is given once. When simultaneous prompting is used, two or more prompts are presented concurrently. In assisting a young child to move into a standing position, for example, a combination of three prompts may be used: A sibling 1) holds the child's hands and nudges her up while a parent 2) provides support at her hips and 3) says, "Up, up, up."

Natural prompts may be paired with artificial ones as a strategy to teach the child to recognize natural ones. For instance, in teaching a preschooler to say "I want water," the natural prompt of "Would you like something to drink?" is immediately followed by the instructional prompt of modeling (saying) the word "water." Pairing natural and instructional prompts is a particularly valuable strategy for teaching in natural situations because the natural prompt will always be present, even when the instructional prompt is not.

A *prompt sequence* is a series of two or more prompts. For example, a three-step sequence consisting of verbal direction, modeling, and physical guidance may be used to teach a toddler the initial step of putting on a T-shirt. The sequence begins with the teacher saying "Hold your T-shirt at the bottom." A second prompt is provided by modeling how to hold the T-shirt. If the child does not imitate the model (demonstrating the desired response), a third prompt is given as a correction by guiding the child's hands to grasp the shirt. The verbal direction and model provided prior to the response are a two-step prompt sequence; the physical guidance in the correction procedure creates a three-step prompt sequence. The prompt sequence is always implemented in the same manner.

Prompt Hierarchies

A prompt hierarchy is a prompt sequence ordered according to the amount of assistance provided by each. The hierarchy can range from least to most assistance ("increasing assistance") or from most to least ("decreasing assistance"). An example of a four-step hierarchy is as follows:

1. Verbal: Mother or father says, "Show me the toy."
2. Gestural: Mother or father points to the toy.
3. Partial physical assistance: Mother or father sets the toy on Lily's hand.
4. Full physical assistance: Mother or father sets the toy on Lily's hand and guides her hand forward.

If the above hierarchy begins with the verbal prompt, it is a least-to-most hierarchy; if it begins with full physical assistance, it is a most-to-least hierarchy. In implementing a least-to-most assistance hierarchy, the first prompt is always the least intrusive prompt of those in the sequence. If the child does not respond as desired within a specified time period (e.g., 5 seconds), the caregiver or teacher proceeds through the prompt hierarchy, providing the next prompt and waiting the specified length of time. When the desired response is demonstrated, the child is reinforced. The least-to-most hierarchy provides only as much assistance as the child needs. More intrusive prompts are automatically faded (used less often—see the section on fading below) as the child responds to the less-intrusive prompts. Thus, the least-to-most assistance hierarchy is minimally intrusive.

Some young children, however, become "prompt dependent" when a least-to-most hierarchy is used. They wait for prompts that provide more assistance because they learn that eventually they will be given help (Glendenning, Adams, & Sternberg, 1983). Another problem with least-to-most hierarchies is that prompts that provide minimal assistance allow for errors (Csapo, 1981; Day, 1987).

A most-to-least assistance hierarchy may eliminate the problems of prompt dependency and high error rates associated with the least-to-most hierarchy. In a most-to-least hierarchy, the prompt that provides the most assistance is used first. When the child demonstrates the response at a criterion level (e.g., a specified number of times), instruction proceeds to the next prompt assistance level. When an error occurs, the previous prompt level is implemented as a correction. If the criterion for progressing through each level is more conservative than necessary, instruction is not efficient. Errors, however, are kept to a minimum.

As noted earlier, not all prompts are equally effective for all infants and young children; some children will not use particular prompts. Prompt hierarchies, therefore, are formulated on an individualized basis. For example, a young child who is irritated by touch does not respond well to physical guidance. Such prompts are not included in prompt hierarchies for her. Or, for some children, a verbal prompt provides a great deal of assistance, and a slight gestural prompt provides less assistance. Furthermore, while combining prompts increases the intensity of prompting (Skinner, 1938), there is some evidence that single or simultaneous prompts result in more efficient learning than prompt hierarchies or prompt sequences (Wolery, Ault, & Doyle, 1992).

Graduated Guidance

A less structured prompting strategy, but one that is responsive at the moment to the child's performance, is graduated guidance, also referred to as *flexible prompt fading* (Soluaga, Leaf, Taubman, McEachin, & Leaf, 2008). In graduated guidance, the teacher or parent/caregiver watches as the child attempts a skill and determines how much assistance is needed. Initially, much assistance is provided to ensure success. As the child acquires the skill, the amount of assistance is reduced. This procedure is similar to the most-to-least prompt hierarchy, because the amount of assistance is gradually reduced. The actual amount and type of assistance, however, differs from the most-to-least assistance prompt hierarchy because the amount is sometimes increased. Furthermore, the amount and type of assistance is determined *while* the child is attempting the response, rather than being predetermined (Snell & Brown, 2011). In using graduated guidance to help an infant place toys in a container, the infant specialist sits close by and watches. The infant's hand is guided to the container when it appears that he will miss it. More assistance is provided when it appears that he might drop the toy. When graduated guidance is properly implemented, errors rarely occur and only the least amount of assistance necessary is provided (Soluaga et al., 2008).

Cues

A cue is a prompt that directs attention to a particular dimension of a stimulus or task. For example, pointing and saying "Pick up your spoon" is a cue because it directs the child to a specific object. The most effective cues are ones that direct attention to the most important features of a stimulus. Pointing to the handle rather than the bowl of the spoon is a more precise cue, and it is potentially more effective because it informs the child where to place his hand. Skilled teachers are keen observers of young children, noting when cues are needed to direct attention to important stimulus features. Like prompts, cues can be of various forms: verbal, tactile, physical, movement, or spatial, for instance.

Errorless Procedures

As previously mentioned, the most desirable assistance procedures use highly effective (*controlling*) prompts that minimize errors. Some instructional procedures are virtually error free. *Time delay* (Snell & Gast, 1981; Touchette, 1971) is an errorless procedure in which an instructional prompt is paired with a natural one. Over successive trials, the time interval between the natural prompt and the instructional prompt is gradually increased until the child responds to the natural prompt alone. A mother may use time delay, for example, to teach her child to ask for help with activating a toy. When he is attempting to activate a toy and is not having success, she says, "Do you want me to help you?" (the natural prompt) and models (the instructional prompt), "Help please." She repeats this 0-second delay procedure several times over the next 2 days whenever her son appears to need assistance. On the fourth day, when he appears to need help, she says, "Do you need help?" and then pauses for 2 seconds. This pause gives her son a chance to say, "Help please" without the model. If he does, she immediately provides the necessary assistance. If he does not say, "Help please" within 2 seconds, she provides the model for him. She uses this 2-second delay procedure for 2 days. Every 2 days the interval increases by 2 seconds. Eventually her son says "Help please," responding independently to the natural prompt, "Do you need help?"

Several types of delay schedules have been shown to be effective (Snell & Brown, 2011). *Progressive schedules* begin with a 0-second delay (the natural and instructional prompts are paired), and the delay increases a fixed amount each trial (0 sec, 1 sec, 2 sec, 3 sec, and so forth; or 0 sec, 2 sec, 4 sec, and so forth). In *blocked schedules*, the initial trial is at 0 seconds, and all subsequent trials are at a fixed interval (0 sec, 0 sec, 0 sec, 0 sec, 4 sec, 4 sec, 4 sec, 4 sec,

4 sec, and so forth). This schedule is easier to implement accurately than the progressive schedule. A *blocked and progressive schedule,* the third alternative, begins with several trials at 0 seconds and then progresses through a schedule of increasingly longer delays, with several trials at each level (0 sec, 0 sec, 0 sec, 2 sec, 2 sec, 2 sec, 4 sec, 4 sec, 4 sec, and so forth). The progressive delay schedule moves through the delay sequence very quickly and may result in errors for young children who have severe disabilities and don't catch on to the strategy. The blocked or blocked-and-progressive schedules provide a longer opportunity to learn to wait for prompts when the correct response is not known and thus minimizes errors.

In time delay, correct responses following the instructional prompt are *waited corrects,* and correct responses following the natural prompt are *anticipated corrects.* Both types of correct responses are reinforced. This decreases the likelihood of the child responding incorrectly during the delay: If the child does not know the correct response, she waits through the delay period for the instructional prompt, responds correctly, and receives reinforcement.

If an error occurs, a correction procedure is implemented. A typical correction procedure for time delay is to guide the correct response and return to the previous delay for a few trials. If several errors occur, the instructional plan is evaluated and modified. If the errors are occurring before the instructional prompt (*nonwaited errors*), a more powerful reinforcer may be needed. Sometimes nonwaited errors occur because the child doesn't realize that if she waits, a prompt will be provided to help. Waited errors suggest that the instructional prompt is not effective and a different prompt is needed.

Recent research has indicated that using instructional feedback concurrently with progressive time delay can increase the efficiency of learning (Reichow & Wolery, 2011). Instructional feedback is provided immediately after each anticipated and waited correct response. If time delay is being used to teach a child to point to her toys, for example, when the child points correctly (before or after the instructional prompt), the teacher responds with, "Yes, that coloring book is yours." No feedback is provided when errors occur.

Stimulus shaping and fading procedures are errorless prompting strategies in which an easily recognized prompt is gradually altered (stimulus shaping) or reduced (stimulus fading) until its appearance matches that of the natural prompt. If materials such as pictures are used, a series of prompts are prepared prior to implementing this procedure, with slight modifications to each stimulus (picture). Modifications from one stimulus to the next are subtle so that the child responds correctly as the prompt gradually changes to approximate the natural one. Figure 6.1 illustrates materials for stimulus fading and shaping.

Guidelines for Effective Prompting

As noted, systematic instruction must be implemented accurately and consistently, regardless of which prompting procedures are used. Too often, prompts are repeated even though an instructional plan specifies that the prompt be given once. If the child does not respond or responds incorrectly, the correction procedure specified in the instructional plan should be implemented—the

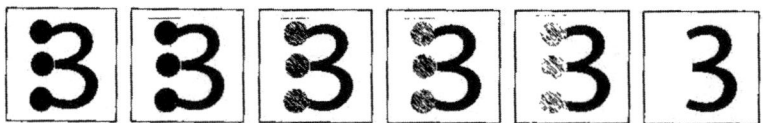
Stimulus fading to teach a number concept

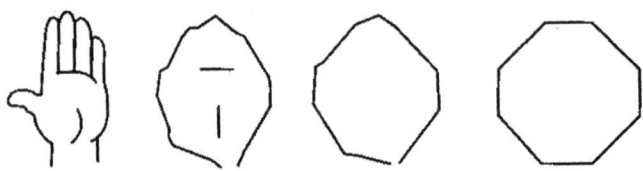
Stimulus shaping to teach the stop sign

Figure 6.1. Sample materials for stimulus fading and stimulus shaping.

prompt is *not* repeated (unless that is the correction procedure). Repeating prompts often leads to prompt dependency, the situation in which the child learns that not attending or not responding will result in receiving more help. Caregivers should adhere to the following guidelines for prompting:

- Implement prompting procedures as specified in the instructional plan. Do not repeat prompts unless indicated in the plan.
- Be certain that the child is attending to them or to the relevant stimuli (e.g., task materials) *before* implementing the prompt.
- Deliver prompts so that they are clear and easily recognized.
- Select prompts that are least intrusive, yet effective enough to minimize errors.
- Change the prompt if the prompt is ineffective (the child makes several errors).
- Use prompts and cues that help the child notice the naturally occurring ones. Natural and instructional prompts can be paired.
- Use cues that focus attention on the most relevant characteristics of the stimuli.

Fading Prompts and Cues

Instructional prompts must be eliminated for the child to respond under natural conditions (Wolery & Hemmeter, 2011). A good instructional plan is one that provides the assistance necessary for correct responses and gradually eliminates assistance while maintaining correct responding. Prompt fading procedures all have one thing in common: They result in the instructional prompt becoming less noticeable. One method of fading is to decrease intensity. The intensity of a verbal prompt can be faded by speaking more and more softly (as in "Take another bite"). Physical assistance can be faded by gradually distancing the assistance (helping a child hold a crayon with hand-over-hand assistance can be faded by moving guidance from the hand to the wrist, the wrist to the forearm, to the elbow, and so on). Physical guidance is also faded by decreasing pressure (the touch associated with hand-over-hand assistance gets increasingly lighter until eliminated) or time (hand-over-hand assistance is first provided the entire time the child is coloring, then 90% of the time, 80% of the time, and so on).

Prompt fading strategies are related to the type of prompt: Auditory prompts become quieter, spatial and movement prompts become smaller, visual prompts become lighter. The key is to make the prompt less noticeable in a subtle manner so that the child responds correctly as he or she did to the original prompt. Note that the most-to-least and least-to-most prompt hierarchies are complete prompt fading strategies when the least intrusive prompt of the hierarchy is a natural one.

Errorless prompting techniques (time delay, stimulus shaping, and stimulus fading) incorporate prompt fading as part of the strategy. In time delay, the instructional prompt is faded temporally; in stimulus shaping and fading, characteristics of the task materials/stimuli are gradually altered/reduced until only the natural ones remain.

EFFECTIVE MOTIVATION: ENCOURAGEMENT

Encouragement, the motivational component of systematic instruction, is provided through reinforcement procedures *after* the child demonstrates the desired response. Motivation is also addressed *before* the response is expected, using interesting or enticing materials, settings, activities, or situational arrangements. Selecting objectives or skill steps that are challenging also provides motivation prior to response. Well-formulated systematic instruction includes procedures that provide assistance and encouragement before and after the child's response.

When encouragement is provided after the opportunity for demonstrating the response, it is usually *positive reinforcement*. Desired responses may also be encouraged by selectively reinforcing approximations of the response with shaping strategies. Motivational procedures implemented before a response are usually *environmental arrangements* that can provide motivation when they create a more interesting or challenging task, such as selecting attractive materials or teaching a basic skill in a favorite play situation.

Positive Reinforcement

Positive reinforcement is a consequence that increases the likelihood of a response being repeated. It is defined by its effect. Something that is reinforcing for one child or one situation may not be reinforcing for another child or another situation. Most young children live in environments rich with positive attention from family members and caregivers. Parents respond to children with smiles, praise, frequent physical contact, and attention for almost everything the children attempt or accomplish. For young children with disabilities, however, such naturally occurring encouragement may not be adequate to promote development or to teach new skills. The children may not notice the encouragement, or the encouragement may not be powerful enough to motivate a child to learn a relatively difficult skill. When encouragement is not effective, the child is not receiving positive reinforcement. (Remember, positive reinforcement is defined by its effect.)

Young children with special needs who have difficulty acquiring new skills or do not recognize naturally occurring encouragement should be provided with *instructional positive reinforcement.* Instructional positive reinforcement is in addition to any natural reinforcement that may be associated with a response. It is provided as part of systematic instruction to address a specific skill need. Instructional positive reinforcement may include verbal praise ("Good, you got your toy!") or nonverbal praise such as hugs, smiles, and pats on the back. It may also include highly desired objects or actions (favorite toy or food, clapping). Ideally, instructional positive reinforcement is paired with naturally occurring reinforcement to help the child recognize naturally occurring reinforcement. For example, when an infant is learning to grasp objects, the natural reinforcement is obtaining the object and having it available for play. Instructional positive reinforcement might include verbal praise ("Hurray! You touched it!") and smiles, plus assistance to shake and play with the toy. Note that whatever is selected as instructional positive reinforcement must be considered potentially positive reinforcement. If learning does not occur, or if it occurs much more slowly than expected, a different or more powerful potential instructional reinforcer may be required. The effectiveness of a reinforcer is most evident when learning occurs.

When a child is first learning a skill, instructional positive reinforcement should be provided every time the response occurs. This is a continuous schedule of reinforcement. As the child progresses in learning the skill, instructional positive reinforcement is provided less often: for example, every second or every third response (a *fixed ratio schedule*) or perhaps every 30 seconds or every minute (a *fixed interval schedule*). As the child approaches mastery of the skill, the instructional positive reinforcement is faded so that it is less recognizable. It is provided on a *variable interval schedule* (approximately every 2 minutes). Variable schedules of reinforcement are more resistant to extinction compared to fixed (and predictable) schedules of reinforcement; they are strong schedules of reinforcement that promote maintenance of new skills. (When reinforcement is withheld from a previously reinforced behavior, the behavior is eventually eliminated. This is called *extinction.*)

Effective instructional positive reinforcement highlights naturally occurring reinforcement and is gradually faded. When instructional reinforcement is eliminated, natural reinforcers maintain the behavior. Reinforcement is gradually faded by changing the reinforcement schedule. Reinforcement may also be made less noticeable by decreasing its intensity or quantity or by delaying when it is delivered.

Shaping and Selecting Reinforcement

Positive reinforcement provided contingent on an approximation of a desired response is called *shaping*. For example, any vocalization beginning with "b" is reinforced as an approximation to "bottle." As the toddler achieves success, more of an approximation—the first syllable, "bah," rather than just the initial consonant—is required for reinforcement (other vocalizations beginning with "b" are ignored). This encouragement strategy is *reinforcing successive approximations or selective reinforcement.*

Shaping, or reinforcing successive approximations, can be implemented systematically by using a *changing criterion design.* In a changing criterion design, a response is reinforced when it meets a particular standard (criterion). The standard gradually changes (increases or decreases) until the desired standard is achieved. For example, a preschooler is reinforced for playing independently for 30 seconds. When the preschooler demonstrates 30 seconds of independent play on three occasions, the criterion is raised to 45 seconds. Each time the preschooler meets the criterion three times, it is increased by 15 seconds, until the objective of 5 minutes of independent play is achieved. The changing criterion design is effective because the reinforcement schedule remains predictable, even though it is thinned. Furthermore, natural reinforcers assume a more powerful role as the child learns a functional behavior and instructional reinforcers are delayed (e.g., as the preschooler learns to play, the natural enjoyment of play is reinforcing).

If the criterion in the changing criterion design is altered too drastically or too quickly, extinction may inadvertently occur because the child does not receive or anticipate reinforcement. Returning to the example of the preschooler learning to play, if the initial criterion of 30 seconds of play was doubled and raised to 1 minute (instead of 45 seconds), the child might give up after about 45 seconds, not realizing that there is still an opportunity for reinforcement. After several occasions of playing alone for brief periods of time and not being reinforced, the child's independent play is extinguished.

Environmental Arrangements

As previously noted, environmental arrangements can provide encouragement. Environmental arrangements that can be modified to encourage learning include the instructional situation, materials, and style of presentation. The *instructional situation* is the context of instruction—the where, when, why, and with whom. The place and time are the where and when of instruction. Natural places and times ensure a real need for the skill and that natural reinforcers are available. For example, teaching Malia, a preschooler, dressing skills weekly at the public swimming pool is a very motivating time and place: Malia needs to put on her swimsuit before she can enter the pool, and Malia is taken into the pool (natural reinforcer) as soon as she has dressed herself in her swimsuit. The why of instruction refers to the activity used for teaching. A meaningful activity teaches the purpose of a skill and thus provides motivation. Functional skills, such as dressing, are taught when activities that require the skills typically occur. Referring to the dressing example, there is no need to contrive opportunities to teach dressing. Morning and evening routines, and activities such as swimming, provide natural and motivating times for instruction. Basic skills, such as vocalizing, sitting, and reaching, should also be taught within meaningful activities. The "with whom" of instruction involves the teacher or parents/caregivers as well as other individuals. Including preferred people, such as parents, grandparents, siblings, or peers, in an instructional situation increases motivation. A toddler, for example, is highly motivated to "be like his big brother" and makes more of an effort to work on his sitting skills while playing with his brother.

Materials provide another opportunity for enhancing motivation. Attractive, age-appropriate, and interesting materials are more appealing than drab materials. New or different materials increase motivation because they are novel (Dunst, 1981). And materials that correspond to the physical and intellectual capabilities of the child hold the child's attention because they will facilitate the child's participation in a task or activity.

Style of presentation involves the affective characteristics of instruction. Most of what infants and young children do should be fun, and that requires the instructional style to be enthusiastic, playful, and appropriate to the activities in which they occur. If instruction is enjoyable, the level of task difficulty must be appropriate to the child's current levels of performance. An appropriate level of task difficulty is one in which the task is slightly beyond the child's present ability so that it is challenging. The task is not so easy that it is boring or so difficult that it seems insurmountable.

When a task is too difficult, it may be broken down into component steps through *task analysis*. A task analysis is constructed by thinking through the steps of a task, a caregiver doing the task oneself, or observing a competent adult/child doing the task. Table 6.1 illustrates a task analysis that was constructed by observing a competent 2-year-old demonstrate the task. Task analyses should be individualized to the child and include more and smaller steps for difficult tasks or difficult portions of tasks and fewer and larger steps for easy tasks or easy portions of tasks (Gold, 1980).

Instructions for a skill that has been task analyzed is implemented one step at a time until each step is mastered or until it occurs for all steps concurrently (*total task*). The total-task approach is more efficient than teaching one step at a time (Snell & Brown, 2011). But if the skill is too difficult or complex for the total-task approach, it is taught one step at a time. There also is the option to forward chain or backward chain the steps. In *forward chaining*, the first step is taught until it is learned, and then the first step plus the second step are taught until learned, until the entire sequence is taught. In *backward chaining*, the last step of the task analysis is the first step taught. When it is learned, the last step plus the second last step are taught, until the task analysis is completed. When forward or backward chaining is used, the child may be assisted to complete all the steps in addition to the step(s) being taught, or someone else may complete the steps.

Table 6.1. Example of a task analysis for putting on shorts (constructed by observing a competent 2-year-old perform the task)

1. Grasp shorts at the waistband with hands on either side.
2. Look for label on inside of waistband; if necessary, turn shorts so that label faces the back.
3. Squat and hold shorts close to floor.
4. Insert left foot into left leg of shorts.
5. Insert right foot into right leg of shorts.
6. Pull up shorts to hips, pulling up one side at a time until reaching the hips.
7. Grasp shorts at back of waistband and pull up over buttocks.
8. Grasp front of shorts and pull up to waist.

Total task
Grasp spoon
Scoop food
Lift spoon to mouth
Open mouth
Insert spoon in mouth

Forward chaining:	Backward chaining:
1. Grasp spoon	1. Insert spoon in mouth

2. Grasp spoon
   Scoop food
	2. Open mouth
	   Insert spoon in mouth

3. Grasp spoon
   Scoop food
   Lift spoon to mouth
	3. Lift spoon to mouth
	   Open mouth
	   Insert spoon in mouth

4. Grasp spoon
   Scoop food
   Lift spoon to mouth
   Open mouth
	4. Scoop food
	   Lift spoon to mouth
	   Open mouth
	   Insert spoon in mouth

5. Grasp spoon
   Scoop food
   Lift spoon to mouth
   Open mouth
   Insert spoon in mouth
	5. Grasp spoon
	   Scoop food
	   Lift spoon to mouth
	   Open mouth
	   Insert spoon in mouth

Figure 6.2. Example of total task, forward chaining, and backward chaining.

The decision to use forward or backward chaining is based on the child's present level of performance. Begin the task analysis on a step in which the child demonstrates partial acquisition (the steps may be easier and thus more motivating). If the level of task difficulty is similar throughout the task, backward chaining is the procedure of choice because of its motivational value. The last step of a task yields a functional outcome and immediate reinforcement. Figure 6.2 illustrates these approaches to chaining with a skill that has been task analyzed.

Guidelines for Effective Encouragement

Infants and young children with special needs can be encouraged to learn by including motivational strategies within systematic instruction. Encouragement procedures are provided during two points of instruction: 1) in response to the child's attempt to demonstrate the desired response (reinforcement procedures) and 2) prior to the child's attempt at the response (environmental arrangements). The following are guidelines for using encouragement procedures:

- Provide instructional reinforcement on a continuous schedule for new skills.

- Monitor the child's affective reaction to reinforcement and his or her skill acquisition to be certain that it is effective.

- Pair instructional reinforcers with natural ones. Whenever possible, use the instructional reinforcer to highlight or accentuate what typically functions as a natural reinforcer.

- As the child learns a new skill, change the reinforcement schedule to a less frequent and less predictable schedule or change the reinforcer to a less intense or noticeable one.

- Use selective reinforcement to encourage increasingly closer approximations to the desired skills (shaping, reinforcing successive approximations, and changing criterion design).
- Carefully select the setting, time, activity, and participants to make instruction as functional, interesting, and challenging as possible.
- Use materials to aid in maintaining the child's attention. Remember that novel materials are often effective in maintaining/increasing attention.
- Be certain that task difficulty corresponds to the child's present level of performance: not too easy, not too difficult, but just difficult enough to be challenging.
- When a task is too difficult, use task analysis to identify the steps of the task. Teach the task-analyzed skill one step at a time or use a total-task approach. Select a forward or backward chaining technique to teach the child to perform the steps of the task successively.
- Teach skills in sequences with other functional skills to enhance meaningfulness.

PROMOTING GENERALIZATION

The goal of the naturalistic curriculum model is to improve or increase participation and interaction in natural experiences. The opportunities and needs for this are innumerable, and there is not enough time to teach the endless number of skills required to address them all. Rather than teach a few isolated skills that are useful, the naturalistic curriculum model emphasizes instruction that promotes skill generalization.

There are two types of generalizations: stimulus and response. *Stimulus generalization* occurs when a response is demonstrated across one or more noninstructional situations. For example, the child is taught to say "please" to his preschool teacher (instructional situation) and then uses the skill at home with his mother and his father (noninstructional situations). Generalization across persons, settings, activities, conditions, or time are all considered stimulus generalization. The group of stimuli that signals a particular response is referred to as a *stimulus class*.

Response generalization occurs when a child demonstrates a response that is slightly different from the newly learned skill. For example, if the child is taught to grasp her cup by the handle (newly learned skill) but later grasps it with one hand around the base of the cup or with both hands around the cup, she demonstrates a generalized response (slightly different than what was taught). Slight variations in form among responses that serve the same function constitute a *response class*. Frequently, stimulus generalization and response generalization occur together. A child may learn to unscrew container lids and demonstrate variations of grasping and turning when given a tube of toothpaste, peanut butter jar, and thermos.

The usefulness of a skill is often dependent on whether it is generalized or not. If an infant lifts her head only when receiving physical therapy, her ability to lift her head is not very useful. Likewise, the preschooler who says "mama," "ball," and "cup" when shown photographs but does not use the words to make his desires known, lacks functional use of the words. Early intervention goals and objectives in the naturalistic curriculum model, therefore, are ones that target generalized skills and specify the parameters of the respective stimulus and response classes. They are referred to as *general case objectives* (Horner, Sprague, & Wilcox, 1982).

Formulating General Case Objectives

Writing an instructional objective that addresses generalization relies on a procedure called *train sufficient exemplars* (Stokes & Baer, 1977). In using the sufficient exemplar procedure, the target skill is taught across several examples of stimuli that typically occasion the target skill. For example, in teaching a young child to identify "cup," a small plastic cup, a coffee mug, and a toddler "sippy cup" may be used as exemplars. The exemplars are trained concurrently rather than sequentially. The term *sufficient* suggests that an adequate, yet efficient, number of stimuli are selected (Anderson & Spradlin, 1980). Too few stimuli would not be likely to yield generalization; too many stimuli are unnecessary, inefficient, and fail to take advantage of the strategy. Horner et al. (1982) suggested that enough exemplars be selected to represent the common and diverse characteristics of the stimulus or response class targeted for generalization.

The response or stimulus class selected for generalization is the *instructional universe* (Becker, Englemann, & Thomas, 1975). Returning to the example of teaching a child to generalize the skill of identifying "cup," the instructional universe (the stimulus class of cups) and its features are identified. Note the variety of cups the child encounters at home, in child care, and in the community. For example, the instructional universe might include a mug, a child's small cup, a "sippy cup," a Styrofoam cup, and a soft drink cup. The features of the instructional universe are as follows:

- *Material:* ceramic, glass, plastic, Styrofoam, paper
- *Breakability:* breakable, nonbreakable
- *Handles:* no handle, one handle, two handles
- *Size:* small, medium, large
- *Weight:* heavy, moderate, light
- *Color:* white, yellow, blue, and so forth; solid, multicolored

In selecting exemplars from the instructional universe, a few cups that best represent the range of features are chosen. Choosing the mug (large, one handle, heavy, solid color, breakable), plastic cup (small, no handles, lightweight, solid color, nonbreakable), and "sippy cup" (medium size, two handles, medium weight, multicolored, nonbreakable) samples most of the features of the stimulus class. If the child learns to recognize the three exemplars as cups, she is likely to generalize and identify a Styrofoam cup as a cup, an example that was not included in the instruction. Sufficient exemplar instruction is not limited to stimuli that are objects. It can be applied to people, places, times, situations, words, or activities. It may be used to promote response generalization by applying the same strategy of identifying the instructional universe (a response class, in this instance) and the range of features to which one wishes to generalize.

To formulate a general case objective, one defines the instructional universe: identify the extent to which the skill will be generalized and whether the skill involves stimulus generalization, response generalization, or both. The scope and size of the instructional universe is a judgment based on the exemplars likely to be encountered by the child, and the extent to which the child is likely to generalize (appropriate level of task difficulty). Then one writes the behavioral objective (conditions, behavior, and criterion) with selected exemplars in parentheses. Below are examples of general case objectives.

Stimulus generalization

Conditions: When a familiar person* (infant specialist Tina, Grandma, Daddy) asks the child if he'd like to be picked up

Behavior: Arman will vocalize

Criteria: Within 10 seconds for three consecutive opportunities

(* Instructional universe of familiar persons: Mom, Daddy, Grandma, Grandpa, cousin Tom, Uncle Kimo, Auntie Sue, neighbors Tom and Julie, infant specialist Tina)

Response generalization

Conditions: When the child crawls to her toy box

Behavior: LiAn will request* a toy (by pointing to a toy in the toy box, by saying "toy," or by saying "please")

Criteria: On four consecutive opportunities

(* Instructional universe of requesting responses: reaching, pointing, vocalizing, naming, saying "please," saying "more")

Stimulus and response generalization

Conditions: When given finger foods* (crackers, raisins, sandwich pieces)

Behavior: Darryl will grasp** the food, pick it up, and feed himself

Criteria: At least five times per meal, four of five lunchtimes

(* Instructional universe of finger foods: cookies, crackers, cereal, banana slices, orange slices, raisins, sandwich pieces)

(** Instructional universe of grasping: light grasp, firm grasp, fine pincer, gross pincer, rake)

When general case objectives need to be simplified to correspond to the child's current level of performance, two or more short-term general case objectives can be formulated. It is important to include the multiple exemplars in each short-term objective; otherwise, instruction will not be promoting generalization. Examples of three short-term general case objectives for the self-feeding objective are as follows:

Short-term general case objective 1

Conditions: When given finger foods (crackers, raisins, sandwich pieces)

Behavior: Darryl will grasp the food

Criteria: At least three times per meal, three consecutive lunchtimes

Short-term general case objective 2

Conditions: When given finger foods (crackers, raisins, sandwich pieces)

Behavior: Darryl will pick up the food and raise it to his mouth

Criteria: At least three times per meal, four of five lunchtimes

Short-term general case objective 3

Conditions: When given finger foods (crackers, raisins, sandwich pieces)

Behavior: Darryl will pick up the food and feed himself

Criteria: At least five times per meal, four of five lunchtimes

Note that the last short-term objective is identical to the long-term objective.

General Case Instruction

General case instruction adheres to the guidelines specified earlier in this chapter for systematic instruction. Assistance and encouragement procedures are stated in an instructional plan and implemented exactly as stated. When an instructional plan is developed for a general case objective, the stimulus and/or response exemplars are specified. The plan is designed so that exemplars are taught concurrently rather than separately. For example, for the short-term objective in which Darryl grasps raisins, crackers, and pieces of sandwich, the instructional plan includes daily opportunities for instruction with the three types of finger foods and the three types of grasp (this is in contrast to teaching Darryl to grasp raisins until the skill is mastered, then to grasp crackers until grasping crackers is mastered, and so on). Figure 6.3 is a general case instructional plan for this objective.

Other Generalization Procedures

A number of other methods have been demonstrated to facilitate generalization (Stokes & Baer, 1977). These methods can be incorporated into general case instructional plans to increase the likelihood of generalization. There are five generalization procedures in addition to the sufficient exemplar strategy:

1. Program common stimuli
2. Introduce to natural maintaining contingencies
3. Use indiscriminable contingencies
4. Mediate generalization
5. Train loosely

Child: Darryl Objective: Finger feeding (grasping finger food) Conditions: When given finger foods (crackers, raisins, and sandwich pieces) Response: Darryl will grasp the food Criterion: At least 3 times per meal, 3 consecutive lunchtimes		Date begun: 9/27/13 Date completed: Interventionist(s): Anna and Mom
Intervention context	Prompting/ facilitation techniques	Consequences

Setting(s):
   Mondays: infant center
   Others days: home
Routine(s)/activity(ies):
   Lunch
Skill sequence(s):
   Makes choice
   Grasps food
   Asks for more
Occasions for incidental intervention
   n/a
	Positioning and handling special equipment/materials:
	   Seated in adaptive high chair with tray
	   Crackers, raisins, sandwich pieces
	Environmental modifications:
	   Place finger foods on plate with high lip.
	Prompting/facilitation:
	   Guide Darryl's hand as needed toward food; wait 6 seconds.
	Additional generalization procedures
	   Use same plate at home and infant center (program common stimuli).
		Reinforcement:
		   Verbally praise Darryl for picking up food.
		   Provide physical assistance to help Darryl get food to his mouth.
		Corrections:
		   Place Darryl's hand on top of the food piece; wait 6 seconds. If he grasps the food, provide full physical assistance to help Darryl get his food to his mouth. If he still does not grasp the food, provide full physical assistance.

Figure 6.3. Instructional plan incorporating generalization procedure (program common stimuli).

Program Common Stimuli In this technique, materials or stimuli from the generalization situations are used in the instructional situation. For example, if a preschooler must learn to drink with a straw from a milk carton for school, the family may assist the child in learning the skill at home. They implement the program common stimuli technique by using the same types of milk cartons and straws at home that are used at the preschool. When the child learns to drink from the milk carton at home, he or she is likely to generalize and demonstrate the skill at school where the same stimuli are present. The program common stimuli technique is also a good generalization technique when instructional objectives address skills needed in subsequent environments (e.g., teaching cutting in preschool with the same types of scissors that will be used in kindergarten).

Introduce to Natural Maintaining Contingencies *Natural maintaining contingencies* refer to the reinforcers and schedules of reinforcement that occur in settings in which skills are needed. In this strategy, generalization is promoted by gradually shifting from instructional reinforcers and reinforcement schedules to natural ones. Natural and instructional reinforcers initially are paired, and then the instructional ones are faded. When assisting a toddler to pull her panties and shorts up, for example, a parent's verbal praise and hug are immediately followed by allowing the child to leave the bathroom and return to play. Verbal praise and the hug are gradually eliminated, and returning to play (the natural reinforcer) continues to reinforce pulling her pants up. This natural contingency is in effect at child care and at grandma's house, and thus generalization is likely.

Use Indiscriminable Contingencies The term *indiscriminable* means "difficult to notice" or "not too obvious." Reinforcers that are instructional are often obvious and contrived. Very noticeable instructional reinforcers may be necessary in the early phases of learning, but they interfere with generalization to other settings in which the skill is needed and similar reinforcers are not available. Gradually decreasing the obtrusiveness of an instructional reinforcer increases the likelihood of generalization. As noted earlier in this chapter, reinforcement is faded by decreasing its intensity (making verbal reinforcement quieter) or frequency (shifting to leaner and less predictable schedules of reinforcement, such as a variable interval schedule). For example, in assisting a preschooler to learn turn-taking in a game with a peer, the teacher initially sits close and briefly rubs the child's back as reinforcement. This is minimally intrusive because it does not interrupt play. As the child learns to take turns, the teacher rubs her back more briefly and only every other time the child takes a turn. Eventually, she simply touches the child's back a couple of times during a play session when the child is taking turns. Finally, the teacher moves away and withdraws the instructional reinforcement completely, as playing operates as the natural reinforcer of turn taking.

Mediate Generalization In this technique, a strategy is taught. Examples include naming the letters of the alphabet by singing a song or saying a poem to remember which months of the year have 30 days and which have 31. These are cognitive strategies and are applicable to toddlers and preschoolers. Other types of strategies could be included as mediational techniques. For example, teaching a child to put on his shirt by first laying it out on a flat surface such as the bed is a strategy that he can use across environments. Or teaching a child with cerebral palsy to hold a peg on her wheelchair tray to stabilize movements is a mediational strategy that she can use across tasks requiring controlled fine motor movements (e.g., self-feeding, art activities, communication board use).

Train Loosely In the train-loosely technique, generalization is facilitated by relaxing systematic instruction that is typically implemented in a highly consistent manner. Instead of providing precisely the same prompt, reinforcement, and correction procedure each time instruction is conducted, the components of the instructional plan vary slightly from time to time. What constitutes an acceptable response may also vary, but the variation must not extend outside the response class. Minor variations in prompting, reinforcement, corrections, and acceptable responses increase the likelihood that when a similar, noninstructional situation is encountered, generalization will occur. There is a caution, however, that if the instructional plan is implemented too loosely the child will fail to acquire the skill because the benefits of the systematic instructional plan are eliminated (i.e., a predictable prompt-response-consequence relationship is no longer apparent).

When incorporating the train-loosely strategy in systematic instruction, the plan should specify which components may be loosened, and acceptable examples of the component should be provided. For instance, if the prompt is trained loosely, then the plan might state the following: "Provide a simple verbal direction, such as 'Please come with me,' 'Let's get into the car,' or 'Please sit in your car seat.'" In implementing the plan, any of the sample prompts may be used, or prompts that are similar to the examples may be used. Each component of the instructional plan that is trained loosely should be written in this manner.

One or more of the five generalization strategies described in this section (program common stimuli, introduce natural maintaining contingencies, use indiscriminable contingencies, mediate generalization, and train loosely) may be included in a systematic general case instructional plan to supplement the train-sufficient-exemplar strategy that is the heart of general case instruction. Figures 6.4 and 6.5 demonstrate instructional plans incorporating these procedures.

IMPLEMENTATION OF SYSTEMATIC INSTRUCTION

There are three key variables associated with the successful implementation of systematic instruction: amount of engaged time, contingent arrangement of reinforcement, and errors kept to a minimum.

Child: Anisa
Objective: Signals to continue play
Conditions: Given a pause during a repetitious song or rhyme game (e.g., Pat-a-cake, Peekaboo, "Row, Row, Row Your Boat," and so forth)
Response: Anisa will signal to continue play (e.g., eye contact, vocalizing, reaching out for adult, attempting to begin song/game again, and so forth).
Criterion: 3 times in 2 consecutive play periods

Date begun: 10/15/13
Date completed:
Interventionist(s): Karen, Mom, and Dad

Intervention context	Prompting/facilitation techniques	Consequences
Setting(s): After nap When mom or dad arrives home from work *Routine(s)/activity(ies):* Repetitious songs or rhyme games *Skill sequence(s):* n/a *Occasions for incidental intervention:* n/a	*Positioning and handling; special equipment/materials:* Sit anisa on your lap (legs apart) facing you; support her lower back. *Environmental modifications:* n/a *Prompting/facilitation:* Play several seconds, then stop. Look directly at Anisa and wait 10 seconds. *Additional generalization procedures:* Vary song and rhyme game. Vary verbal corrections: "What?" "Whose turn is it?" "Do it again," and so forth. Accept any signal that seems to be a request to continue (train loosely).	*Reinforcement:* Reinstate game more enthusiastically than before; smile and laugh enthusiastically. *Corrections:* Provide a verbal prompt, such as "Do it again," or "What?" or "Whose turn is it?" Wait 5 more seconds. If she responds–reinforce. If still incorrect, begin a different game and try again.

Figure 6.4. Instructional plan incorporating generalization procedures (train loosely).

Child: Jacob	Date begun: 10/16/13
Objective: Toy play	Date completed:
Conditions: When playing with brother, cousin, or neighbor	Interventionist(s): Rob
Response: Jacob will shake or bang small toys (squeak ball, rattle, wooden spoon)	
Criterion: For 3 seconds or more, 6 times	

Intervention context	Prompting/ facilitation techniques	Consequences
Setting(s): Living room, brother's room, or lanai *Routine(s)/activity(ies):* While brother waits for school bus When mom babysits neighbor and/or cousin *Skill sequence(s):* n/a *Occasions for incidental intervention:* Whenever Jacob laughs at peer's play	*Positioning and handling; Special equipment/materials:* Side lying or prone over a pillow *Environmental modifications:* Toys must be within easy reach. *Prompting/facilitation:* Shake or bang the toy 3 times within Jacob's reach; wait 5 seconds. *Additional generalization procedures:* After 2 consecutive correct, change to FR2 reinforcement schedule; after 2 more correct, change to VR3 (use indiscriminable contingencies).	*Reinforcement:* Praise both children for playing nicely; assist peer to help Jacob bang or shake the toy 3 or 4 more times. *Corrections:* Tap Jacob's arm and say "Play with your toy"; if he does, reinforce as stated above. If he still doesn't shake or bang the toy, physically assist him through a correct response; do not reinforce.

Figure 6.5. Instructional plan incorporating generalization procedure (use indiscriminable contingencies). *Key:* FR2, fixed ratio 2; VR3, variable ratio 3.

Amount of Engaged Time

Engaged time refers to the time in which the child is actively participating in instruction. The more time spent actively engaged in instruction, the greater the amount of learning (Anderson, 1976; McWilliam, 1991; Walker & Hops, 1976). Instruction is more likely to be effective if it is implemented frequently and requires active responding on the part of the child (rather than the child being a passive recipient of instruction).

Contingent Arrangement of Reinforcement

Contingent arrangement of reinforcement means that interesting stimuli are provided immediately and consistently after the child demonstrates an instructional target. It also means that one should use stimulation only contingently. In the past, noncontingent stimulation, such as auditory stimulation (ringing bells), was implemented in an effort to improve or heighten sensory functioning (auditory attending) and overall environmental awareness. Noncontingent sensory stimulation has been shown to be ineffective (Dunst & Trivette, 2009). Instead, specific skills should be taught. For example, rather than have a father hold his 1-year-old daughter on his lap and talk to her for 5 minutes to teach her to attend (noncontingent stimulation), he might bounce his daughter on his knee five times each time she approximates "Again!" (bouncing is arranged contingently).

Errors Kept to a Minimum

Instruction is more effective and efficient when *errors are kept to a minimum* (Bereiter & Englemann, 1966). Effective instructional techniques are those that help a child make a response and then provide reinforcement. If errors occur frequently and the child has few opportunities to experience the correct response and its resulting reinforcement, the instructional plan should be revised. More assistance, a different type of facilitation, or a more powerful reinforcer may be necessary.

There are two concerns related to the exclusive use of errorless instruction. First is the importance of allowing young children to make errors and experience natural corrections. Children should have opportunities to experience naturally occurring corrections, particularly when the corrections include informative feedback. For example, if a toddler takes a toy from her brother without asking, her brother may take it back. The child's ability to use the natural corrections should also be monitored. If the child does not seem to understand them, it would be useful to pair instructional corrections with natural ones and gradually fade the instructional corrections. In the example of the sister taking the toy from her brother, for instance, the sister might look confused when her brother takes it back for himself. An instructional correction prompting the sister to ask her brother for a toy could be paired with the natural correction (the brother taking the toy back). This might help the sister understand why her brother took the toy from her.

The second concern related to errorless instruction is the importance of providing opportunities for young children to self-correct when errors occur (the preschooler whines, but no one comes to help him, so he self-corrects by raising his hand). Corrections should be provided only when no attempt is made to self-correct. There should also be consideration given to teaching young children problem-solving skills that enable them to generate possible solutions (i.e., self-corrections) to minimize their dependence on adults and instructional corrections. Regardless of the specific type of instruction used, the three major variables associated with successful instruction—engaged time, contingent arrangement of reinforcement, and minimal errors—should be addressed.

MONITORING SYSTEMATIC INSTRUCTION

A hallmark of systematic instruction is data-based decision making. A data-based decision is a judgment of whether to change or continue implementing an instructional plan based on data gathered during the instruction. Objective evaluation of instructional effectiveness is determined by collecting data on skill acquisition, graphing the data, and interpreting the graphs. Traditionally, systematic instruction was characterized by extensive data collection (i.e., data were collected continuously throughout all activities on a daily basis). In a naturalistic curriculum model, however, concerns for flexibility and unobtrusiveness must be balanced with concerns for objective evaluation. Recommendations to achieve this balance are discussed following the descriptions of how to develop and implement data collection procedures.

Measuring Instructional Progress

The dimensions on which behavior may be observed and measured were discussed in Chapter 3. There are four types of measurement systems commonly used for monitoring instructional progress: 1) frequency, 2) duration, 3) interval, and 4) time sampling. *Frequency* is a count of each time a behavior occurs. If the opportunities for demonstrating a skill vary from day to day, the data may be reported as a percentage (9 correct responses out of 10 opportunities is 90%). *Duration* is the length of time a behavior occurs (one occurrence of a behavior or the total time of several occurrences of a behavior). *Interval* recording indicates whether the behavior occurs or does not occur during a period of time (e.g., 30-second intervals). In *time sampling*, the data indicate whether the behavior occurs at the moment following a specified time interval (at 30 seconds, at 1 minute, at 1 minute 30 seconds, at 2 minutes, and so forth).

Three other measurement systems are useful for data-based decision making: latency, rate, and permanent product. *Latency* is the time between a prompt (natural or instructional) and the response. For example, it is the time between a father taking a turn at pat-a-cake and his child taking the next turn. Latency is a relevant measure when it affects the usefulness or functionality of a skill. If a child takes too long to respond to his father in the pat-a-cake game, the father assumes that the child is not interested and quits the game. Latency is also relevant when a child's response times are slow due to the effects of a disability. A child with a developmental delay may be slow to initiate her response because it takes her several moments to recognize a prompt and several moments more to determine how to respond. A child may also demonstrate lengthy response latencies because of a physical impairment that interferes with movement. Families and others need to recognize a child's need for longer response latencies and adjust interaction patterns and expectations accordingly.

Rate is a measurement of how quickly or slowly responses occur (also known as *fluency*). For example, an infant may eat 23 spoonfuls of cereal in half an hour, that is, a rate of .76 spoonfuls per minute. Rate is calculated by dividing the number of responses by a unit of time: 23 spoonfuls divided by 30 minutes equals the number of spoonfuls (.76) per minute. Rate is typically reported as the number of responses per minute, per hour, per day, or per week. Similar to latency, rate is a relevant measure when the quickness of a response influences whether it is functional or not. For example, a child feeds himself without adult assistance, but eats only three spoonfuls within 20 minutes. His family may not allow him to feed himself at home because it is impractical to spend so much time to complete a meal. Increasing how quickly this child eats would be a meaningful objective, and rate would be the appropriate measurement system.

Permanent product measures provide lasting evidence of responses and do not require direct observation. In much of general education, written tests provide permanent product measures of school achievement. In early intervention, a physical therapist asks a child to reach as far as possible in different directions and mark on a paper with a magic marker. The marks remain as evidence of the child's range of motion. Videotapes and photographs also provide permanent product data. Permanent product measures are useful because the child's behavior (or the effect of the child's behavior) may be reviewed time and again.

Selecting a Measurement System

The primary consideration in selecting a measurement system is the extent to which the system provides a clear indication of how well a child is performing a target skill relative to the criterion stated in the instructional objective. Matching the measurement system to the criterion is necessary to determine when a child has met an instructional objective. If the criterion states that the child will vocalize the initial sounds of familiar words beginning with "b," "p," and "m" on three consecutive opportunities, then each time the child says a word beginning with a designated consonant sound, his or her response is recorded as correct or incorrect (+ and –). This is event recording. When three consecutive plusses are recorded, the objective has been met.

Identifying Where and When to Collect Data

The where and when of data collection is determined by three factors: 1) conditions stated in the instructional objective, 2) generalization concerns, and 3) practical and naturalistic considerations. The first factor, *conditions stated in the instructional objective*, often indicates what times of day or in what situations the skill is to be performed. For example, an objective may state conditions such as "at breakfast, lunch, and dinner." Data must be collected during all three mealtimes to know when the criterion has been met.

The second factor that will influence where and when data are collected is *generalization concerns*. A general case objective is considered mastered when generalization to one or more noninstructional exemplars from the instructional universe is demonstrated. The child's performance with untrained exemplars is measured with *generalization probes*. Generalization probes are conducted when skill acquisition has been demonstrated with the exemplars specified in the objective. To conduct a generalization probe, the child is presented with a noninstructional stimulus/situation from the instructional universe. The examples of general case instructional plans in Figures 6.3, 6.4, and 6.5 include generalization probe components. Note that generalization probes can also be conducted periodically (e.g., weekly) prior to demonstrating skill acquisition.

The third factor that influences where and when data are collected is *practical and naturalistic considerations*. These considerations go hand in hand. For example, it is impractical and unnaturalistic to expect a family to collect data on how quickly their child eats at every meal. In fact, for many families it is impractical (and inconsiderate) to ask them to collect data at all. Instead, infant program personnel and early childhood teachers should assume primary responsibility for data collection. Practical and naturalistic considerations suggest that a teacher should not have a clipboard and stopwatch in hand during every activity. This would certainly interfere with a teacher's full participation in an activity, and, more important, may interfere with a teacher's ability to provide instructional prompts and other physical assistance that some children may need.

The balance between the need to collect data and practical considerations is achieved by collecting data on a regular basis for the three to five objectives that are each family's highest priorities. When it is impractical to collect data every day on each instructional priority, data are collected every other day, or

Frequency of Shaking or Banging a Toy for 3 Seconds or More

Week of	Monday	Tuesday	Wednesday	Thursday	Friday
10/17/2013	/	//	//	/	/
10/24/2013	/	/	//	///	///
10/31/2013	//	///	///	//	///

Figure 6.6. Sample data sheet for event recording.

once a week. It should be noted, however, that the performance of infants and young children with disabilities varies considerably from day to day. Therefore, the more frequent the data collection, the more likely that the data will provide an accurate measure of child progress and instructional effectiveness (Taber-Doughty & Jasper, 2012). Data should be collected on lower priority objectives every 2 to 4 weeks.

It may be impractical to record data throughout an entire activity. When it is possible to assess the criterion of an instructional objective with brief periods of measurement, it may be more practical to do so. For instance, data may be collected on a child's rate of self-feeding during the first 10 minutes of each meal rather than through an entire meal.

Figure 6.6 is a data sheet for the instructional program presented in Figure 6.5. Tally marks are used to record the frequency of play episodes that last 3 seconds or longer. Another option would have been to record the duration of toy play. Given that the duration criterion is brief (3 seconds), duration does not seem to be the most relevant feature to measure. Instead, the objective is concerned with building the frequency of brief play episodes.

Interpreting Instructional Data

To interpret child progress and instructional effectiveness from data, it is necessary to chart the data on a graph. Because child performance data tend to be variable, it is difficult to judge whether the child is progressing by simply looking at numbers on a data sheet. There are numerous graphing methods, but the most common is a line graph. On a line graph, the horizontal axis (abscissa) usually represents sessions or days, and the vertical axis (ordinate) is labeled with the measurement system (e.g., frequency, percent, latency). Figure 6.7 is a line graph depicting child progress as indicated on the data sheet in Figure 6.6.

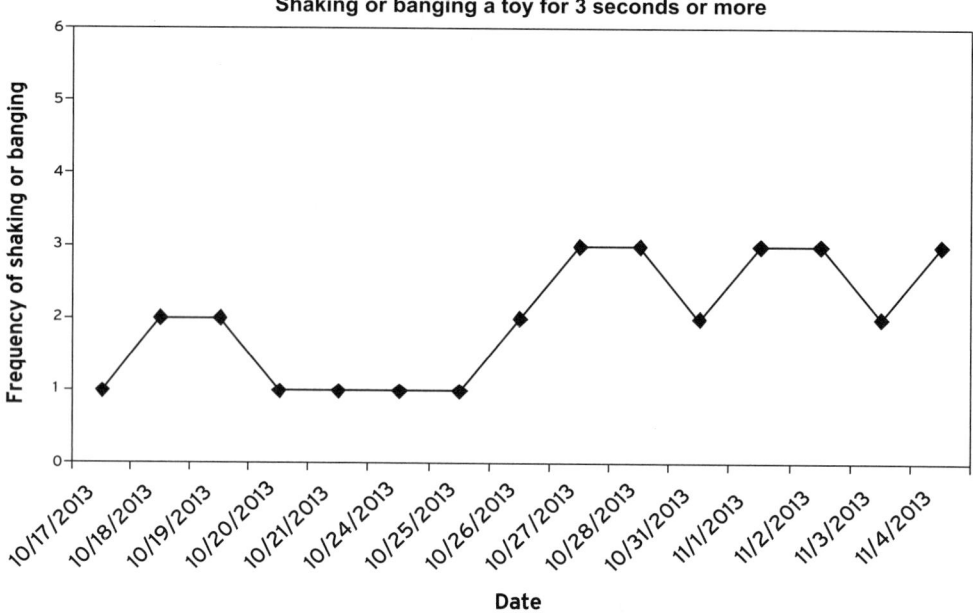

Figure 6.7. Sample graph for data-based decision making (from data sheet in Figure 6.6).

Once the data are graphed, the next step is to judge whether progress is adequate or not. If the child is not progressing or is not progressing as rapidly as desired, the instructional program is changed. The modified program is then implemented and monitoring continues. Graphs should be reviewed every five or six data points. The following guidelines, based on Browder, Demchack, Heller, and King (1989) and Haring, Liberty, and White (1981) should be observed in making data-based instructional decisions:

1. If the graph suggests that the child is approaching criterion, no change should be made to the instructional program.
2. If the child's performance is highly variable and is not approaching criterion, change the instructional program to improve motivation.
3. If the child's performance is fairly steady and is not approaching criterion, change the instructional program to make it easier. For example, use a more detailed task analysis or use a different prompt that provides more help.

In reviewing the data presented in Figure 6.7, Hank's toy play is not improving, and the data are fairly steady. Therefore, recommendation 3 applies: change the instructional program to make it easier. The prompting procedure in the instructional program is "Shake or bang the toy three times within Hank's reach and wait 5 seconds" (see Figure 6.5). A prompt that provides more assistance is one way to make the program easier. For example, a new prompting procedure is "Place the toy in Hank's hand and shake it or bang it several times. Stop in the middle of a banging or shaking motion and wait 5 seconds." This prompt provides more direct practice prior to expecting the response and requires Hank to continue the response after it is started for him.

SUMMARY

Systematic instruction is the consistent application of procedures designed to assist and encourage a child with disabilities to acquire or improve skills needed for participation in natural experiences. Assistance procedures include a wide variety of instructional prompting procedures, such as single prompts, multiple prompts, prompt hierarchies, and errorless procedures. Encouragement procedures are reinforcement techniques and environmental strategies that help motivate a child to demonstrate a desired response. Systematic instruction can be designed to promote generalized skill acquisition by stating instructional goals as general case objectives, applying general case instruction, and/or incorporating additional generalization procedures into the instructional plan. Those generalization procedures include programming common stimuli, introducing natural maintaining contingencies, using indiscriminable contingencies, mediating generalization, and training loosely. When systematic instruction is implemented, the effectiveness of the instructional program is monitored through frequent data collection. Based on the data, program modifications are made when skill acquisition is not as expected.

STUDY QUESTIONS

1. Discuss how it is possible for instruction to be both systematic and naturalistic.
2. Write a definition of *systematic instruction*.
3. Describe at least three situations when it might be beneficial to use *direct instruction*.
4. Define and provide an example of the following types of instructional prompts: indirect verbal, direct verbal, gestural, model, tactile, partial physical assistance, full physical assistance, spatial, movement, visual/pictorial, and auditory.
5. Provide an example of operationalizing a partial physical assistance prompt for helping a child hold a paintbrush.
6. Describe the difference between *most-to-least assistance* and *least-to-most assistance* prompt hierarchies. When is it most appropriate to use a most-to-least assistance prompt hierarchy?
7. Describe the difference between a *prompt* and a *cue*. Provide an example of a prompt and a cue for assisting a child in recognizing her written name.
8. Provide examples of using *time delay*, *stimulus shaping*, and *stimulus fading* for teaching a young child to use a communication board with three line drawings on it.
9. Identify and define the various schedules of *reinforcement*. When is it most appropriate to use a continuous reinforcement schedule of reinforcement? When is it most appropriate to use a variable schedule of reinforcement?
10. Provide an example of how instructional reinforcement can be shifted from a fixed-ratio schedule to a variable-ratio schedule.
11. What is a *changing criterion design*? Describe an example of using the changing criterion strategy in teaching a preschool child a new skill.
12. Discuss how the instructional situation, materials, and style of presentation can be used to provide encouragement (motivation).
13. Write a definition of *generalization*.

14. Define and compare stimulus and response generalization.

15. Write a *general case objective* for the skill of taking turns.

16. Describe the major elements of a general case instructional plan.

17. Define and provide an example of the following generalization procedures: train sufficient exemplars, program common stimuli, introduce to natural maintaining contingencies, use indiscriminable contingencies, mediate generalization, and train loosely.

18. Discuss the following three considerations for implementing systematic instruction: amount of engaged time, contingent arrangement of reinforcement, and minimizing errors.

19. Develop a data collection strategy for teaching a child to play blocks with a sibling or peer. Draft a graph for charting the data.

REFERENCES

Anderson, L.W. (1976). An empirical investigation of individual differences in time to learn. *Journal of Educational Psychology, 68,* 226–233.

Anderson, S.R., & Spradlin, J.E. (1980). The generalized effects of productive labeling training involving common object classes. *Journal of the Association for the Severely Handicapped, 5,* 143–157.

Bambara, L.M., & Warren, S.F. (1993). Massed trials revisited: Appropriate applications in functional skill training. In R.A. Gable & S.F. Warren (Eds.), *Strategies for teaching students with mild to severe mental retardation* (pp. 165–190). Baltimore, MD: Paul H. Brookes Publishing Co.

Becker, W., Engelmann, S., & Thomas, D. (1975). *Teaching 2: Cognitive learning and instruction.* Chicago, IL: Science Research Associates.

Bereiter, C., & Engelmann, S. (1966). *Teaching disadvantaged children in the preschool.* Englewood Cliffs, NJ: Prentice-Hall.

Browder, D., Demchack, M.A., Heller, M., & King, D. (1989). An in vivo evaluation of the use of data-based rules to guide instructional decisions. *Journal of the Association for Persons with Severe Handicaps, 14,* 234–240.

Buysse, V., & Hollingsworth, H.L. (2009). Program quality and early childhood inclusion recommendations for professional development. *Topics in Early Childhood Special Education, 29*(2), 119–128.

Csapo, M. (1981). Comparison of two prompting procedures to increase response fluency among severely handicapped learners. *Journal of the Association for the Severely Handicapped, 6*(1), 39–47.

Day, H.M. (1987). Comparison of two prompting procedures to facilitate skill acquisition among severely mentally retarded adolescents. *American Journal of Mental Deficiency, 91,* 366–372.

Dunst, C.J. (1981). *Infant learning.* Allen, TX: DLM/Teaching Resources.

Dunst, C.J., Bruder, M.B., Trivette, C.M., Raab, M., & McLean, M. (2001). Natural learning opportunities for infants, toddlers, and preschoolers. *Young Exceptional Children, 4*(3), 18–25.

Dunst, C.J., & Trivette, C.M. (2009). Using research evidence to inform and evaluate early childhood intervention practices. *Topics in Early Childhood Special Education, 29*(1), 40–52.

Glendenning, N.J., Adams, G.L., & Sternberg, L. (1983). Comparison of prompt sequences. *American Journal of Mental Deficiency, 88,* 321–325.

Gold, M.W. (1980). *Try another way: Training manual.* Champaign, IL: Research Press.

Grisham-Brown, J., Pretti-Frontczak, K., Hawkins, S.R., & Winchell, B.N. (2009). Addressing early learning standards for all children within blended preschool classrooms. *Topics in Early Childhood Special Education, 29*(3), 131–142.

Haring, N., Liberty, K., & White, O. (1981). *Final report: Field initiated research studies of phases of learning and facilitating instructional events for the severely/profoundly handicapped.* (U.S. Department of Education, Contract No. G007500593) Seattle: University of Washington College of Education.

Holland, J.G., & Skinner, B.F. (1961). *The analysis of behavior.* New York, NY: McGraw-Hill.

Horner, R.H., Sprague, J., & Wilcox, B. (1982). General case programming for community activities. In B. Wilcox & G.T. Bellamy (Eds.), *Design of high school programs for severely handicapped students* (pp. 61–98). Baltimore, MD: Paul H. Brookes Publishing Co.

Leach, D. (2012) *Bringing ABA to home, school, and play for young children with autism spectrum disorders and other disabilities.* Baltimore, MD: Paul H. Brookes Publishing Co.

McEachin, J.J., Smith, T., & Lovaas, O.I. (1993). Long-term outcome for children with autism who received early intensive behavioral treatment. *American Journal of Mental Retardation, 97*(4), 359–372.

McWilliam, R.A. (1991). Targeting teaching at children's use of time. *Teaching Exceptional Children, 23*(4), 42–43.

McWilliam, R.A. (2012). Foreword. In D. Leach, *Bringing ABA to home, school, and play for young children with autism spectrum disorders and other disabilities* (pp. x–xii). Baltimore, MD: Paul H. Brookes Publishing Co.

Reichow, B., & Wolery, M. (2011). Comparison of progress prompt delay with and without instructive feedback. *Journal of Applied Behavior Analysis, 44*(2), 327–340.

Skinner, B.F. (1938). *The behavior of the organism.* Englewood Cliffs, NJ: Prentice Hall.

Snell, M.E., & Brown, F. (2011). *Instruction of students with severe disabilities* (7th ed.). Upper Saddle River, NJ: Pearson.

Snell, M.E., & Gast, D.L. (1981). Applying time delay procedure to the instruction of the severely handicapped. *Journal of the Association for Persons with Severe Handicaps, 6*(3), 3–14.

Soluaga, D., Leaf, J.B., Taubman, M., McEachin, J., & Leaf, R. (2008). A comparison of flexible prompt fading and constant time delay for five children with autism. *Research in Autism Spectrum Disorders, 2*(4), 753–765.

Stokes, T.F., & Baer, D.M. (1977). An implicit technology of generalization. *Journal of Applied Behavior Analysis, 10,* 349–367.

Strain, P.S., Wolery, M., & Izeman, S. (1998). Considerations for administrators in the design of service options for young children with autism and their families. *Young Exceptional Children, 1*(2), 8–16.

Taber-Doughty, T., & Jasper, A.D. (2012). Does latency in recording data make a difference? Confirming the accuracy of teachers' data. *Focus on Autism and Other Developmental Disabilities, 27*(3), 168–176.

Touchette, P.E. (1971). Transfer of stimulus control: Measuring the moment of transfer. *Journal of the Experimental Analysis of Behavior, 15,* 347–354.

Walker, H., & Hops, H. (1976). Increasing academic achievement by reinforcing direct academic performance and/or facilitative nonacademic responses. *Journal of Educational Psychology, 68,* 218–225.

Wolery, M., Ault, M.J., & Doyle, P. (1992). *Teaching students with moderate to severe disabilities: Use of response prompting strategies.* White Plains, NY: Longman.

Wolery, M., & Hemmeter, M.L. (2011). Classroom instruction. *Journal of Early Intervention, 33*(4), 371–380.

7
Specialized Instructional Strategies

Linda McCormick

••••••••••••••••• **FOCUS OF THIS CHAPTER** •••••••••••••••••

- Enhanced milieu teaching procedures
- Activity-based intervention
- Embedded and distributed time delay trials
- High-probability procedures
- Arranging the physical and social environments
- Modifying methods and activities for children with sensory impairments and children with limited motor abilities and/or health impairment

This chapter describes methods to promote engagement, communication, interaction, and play and strategies for adapting classroom procedures and activities to facilitate and support the participation of children with disabilities. These instructional procedures, called *naturalistic intervention* or *systematic naturalistic instruction*, were initially implemented and researched in the context of language intervention. They have been shown to be effective across a range of behaviors (for toddlers through age 5) and in multiple settings (Wolery & Hemmeter, 2011). They are evidence-based practices that have been demonstrated to be effective for teaching communication, social behaviors, and self-help skills.

Systematic naturalistic instruction procedures are not a replacement for direct instruction in which specific behaviors are taught in a brief 1:1 format. They augment and consolidate learning. There are variations of these procedures, but for the most part naturalistic instruction is instruction that is provided in the context of routine events and activities in the child's natural environments (e.g., homes, preschools, child care settings) by individuals (teachers, parents, siblings, paraeducators, peers) who have a daily presence in those environments. It addresses functional skills and has immediate application in interactions that are initiated by the child.

Instructional interactions use whatever interests and motivates the child to encourage targeted behaviors *and* as the natural consequences for the child's responses.

This chapter describes four naturalistic instructional procedures: enhanced milieu teaching (EMT) (Kaiser, 2000), activity-based intervention (ABI; Pretti-Frontczak & Bricker, 2004), embedded and distributed trials (Wolery, 2001), and high-probability ("high-*p*") procedures (Santos, 2001). Being enrolled and present, however, does not mean that children with disabilities necessarily have access to and participate in all of the learning opportunities in naturalistic environments. The last major section of this chapter discusses features of the physical environment that can be modified and adapted to help young children with disabilities gain access to and participate in all of the social and curriculum activities and routines that the environment has to offer.

ENHANCED MILIEU TEACHING PROCEDURES

A series of classic studies in the 1960s and 1970s documented the effectiveness of a set of procedures for facilitating children's language and communication skills (e.g., Hart & Risley, 1975). The initial research grew from observations of caregivers interacting with their typically developing infants and young children. These procedures were first called incidental teaching, then milieu teaching, and now EMT. They are the most thoroughly researched of the naturalistic instruction procedures. They grew from research developed and demonstrated to increase vocabulary, linguistic complexity, and use of language in children with speech delays or mild developmental delay (e.g., Hart & Risley, 1995). They are now also used to teach prelinguistic, cognitive, social, motor, and adaptive skills. Our description of EMT in this chapter draws heavily from the work of Ann Kaiser and colleagues (Hancock & Kaiser 2006; Kaiser, 2000; Kaiser, Ostrosky, & Alpert, 1993).

The four original naturalistic instruction procedures were expanded in the first decade of the century to include six strategies. These procedures are well suited to use in the home as well as the classroom and other naturalistic settings. In the course of their research prior to 2002, Kaiser and Hancock (2003) trained over 200 parents to implement EMT procedures at home. Most impressive are the findings that 97% of the families who completed the training reached the preset teaching accuracy criterion and nearly 90% of the children maintained and generalized their language gains. The six strategies are 1) responsive interaction strategies, 2) environmental arrangement strategies, 3) modeling, 4) a mand-model procedure, 5) a time delay procedure, and 6) incidental teaching (Kaiser, 2000).

Responsive Interaction Strategies

The broad goal of responsive interaction strategies is to establish an interactive context. This is accomplished simply by responding to the child's verbal and nonverbal initiations. The focus is on turn taking, sustained interactions, comprehension of spoken language, and spontaneous interactions during activities that the child enjoys. The adult follows the child's lead, responding communicatively to both verbal and nonverbal communication. Specifically, the adult focuses on

- Following the child's attention focus
- Taking turns in whatever interaction can be established
- Maintaining the child's topic
- Talking about what the child is doing and what they are doing together
- Matching the level of complexity of the child's language
- Expanding and repeating the child's utterances

Environmental Arrangement Strategies

Environmental arrangement strategies are nonverbal schemes for eliciting communication. They provide an assortment of opportunities for adults to respond to, expand, and increase child communication. There are six environmental arrangement strategies: 1) providing interesting materials and activities, 2) placing desired materials in sight but out of reach, 3) offering small portions of needed or desired materials, 4) providing many choice-making opportunities, 5) setting up situations in which children need assistance, and 6) creating unexpected situations. The interests and preferences of the child with disabilities are both the natural stimuli for communication and the natural reinforcement for communication. Reaching for an object or otherwise expressing an interest in a particular material is tantamount to designating a reinforcer. The teacher uses one or another of the procedures as prompts.

The reason for providing interesting age-appropriate materials and activities is to maximize incentives for the child to communicate. Placing materials that the child desires in sight but out of reach is a way to prompt requesting. Whenever the child wants something, there is an opportunity for teaching language. Preferred toys may be placed in clear bins (with tight lids), on high shelves, or simply on the far side of a table. When a child has limited motor control, the material or toy is placed at a sufficient distance from other objects so that it is obvious what the child is reaching for or looking at.

Providing small or inadequate portions of materials such as snacks, blocks, or dress-up clothes virtually guarantees that the child will either protest or request more. If, for example, children are provided with an incomplete set of materials (e.g., the toothpaste is missing from the tray with the other toothbrushing materials), there is typically either a protest or a request for the missing object(s). An added advantage is that peers may get involved when inadequate materials are provided. They often prompt the child to communicate (e.g., seeing that Jace has finished pasting the one circle he was given on his clown face, Amelia says, "Tell Ms. Lee that you need more circles to paste"). The adult waits until the children notice that something is missing. When the child says "more" or simply points or extends to an empty container, the adult models and/or prompts more elaborate requesting (e.g., "Want more juice," "Want more circles to paste").

Providing choice-making opportunities (two or more possible materials or activities) encourages a child to use language to choose the item or activity he or she wants. This works best when one of the choices is an item or an activity that is definitely disliked. Similarly, it is possible to prompt requesting by setting up situations in which the child needs assistance. Examples of situations in which the child might need assistance are activating a battery-operated toy, getting on a swing, or putting a straw in a juice container. Most important is for a caregiver to remember not to rush in with assistance and thus preempt the child's request. Finally, the sixth strategy for prompting the child to communicate is creating unexpected situations. A caregiver can create situations that violate the child's expectations in that they are out of order, unexpected, or clearly absurd. Examples are holding a book upside down, wearing unmatched shoes, or providing the child with someone else's coat when preparing for outside play. Children are quick to comment on or protest absurdities and inappropriate actions, thus providing an opportunity to encourage use of language. Calculated "silliness" has the additional advantage of helping children develop a sense of humor.

The six environmental arrangement strategies described set the stage for the four teaching procedures discussed below—modeling, mand-modeling, time delay, and incidental teaching. Each of the procedures has different goals and implementation strategies but they also have commonalities. They all begin by establishing joint attention (the adult and the child attend to each other or simultaneously attend to the same material or activity); they all follow incomplete or incorrect child responses by providing an additional prompt, and they all end every teaching episode with a positive consequence (acknowledgment and expansion of the child's response) and provision of the material, assistance, or activity that the child desires.

Modeling

Modeling is "showing how"—providing a demonstration in order to elicit a verbal or motor imitation. There is a substantial body of research over many decades showing how parents teach language through modeling (e.g., Bates, 1976; Halliday, 1977). The goals of the EMT modeling procedure are to teach turn-taking skills, generalized imitation skills, conversational skills, and basic vocabulary. There are six steps in the procedures:

1. *Note the child's interest (as indicated by his attention):* Jace is looking at the new addition to the aquarium—a turtle.

2. *Establish joint attention:* The teacher kneels beside Jace and also focuses attention on the turtle.

3. *Present a verbal model that labels or describes the focus of interest:* The teacher says "turtle."

4. *When the child imitates the model, acknowledge and expand his or her response and provide access to the material or activity:* "Yes, that is a *turtle*. Here, take the turtle food and sprinkle it on the water."

5. *If child does not imitate the model or responds with an unintelligible, partial, incorrect, or unrelated response, present the model a second time (called a corrective model):* The teacher says "turtle" again.

6. *If the child does not respond or responds incorrectly to the corrective model, then provide corrective feedback and access to the material or activity:* "That's a *turtle*. Here, take the *turtle* food and feed the *turtle*."

When providing the verbal model in step 3, be certain to say only what you want the child to imitate. In other words, say "turtle," not "Jace, say 'turtle.'" Note also that the procedure begins with identifying an appropriate teaching opportunity and by establishing joint attention. The model procedure tells the child exactly what he or she is expected to say, so it is especially appropriate for skills that a child is just beginning to learn. Once the child demonstrates progress using the model procedure, the mand-model procedure is used.

Mand-Model Procedure

While the modeling procedure teaches new forms, the goal of the mand-model procedure is to prompt the child to use existing language across activities and environments. A *mand* is a directive or an indirect prompt ("Tell me what you want"). It is used when the child has previously demonstrated the ability to perform the expected response. The steps in the mand-model procedure are as follows:

1. Note the child's interest (as indicated by his or her attention).

2. Establish joint attention.

3. Present a verbal mand. Examples: "Tell me what you want" or "Tell me what you want to do."

4. If the child responds correctly, acknowledge and expand his or her response and provide access to the material or activity. Example: "Oh, you want to feed the turtle. Here's the turtle food."

5. If the child does not provide a correct response or responds with an unintelligible, partial, incorrect, or unrelated response, present a second mand or present a model if the child's interest is waning or a response is not forthcoming. Example: "Tell me..."

6. When the child responds correctly to the mand or model, acknowledge and expand his or her response and provide access to the material or activity. Example: "Oh, you want to feed the turtle. Here's the turtle food."

7. If the child does not respond or responds incorrectly, provide corrective feedback and access to the material or activity. Example: "You need to tell me that you want to feed the turtle. Here's the turtle food."

Time Delay Procedure

The purpose of the time delay procedure is to get the child to initiate communication rather than simply respond to another person's initiations. It is used when there is evidence that the child knows the response but does not produce it consistently. Similar to the modeling and mand-model procedures, environmental stimuli become occasions for communication. Time delay is systematic use of "wait time." It is allowing time for the child to respond before a mand or model is given. There are no verbal or gestural prompts: just look at the child and wait. The following are the steps to use time delay:

1. *Identify or create occasions when the child needs or want materials, assistance, or access to an activity.*

2. *Establish joint attention:* Jace is looking at his favorite music box, which is on a shelf he cannot reach. The caregiver kneels beside Jace and also focuses attention on the music box.

3. *Introduce time delay:* The caregiver looks at Jace and waits expectantly.

4. *If the child responds correctly, provide material, assistance, or access to an activity:* The caregiver says, "You want your music box. Here it is."

5. *If the child does not provide a correct response, present a mand or model:* The caregiver says, "Tell me what you want" and/or says, "music box."

6. *When the child responds correctly to the mand or model, acknowledge and expand the child's response, and provide access to the material or activity:* The caregiver says, "You want your music box. Here it is."

Incidental Teaching Procedure

The goal of the incidental teaching procedure (sometimes called *milieu teaching*) is to teach more elaborate language and improve conversational skills. This entails providing prompts for longer and more complex phrases and sentences. It is used after the child has produced a more sophisticated response than simple looking at or moving toward a desired object or activity. The child's verbal, vocal, or gestural request is followed with a model, mand-model, or time delay to encourage the use of more advanced productions and continuing conversation.

This procedure begins the same way as the other EMT procedures (create a situation to promote communication or identify the occasion for instruction and establish joint attention). The steps are as follows:

1. Identify or create occasions when the child needs or wants materials, assistance, or access to an activity.

2. Establish joint attention.

3. When the child initiates a request, teach more intelligible, complex, or elaborate language by

    - Modeling a new or more difficult form of the request
    - Using the mand-model procedure to encourage conversation
    - Using time delay to encourage the child to produce more advanced language.

4. Provide the requested materials, assistance, or access to the activity.

Application of EMT requires some planning, preparation, and practice, but in a very short time it becomes part of the routine. The natural environment is altered to engage the child's attention and thus teach desired behaviors. The procedures can be as readily applied and effective with children who use alternative and augmentative communication as with those who use the verbal modality as their primary means of communication.

Also, as has been pointed out in the descriptions of the procedures, peers can play an important role in EMT. As in the example above with Amelia and Jace, they may inadvertently prompt a communicative response. Or teachers may prompt one peer to cue another. For example, the teacher might say to Amelia, "Tell Jace that he needs to say 'My turn' to let you know what he wants."

ACTIVITY-BASED INTERVENTION

The core belief underlying ABI is that embedding instruction into routine, planned, and spontaneous activities is an effective way to teach function skills (Macy & Bricker, 2007; Pretti-Frontczak & Bricker, 2004). Other terms associated with this approach are *embedded intervention/instruction, routines-based intervention/instruction,* and *integrated therapy*. As these terms imply, ABI is essentially dispersal of teaching trials within the series of actions that make up daily activities. Similar to EMT, there is a substantial body of research supporting the use of ABI with young children with disabilities. A few examples of skills that can be taught at snack time with ABI are "eating independently," "pouring juice," and "requesting more." The basic premises underlying ABI are as follows:

- Child-initiated activities and actions are most likely to hold the child's attention.

- Daily routines and planned or child-initiated activities are opportunities for instruction of individualized family service plan (IFSP) and individual education program (IEP) goals and objectives.

- Instruction should use naturally occurring antecedents (materials, prompts) and consequences (logical outcomes).
- Instruction should develop skills that will enable the child to become more independent in current and future environments and skills that will generalize to a variety of settings (Bricker, Pretti-Frontczak, & McComas, 1998).

The first step in ABI is to select the activities within which the teaching episodes will be embedded. Bricker et al. (1998) define an activity as a sequence of events that has a beginning and a logical outcome and requires a variety of both initiated and reciprocal actions by the child. Table 7.1 provides suggestions for selecting activities to provide opportunities for a child to learn and practice specified objectives. The majority of activities in preschool and child care programs are appropriate contexts for ABI.

After selecting appropriate activities, the next step is to decide how the targeted skills will be taught. In ABI, as in EMT, the teaching episode is generally child-initiated. However, it is the adult's responsibility to ensure that there are frequent teaching opportunities throughout the day. When the child initiates an interaction the adult responds in a reciprocal manner to the initiation and joins the child in the activity. Teaching episodes may also be initiated by other adults or peers, using a variety of antecedents to evoke the target behaviors if the child does not initiate an interaction. The consequences are inherent in the activity as they are the logical outcomes of the interaction.

Among the other approaches that are in the same genre as ABI are routines-based intervention (RBI) (McWilliam, 2010) and embedded learning opportunities (Sandall & Schwartz, 2008). They are similar to ecological assessment and planning as described in this text in that they facilitate identification of the intervention/instructional target and embed these objectives into the day-to-day routines and activities of infants and young children with disabilities. They embed strategies that have been demonstrated to be effective into naturally available learning opportunities in the home, classroom, and other settings.

Table 7.1. Suggestions for selecting activities for activity-based intervention

1. Select activities that group similar objects for different children. For example, telling stories with puppets is an activity for circle time that lends itself to teaching "identifying objects by their function."
2. Select activities that group different goals and objectives for the same child. For example, Jace has three objectives that can be taught in the context of snack preparation: a language objective (naming objects), a cognitive objective (matching colors and shapes), and a fine motor/self-care objective (pouring).
3. Select activities that can be adapted for varying ages and skill levels. For example, an activity such as "Yes, you can," which teaches children to help with simple tasks, can easily be adapted to different ages and skill levels; Jace is assigned tasks that are equally important but less physically demanding.
4. Select activities that require minimal adult direction and assistance. For example, most free-play activities and some clean-up routines require minimal direct assistance from adults once they begin.
5. Select activities that provide many opportunities for child initiations. For example, the activity "Up, up, and away" requires children to name a peer and then pass a balloon to that peer. Each game provides numerous opportunities for children to initiate to peers.
6. Select activities that are motivating and interesting. Routines and activities that are fun and inherently reinforcing are more likely to keep children engaged and therefore learning.

Source: Bricker, Cripe, and Norstad (1990).

EMBEDDED AND DISTRIBUTED TIME DELAY TRIALS

There is considerable overlap between EMT and ABI in that both provide trials within daily routines and activities. However, neither one systematically plans for and uses time delay trials to help children learn to perform new behaviors independently. While time delay is one of the six procedures in EMT, it is not used to teach new behaviors but rather it is used when the child knows the response but has come to rely on a prompt before producing it.

The terms *embedded* and *distributed* refer to when the teaching trials are provided. They are inserted or embedded into naturally occurring activities and routines and distributed rather than provided as a set, one right after another. There are opportunities for the child to perform other behaviors between the instructional trials. There is now a body of research documenting the effectiveness of embedded and distributed time delay trials (e.g., Wolery, 1994, 2001; Wolery, Ault, & Doyle, 1992).

Wolery (2001) describes the steps to embedding and distributing time delay procedures in classroom activities. The example Wolery provides for application of the procedures is with a preschooler named Isaiah.

Step 1: Identify the Specific Skills to Be Taught

Time delay can be used to teach any type of skill. The three skills that have been identified for Isaiah are using words to request, using action words to describe his play, and pushing down and pulling up his pants during toileting routines.

Step 2: Identify Activities and Routines When the Skills Will Be Taught

The procedures may be implemented during only one activity, during multiple activities, or during transitions between activities. Decisions about when to embed time delay depend on what is being taught, how many teaching opportunities are possible, and teacher responsibilities.

Isaiah's teachers decide to teach the first skill (requesting) during snacks and meals and free play. The second skill (using actions words) will be taught during free play and outdoor play, and the third skill (getting pants up and down) will be taught during toileting routines.

Step 3: Decide How Many Trials Will Be Given and How Often

Wolery suggests aiming for approximately five trials per day for each skill. Set a minimum and a maximum time between trials. For example, one might decide on at least 2 minutes and no more than 10 minutes between trials.

It was decided that Isaiah's first skill (requesting) would be taught each time he made a nonverbal request and whenever he was given a choice. If Isaiah did not make a verbal request in 3 minutes, the teacher asked him if he wanted something. For action words, the teacher used the rule "at least 2 minutes but no more than 10." The skill "pushing down and pulling up pants" was taught each time Isaiah was taken to the bathroom.

Step 4: Select a Time Delay Procedure

Decide whether to use constant time delay or progressive time delay. Both begin with 0-second trials. With constant time delay (which is somewhat easier to use), the response intervals of delay trials are all the same length. With progressive time delay, the response intervals gradually increase over trials or days. Whether to use constant time delay or progressive time delay depends on the child. If the child waits for help and is attentive, then the constant time delay procedure is the best choice. With children who have difficulty waiting, use the progressive time delay procedure.

With Isaiah, the decision was to use constant time delay for requesting (because he attends and waits for what he wants), progressive time delay for using action words, and constant time delay for pushing down and pulling up his pants.

Step 5: Identify a Task Cue and a Controlling Prompt

A task cue is a question, a command, or a naturally occurring situation that signals the child to perform the target behavior. This response signal at the beginning of the trial is called the *discriminative stimulus*.

For the first skill, Isaiah's obvious interest in a material or activity (a naturally occurring situation) was the task cue for him to request. For the second skill, using action words, the task cue was an adult asking, "What are you doing?" For the third skill, pushing down and pulling up his pants during toileting, standing in front of the toilet (a naturally occurring situation) was the task cue. It is also important to identify controlling prompts. Because Isaiah is a good imitator, it was decided to use a verbal model (e.g., "Want milk") as the prompt for requesting. The prompt for action words (e.g., "running," "throwing") was also a verbal model. Physical prompts were used for the toileting routines.

Step 6: Select a Reinforcer

The range of potential reinforcers for preschoolers is virtually unlimited. Possibilities include activities, brief play or just "hanging out" time with favorite adults, or toys. As noted above, one of the strengths of naturalistic instruction is that activities and materials in the environment that the child finds interesting and fun serve as both the antecedents and the reinforcers for targeted skills.

Where Isaiah is concerned, seeing a food, drink, or toy he wants is the antecedent for requesting, and receiving the desired food, drink, or toy is the reinforcer for requesting. Allowing him to continue with his play and acknowledgment are the reinforcers for using action words. Adult interaction is the reinforcer for pushing down and pulling up his pants during toileting routines.

Step 7: Determine the Number of 0-Second Trials to Use

The purpose of the initial 0-second trials is to establish the all-important relationship between the task cue and the response. In order to accomplish this, it is important to offer the prompt *immediately* after the task cue and then provide reinforcement *immediately* after the response. It can take as long as

5 days at the 0-second delay level, but usually 2 or 3 days are enough time for the child to learn the relationship.

Isaiah's teachers will provide 2 days of 0-second trials at snacks and lunch for requesting, 4 days of 0-second trials for action words, and 3 days of 0-second trials for managing his pants.

Step 8: Determine the Length of the Response Intervals

The length of the response interval is increased by 1 or 2 seconds every 2 or 3 days. A child who is slow to respond will need a longer interval. There is no need for a stopwatch: Simply counting "1001, 1002," and so forth (silently) is accurate enough.

The decision for Isaiah is to provide a 4-second interval for requesting and for managing his pants. The interval for using action words will be increased by 1 second every 2 days.

Step 9: Select a Monitoring System

Data collection is critical to determining whether the program is working as intended. There are three possible responses with 0-second trials: correct, incorrect, or no response. An incorrect response on 25% or more of the trials for 2 or more days suggests the need for a more controlling prompt. A "no response" on 25% or more of the trials suggests the need for a better reinforcer.

There are five response possibilities with the delay trials: 1) a correct response *before* the prompt, 2) a wrong response *before* the prompt, 3) a correct response *after* the prompt, 4) a wrong response *after* the prompt, and 5) no response. A wrong response before the prompt on 25% or more trials for 2 or more days indicates a need to teach the child to wait. The procedure for teaching the child to wait is as follows:

- Assemble a set of small cards with abstract symbols on them.
- Show the child a symbol card and ask "What's this?"
- Wait about half a second and give the child a made-up name for the symbol (e.g., "a flob").
- Immediately reinforce the child for imitating the name.
- Gradually lengthen the time before naming the symbol. (The child must wait for the symbol to be named before he can imitate and claim the reinforcer.)
- If necessary, gently place fingers to the child's lips as an additional cue to wait.

If the child is wrong *after* the prompt on 25% or more trials for 2 or more days, a more controlling prompt is needed. A "no response" on 25% or more trials for 2 or more days indicates the need for a better reinforcer. Similarly, the reinforcers should be modified when the child is correct only after the prompt on 90% or more trials for 3 consecutive days. Begin to provide a more desirable reinforcer for correct responses before the prompt than for those after the prompt.

Step 10: Implement the Plan and Monitor Its Use and Effects

The importance of planning and rigorous application of the procedures cannot be overemphasized. In addition to reviewing the procedures frequently to ensure that they are implemented precisely as planned, it is important to pay careful attention to the child's behavior after every embedded trial to be sure that he or she continues to participate in the activity. Aim for relatively the same number of trials each day.

HIGH-PROBABILITY PROCEDURES

The high-probability request sequence is a proactive antecedent teaching strategy that has been demonstrated to effectively increase compliance as well as a range of functional skills (Santos, 2001). The high-probability (high-*p*) request sequence involves the presentation of a sequence of easy and favorite requests *immediately* before a request that is not typically performed—the low-probability (low-*p*) request.

Why is presenting a sequence of requests for performance of a skill or skills that are already in the child's repertoire (that the child easily and consistently performs) followed by a request for performance of a new skill that the child does not (or cannot) perform on a consistent basis effective? There are two possible explanations. One is that the experience of compliance (with reinforcement) to preferred instructions may produce a generalized class of compliance to instruction that includes less preferred activities. Another possible explanation is that the effectiveness of the high-*p* request sequence can be explained by behavioral momentum: Delivering the high-*p* request immediately followed by a low-*p* request establishes a momentum of compliant behavior.

Behavioral momentum procedures rely on delivering a set of simple requests (usually 3 to 5) to which there is a high probability that the child will respond, followed immediately by a request to which the child is not likely to respond. Examples include teaching social skills, responding to indirect questions and comments, and increased use of augmentative communication devices.

Santos (2001) provides a detailed description of the three major steps in the high-probability procedure and examples of application of the procedure in the classroom and at home.

Step 1: Identify High-*p* and Low-*p* Requests

Identify a series of requests that the child is likely to respond to consistently and fluently (the high-*p* requests) and a low-*p* request that the child either does not respond to or responds to inconsistently. The high-*p* and low-*p* requests may require either motor or language responses. Requests during transition times may require motor response (e.g., "Please return the crayon and scissors boxes to the shelf," "Please get your backpack," "Please put on your jacket"). Requests during other activities may require verbal or augmentative communication responses. These requests may ask the child to name or label an object, person, or activity (e.g., "What are you making with those beautiful colors?" "Who is your partner on this project?"); select from an array of items (e.g., "Would you like _____ or _____ today?"); or describe objects or events/activities (e.g., "What color is _____?" "How do you _____?").

Santos (2001) used the example of Adrian. His mother says that he responds to requests to identify or name objects (e.g., "What is this?") 80% of the time. However, he has difficulty responding to his mother's specific request to put away his toys when he is finished with them. His mother decides to use labeling objects as her high-*p* request to encourage Adrian to begin responding to the low-*p* request, "Let's put your toys in the toy box."

Step 2: Use Routines, Activities, and Materials in the Environment

Observe the child to identify favorite toys and materials and preferred routines and activities. These high-interest stimuli, routines, and activities are the ones to incorporate into high-probability procedures.

Adrian's favorite toys are those that he can pull apart and put together such as Mr. Potato Head. His favorite activities are art activities. He especially enjoys using markers, paint, glue, construction paper, and crayons to create pictures that he can take home. Adrian's teacher and his mother plan to use these preferred toys and materials and activities as the context for high-probability procedures.

Step 3: Deliver Three High-*p* Requests and One Low-*p* Request

Actual implementation of the high-*p* procedures in a classroom routine or activity takes only 1 to 2 minutes. It is comparable to the game Simon Says. The teacher delivers the sequence of high-*p* requests (e.g., "Pat your tummy," "Raise one knee," "Put your hands on your head"), followed by the low-*p* request ("Sit on your carpet square"). High-*p* procedures can be used with the other naturalistic instructional procedures described in this chapter.

See Table 7.2 for an example provided by Santos (2001) of high-*p* procedures used with Adrian during tabletop activities. The goal is for Adrian to respond consistently to the teacher's comments. The teacher uses a silly comment (calculated silliness as in EMT) in the first low-*p* request. Adrian's picture has a *red* bird.

One caveat: If it is not possible to identify a set of directions or requests to which the child consistently complies (high-*p* requests), then it may be necessary to provide discrete trial training (described in Chapter 6) to increase compliance before beginning the high-*p* teaching sequence.

Timing of the delivery of the requests and the reinforcement is crucial: The goal is to build momentum. The high-*p* requests must be delivered in rapid

Table 7.2. Example of high-*p* procedures used with Adrian

	High-*p* request	High-*p* request	High-*p* request	Low-*p* request
Teacher *requests*	"Adrian, what are you making?"	"Who's that?"	"What's that on top of the house?"	"That looks like a *yellow* bird."
Adrian *responds*	"My house!"	"Adrian and Mommy."	"A birdie."	"No, it's a red bird!"
Teacher *praises*	"Oh, that's a beautiful house."	"That's really nice."	"You drew a pretty bird on the house."	"Oh, that's right. It is a *red* bird."

Source: Santos (2001).

succession, followed immediately by appropriate reinforcement. High-*p* procedures are best used as a short-term intervention. If the game goes on too long, it could become predictable and tiresome for the child, resulting in challenging behaviors to escape or avoid having to respond to the adult.

ARRANGING THE PHYSICAL AND SOCIAL ENVIRONMENTS

As discussed in Chapter 1, access goes beyond the concepts of inclusion or mainstreaming. It involves removal of physical barriers and provision of instructional formats and activities that maximize the development and learning in all infants and young children in early intervention and early childhood environments (DEC/NAEYC, 2009). This section describes elements in the environment that influence children's access to activities and routines. These are variables that can either contribute to or impede learning, independence, social interactions, and communication.

The physical environment includes the spaces, both indoors and outdoors, that should allow for positive interpersonal interaction and socialization among children of different abilities and both genders in dyads and small and large groups. Access requires careful attention to the layout of these spaces, materials, equipment, noise levels, lighting, accessibility of materials, and technology.

Two of the practices that are central to access are universal design for learning (UDL; CAST, 2011) and assistive technology (AT; National Professional Development Center on Inclusion, 2011). As noted in Chapter 1, UDL has its roots in architecture and urban planning: specifically, a concern for designing buildings and outdoor environments in such a way as to make them accessible for persons with disabilities. It is a concept that generates principles and practices to enable access *for* all and *to* all aspects of the individual's physical, social, and instructional environments. Universal design led to inclusion of ramps, automatic doors, and curb cuts in urban planning in order to provide access to people with physical disabilities. It was soon apparent that these design features eased access for all members of the community. One has only to remember using a ramp for a stroller or wheeled luggage to corroborate that finding. The essential point about UDL is the focus on designing accommodations that are incorporated at the planning stage rather than after the fact.

Universal design and AT are similar in that both focus on access and both provide a variety of planning tools for making necessary adaptations. Assistive technology includes both high-tech and low-tech devices, ranging from pens and papers and inexpensive adaptations of toys, books, and eating utensils to computer-based literacy tools, voice output communication aids, speech-generating devices, hearing aids, powered scooters, and custom-fitted wheelchairs.

The three basic UDL concepts—*multiple means of representation, multiple means of engagement*, and *multiple means of expression*—refer to design of all aspects of the physical space as well as the daily schedule, classroom routines, curriculum, and teaching strategies (CAST, 2011). The goal is to maximize every child's access to learning in the same way that curb cuts and ramps provide access to the physical environment. Examples of the application of

UDL concepts in early childhood settings include adding handles, buttons, and knobs for easier use of materials; stabilizing furniture and equipment to keep them from sliding or tipping; and providing blocks that have texture, make sounds, and can be color coded.

Layout

Most early childhood classrooms include, in addition to a children's bathroom and a storage area, a block center, a writing center, an art center (with sink and storage), a housekeeping center, a discovery learning area, and a quiet reading area. These areas, their number and size, the way the materials are arranged, and the rules of access all take into consideration the fact that children come in a variety of sizes. If the layout is arranged with the intention of accommodating everyone, it will not need to be modified for a child with disabilities. The rule is to modify only if it is clear that the child cannot participate in the activity center even partially or at a less sophisticated level unless the space is rearranged or modified (McCormick & Feeney, 1995).

The variable to consider when planning the room layout is sufficient space for a wheelchair, a walker, or some other method of mobility. These often require wide routes to activity centers, the bathroom, the cafeteria, and the playground. Also, arrival and departure areas need to be clear of furniture, equipment, and carpet and should allow wheelchair mobility and access.

Materials

The available materials in a setting will depend on the ages and range of ability levels of the children. Preschool settings typically include at least the following materials:

- Low-tech tools (e.g., crayons, chalk, chalkboards, magic markers, bulletin boards, poster paper)
- Natural materials (e.g., sand, clay, water, live specimens, magnets)
- Active play materials (e.g., tires, seesaws, tricycle)
- Construction toys (e.g., blocks, LEGOs, Lincoln Logs, Tinker Toys) and manipulatives (e.g., puzzles, beads, pegboards, games)
- Creative materials (e.g., play dough, scissors, paint, crayons, glue, clay)
- Literacy materials (e.g., books, tapes, flannel board, CDs, interactive software)
- Dramatic play materials (e.g., dolls, puppets, dress-up clothes, child-size kitchen furnishings, kitchenware) and furnishings and materials for themes such as store, bus, or restaurant

Engagement is an important consideration when selecting materials. For children to benefit from an activity, the materials and objects that are part of the activity must be developmentally and contextually appropriate for everyone. They should be interesting and appealing, because young children are more likely to attend to and manipulate complex and colorful materials and objects. Also, children are more likely to initiate communication when they are engaged with preferred materials. Thus, increasing interactions with materials enhances use of language.

The description of toy characteristics provided by Sadao and Robinson (2010) is valuable when evaluating and buying toys for any setting that includes infants and young children. Again, the central concern is access—whether the child will be able to touch, see, and initiate interaction the toy. In addition to considering the size, shape, and weight of toys, teachers should keep in mind that children learn about the properties of objects by mouthing, shaking, throwing, and pounding with them. They must be durable.

Children's developmental needs and interests also influence toy selection. Cause-and-effect toys are most appropriate for young children who are exploring object properties and functions as well as their own sensory and motor capabilities. At this stage they need toys that they can grasp, shake, stack, and hug. Building toys such as blocks, tracks, playdough, and beads and pretend toys such as dolls, shopping baskets, pretend food, and dress-up clothes encourage socialization, communication, cooperation, and creativity. Dress-up clothes should have large neck and arm openings and simple closures.

The National Lekotek Center website is an especially good resource when selecting toys for infants and young children with disabilities (http://www.lekotek.org). It suggests the following considerations:

- Does the toy appeal to the senses (e.g., lights, sounds, movement, color, texture)?

- How is the toy activated (e.g., requiring force, complexity)?

- Can the toy be used in a variety of positions (e.g., sidelying on a wheelchair tray)?

- Is play with the toy open ended (no right or wrong method)?

- Is the toy popular with same-age peers (helps the child feel "like the other kids")?

- Does the toy allow for creativity and choice making?

- Is the toy adjustable (height, sound, speed, level of difficulty)?

- Is the toy both developmentally and chronologically age appropriate?

- Is the toy safe and durable (moisture resistant, appropriate size, easy to clean)?

- Does the toy encourage social interactions?

Engagement can be increased by providing a supply of preferred materials and rotating them in and out of play areas so that they continue to be novel and appealing. The benefits of toy rotation are increased engagement, more varied play skills, and increased sharing. To implement a toy rotation plan, toys and materials that will be rotated should be coded according to the dimensions of size, complexity, developmental level, category, and sensory quality. Then they should be divided into toy and material sets with at least one item in each set reflecting the different dimensions. For example, each set should have at least one item from each of these categories: manipulatives, building materials, dramatic play objects, and visual motor toys. Each set should also have toys addressing the different sensory modalities. Once the toys have been sorted, the sets are numbered and stored. The toy rotation program begins with the provision of two sets. At the end of the first week, set 1 is replaced with set 3. At the end of the second week, set 2 is replaced with set 4. Thus, half of the toys are "new" each week.

Toy rotation does not include all toys and materials. Some items, such as dolls, dress-up clothes, books, and blocks, are always available. Engagement with the permanent toys and items increases with the toy rotation play, because there is a potential to use them in new ways as the sets are rotated.

Equipment

Under the heading of equipment is furniture (shelves, tables, chairs, desks, easels) and what might be considered high-tech items such as laser disc players and tape recorders, VCRs, slide projectors, overhead projectors, and computers (with interactive software). The first consideration when purchasing equipment is safety, then design and attractiveness. Well-designed equipment helps children develop large and small muscle coordination, concepts about the physical world, creativity, social skills, and self-awareness. Like materials, equipment should have sensory appeal (color, design, texture, sound) and be an appropriate size. All areas (e.g., toy shelves, bookcases, coat hangers, sensory tables, activity centers) should be accessible to all children. There should be some tables (including computer tables) and easels in the classroom that are high enough for a wheelchair to fit underneath. Shelves should be at a height that allows materials to be easily retrieved and replaced by all children.

In early childhood special education, technology is a tool for learning, communicating, and participating in daily routines and activities. Augmentative communication is discussed at length in Chapter 13. Computers and adaptive devices (e.g., switches, alternative keyboards, touch tablets) encourage autonomous behavior and increase possibilities for children with disabilities to interact with the environment. The computer center should be designed to accommodate children working individually or with a partner or in a small group.

Group Size

Social density refers to the number of children present in an activity area, and spatial density refers to the amount of space available to those children. They are interrelated aspects of group size. Modifications of either factor can affect the degree of crowding in an area or a classroom, which, in turn, affects classroom dynamics (specifically, the social interactions) (Zirpoli, 1995). Reducing the size of activity areas has been shown to increase social interactions among preschoolers (Rubin & Howe, 1985), but they should not be so small that there is crowding. During storytime, children will be more attentive if they are spaced equidistant from one another (in chairs or on the floor) rather than allowed to arrange themselves (Krantz & Risley, 1977).

Scheduling

Preschool programs typically have routines associated with arrival, self-care, mealtimes, snacks, rest time, and departure. There are several fairly large blocks of time (indoors and outdoors) when children choose their own activities and other blocks of time designated for teacher-guided large-group activities. Hart (1982) noted that the best schedules list approximate time periods. Rosegrant and Bredekamp (1992) agreed, suggesting a general time schedule that can easily be adapted when children become thoroughly engrossed or when they show evidence of losing interest. All children follow the same consistent schedule and daily routines, which are displayed on the wall with photographs or pictures.

Activity time blocks are linked by transitions—movement from one activity or routine to another. There is a high probability for disruptive behavior before, during, and after a transition, because transitions are typically less structured and more difficult for children to understand. Three sets of circumstances increase the probability for disruptive behavior during transitions: 1) if children are not sure what to do next, 2) if children do not have adequate time to end one activity and clean up before preparing for the next activity, and 3) if there is not ample warning before a bell or buzzer (or other warning) announces that it's time to move to another activity. Table 7.3 provides suggestions for smooth transitions. There are many opportunities to teach new skills during these times (Sandall & Schwartz, 2008).

Assigning teachers to areas and activities (called *zones*) rather than to children is one method to increase engagement and decrease waiting times. For example, a teacher is assigned to the housekeeping area during indoor free play or to the wheel-toy area during outdoor play in the same way that a teacher would be assigned to provide music or read a story. The teacher is responsible for teaching and supervising children in the assigned area.

Zone assignment significantly reduces waiting time (waiting has no positive benefits for children). There are no learning or engagement opportunities and a high probability for disruptive behavior when children are standing or sitting in line. To maximize engagement and minimize disruptions, every child should proceed independently, when ready, from one program activity to the next. As soon as children finish their art projects, for example, each one cleans up, proceeds to the sink to wash hands, and then moves to the story circle area and sits down. A teacher is sitting in the story circle area talking about and showing pictures in the book they will read when everyone assembles.

Table 7.3. Suggestions for smooth transitions

- Give several notices that the activity will end shortly and reiterate what the next activity will be.
- Point to the next activity on a large visual schedule that is posted where everyone can see it.
- Allocate sufficient time to end an activity and clean up before beginning preparation for the next activity.
- Have self-directed activities available and allow children to move to those activities independently if they finish early.
- Use the time productively when waiting for the children to assemble for a large-group activity (e.g., sit and look at pictures in a book or talk with children already assembled).
- Provide specific instructions and practice with transition behaviors: for example, where and how to line up, where and how to put away materials, what to do as acceptable quiet activities while waiting, and so forth.

MODIFYING INSTRUCTIONAL METHODS AND ACTIVITIES

The first task when facilitating access to the curriculum for young children with disabilities is to identify the critical skills and concepts in the general curriculum that all children are expected to learn. The second task is to individualize methods of instruction to accommodate their differences in learning styles and abilities in order to teach these skills and concepts. Even when the UDL framework has been used to design the general curriculum, there will be a need for accommodations and modifications to meet the individual needs of particular children (CAST, 2011). There is no one instructional method that can be effective with all children (with or without disabilities) *or* with all skills. At one time or another all children require prompts, repetitions, and some systematic instruction to learn a new skill or follow through with a routine. The major difference for children with disabilities is that they typically need more prompts, more repetitions, and systematic instruction. Table 7.4 provides some general suggestions for accommodations and modifications. The learning styles of children with sensory impairments and children with limited motor abilities and health impairments are most disparate.

Table 7.4. Suggestions for adapting methods and activities for all children

To help children learn to attend
- Position the children in a circle for group activities so that they can see one another.
- Teach the children to look at the speaker when being spoken to.
- Recognize that some children with disabilities will not be able to block out background sounds, so pair auditory communication with visual communication (gestures, symbols, and pictures).

To help children learn to follow directions
- Show the children that following directions is appreciated by saying "Thank you for (and repeat the direction)" when they comply.
- Ask the children to listen while you describe the steps in the task and then provide the directions one step at a time.
- Provide easily recognizable visuals showing the steps in the activity.
- Provide examples and demonstrations (e.g., an example of a possible product so that the children understand the goal of the activity).
- Be sure that instructions are relevant and specific and use terms that you are sure the children understand.

To teach children to succeed
- Point out cause-and-effect relationships ("Yes, it will start if you hold down the switch") to help the children feel confident that they will be successful.
- Provide specific feedback so that the children do not have to guess whether they are doing what is requested.
- Be sure that your verbal and nonverbal behaviors are consistent—that confirmation and appreciation are delivered in an enthusiastic tone. Children respond to tone and facial expressions.
- Be sensitive to fatigue—even the simplest tasks often require exceptional effort for children with disabilities.
- Provide specific practice on expected behaviors: Learning is less likely to occur incidentally for children with disabilities.
- Talk the child through the activity.
- Post easy-to-understand visual schedules showing the sequence of daily routines and activities in line drawings or photographs.

Children with Sensory Impairments

Hearing and vision impairments are common among children with severe disabilities. Although the majority of children identified as deaf-blind or having dual sensory impairments have some vision or hearing, the combined effects of the impairments severely impede the development of communication and social skills. They can make use of some information presented through the visual and auditory modalities, but the stimuli need to be enhanced and supplemented with tactile teaching methods. Early development of meaningful communication and appropriate social skills are primary goals for toddlers and preschoolers with sensory impairment (as for their peers).

Deaf or Hard of Hearing Hearing impairment can range in severity from mild to profound and can be bilateral or unilateral. Children with losses in the mild to moderate range are usually called *hard of hearing*; those with hearing loss in the severe and profound range are considered *deaf*. Children who are deaf are unable to process spoken language without amplification (e.g., a hearing aid). Children who are hard of hearing may or may not need a hearing aid to process spoken language. They may have a prelingual hearing loss, meaning that the hearing loss occurred prior to spoken language acquisition, or a postlingual loss, one that occurred after language acquisition. Specialists who work closely with the family and teachers to ensure an understanding of the child's hearing impairment and to maximize language development and communication opportunities throughout the day include an early intervention specialist, an audiologist, a speech pathologist trained to work with children with hearing impairment, a teacher of the deaf, or a deaf mentor.

By the time they reach preschool age, most children with hearing loss have been fitted with a hearing aid if they need one. Amplification devices are provided as soon as possible in infancy to maximize the use of residual hearing. The audiologist, family, and teachers work as a team to support optimal use of the device. The audiologist and the parents familiarize the teachers with the specifics of the child's hearing device, which may be a hearing aid or a cochlear implant. Then it is the teacher's responsibility to 1) ensure that the child wears the aid consistently, 2) inspect the cords regularly for wear, 3) keep the earmolds clean, 4) ensure that the receiver does not get wet, 5) check the batteries daily, and 6) replace batteries as needed. (Teachers should always have extra batteries on hand.)

When the deaf child is in preschool, the family has made the important decision about how their child will communicate—whether with signs or speech. Approaches that emphasize speech (sometimes called "oral approaches") stress the importance of teaching the child to produce intelligible speech and to be able to understand spoken language (with amplification and lipreading). Those who advocate approaches that emphasize signing, or "manual communication," believe that manual communication is a more fully accessible and naturally acquired language for children with significant hearing losses. The early childhood special education teacher's role is to understand and support whichever approach the family has decided on.

The world of the child with limited hearing is a purely visual world. Sound has little or no meaning; sight, movement, touch, and smell are the experiences through which learning occurs. Children with hearing impairment represent as diverse a group as children in any other disability category, but there are some considerations that are common to most children with hearing impairment. The following accommodations are recommended for children with mild-to-moderate hearing impairment, but they are also useful for children with language/communication disorders and attention deficits, and for those who are learning English as a second language:

- *Seat the child in front of the speaker in circle activities:* Placement near the speaker maximizes hearing and enables the child to read speech and see facial expressions.
- *Speak in a normal teaching voice:* There is no need to enunciate or speak loudly. Use natural gestures and visuals (e.g., photos, pictures, symbols, objects) to supplement oral presentations.
- *Speak the child's name when addressing him or her:* Wait until he or she is looking at you before speaking.
- *Indicate the referent:* When referring to someone or something in the immediate environment, touch, point, or nod in the direction of the referent.
- *Do not stand in front of a strong light source when speaking to the child:* The child is deprived of important visual cues when your face is in the dark.
- *Teach peers attention-getting techniques and remind them to speak one at a time and to look at the child when addressing him or her:* Even preschoolers learn very quickly to touch the student lightly on the shoulder and look him or her in the face while talking.
- *Learn and use as many signs as possible:* If the child signs, learn and use functional signs (e.g., "all finished," "sit," "toilet") and encourage peers without disabilities to use them also.

For children who are profoundly deaf, additional accommodations may be necessary for full participation and continued exposure to a language-rich environment. Inclusive settings may have co-teachers—one with signing skills or experience working with deaf students. The educational assistant may have special training in working with deaf students, or an educational interpreter may be present in the class part or full time to facilitate communication during storytime or other instructional interactions. These professionals will be able to assist teachers with necessary accommodations.

Because they typically have communication difficulties, young deaf children may be less likely to participate in cooperative play activities that are language or sound based, and when they do participate with peers, they tend to prefer groups of two rather than larger groups. Development of cooperative play can be facilitated by modeling and encouraging use of social play materials (e.g., dolls, blocks, balls) and by coaching peers to include their classmate with hearing impairment in their play routines.

Visual Impairment A child with visual impairment may be identified as partially sighted or blind. The impact of the impairment depends on the age of onset, the amount of functional vision, the etiology (whether it is progressive or nonprogressive), and other disabling conditions. Children with severe visual impairment do not have sufficient visual acuity to easily participate in everyday activities. They experience difficulties with locomotion (crawling, walking), fine motor skills, social interaction, and communication.

Specialists in visual disabilities work closely with the family and with teachers to facilitate optimal adaptations or accommodations for the child with visual impairment. In addition, the team will include an orientation and mobility (O&M) specialist who will work with the child directly and provide consultation to other team members.

Specifically, the O&M specialist teaches the child to use his or her compensatory senses to move around safely and efficiently in the school environment. This professional, together with the specialist in visual disabilities, also works with the teachers and other team members to help them adapt and modify methods and equipment to achieve the child's communication, motor, and sensory instruction goals. Facilitating communication skills is especially important for children with visual impairments. The following are suggestions for working with children with visual impairments:

- *Provide verbal cues for the child as to what is going to happen next:* For example, "Do you smell the orange juice? I'm going to put the juice cup in your hand now. It is half full of orange juice."

- *Provide physical cues about how to carry out a task or activity:* For example, gently guide the child to the housekeeping center; place one hand on a bowl and put a spoon in the other hand.

- *Label actions and objects as they are occurring:* For example, "We are putting the art materials away so that we can get ready to go outside."

- *Ensure exploration and manipulation of all parts of an object:* It is important for the child to understand the relationship of the parts of the object to the whole.

- *Let the child know where you are:* Keep the child informed as to your physical location in the classroom; for example, "I'm leaving the block area now to go and begin preparing for snacks. Peter and Taylor are still here to build blocks with you."

- *Help the child make connections between events:* For example, "When that bell rings, it's almost time to go home—you hear everyone hurrying to put away their materials and get their coats. Then we all stand in line by the door."

- *Provide detailed verbal directions and explanations:* For example, "After you locate your cubby and put away your backpack, walk over to the nearest table and sit down. Ms. Rice will have some of your favorite toys there and you can choose what you want to play with."

- *Show peers how to be friends and helpers:* Teach peers to identify themselves, saying, for example, "It's me, Timmy. I will pull out the chair for you if you want to sit here."

Children with Limited Motor Abilities and/or Health Impairments

Included under the heading of health impairments are asthma, allergies, diabetes, rheumatic fever, leukemia, tuberculosis, sickle cell anemia, epilepsy, lead poisoning, and cystic fibrosis. Whether the impairment is chronic (persisting over a long period of time) or acute (having a short but severe course), these children require medical consultation and dietary supervision. Very often, the medications prescribed for these conditions have an effect on classroom behavior. For example, a commonly prescribed asthma medication is correlated with inattentiveness, hyperactivity, drowsiness, and withdrawn behavior.

Physical impairments include those resulting from congenital anomalies (e.g., absence of a limb) and other causes (e.g., spina bifida, cerebral palsy, muscular dystrophy, spinal cord injury). Physical disabilities affect overall developmental progress as well as participation in the classroom program. There may be many interruptions of home, preschool, and peer group experiences because of repeated and prolonged hospitalizations, surgeries, and illnesses.

The physical and occupational therapists and the parents work closely with the teacher to ensure proper seating and positioning for the child with physical impairment. Proper seating and positioning counteract poor circulation, muscle tightness, and pressure sores. It helps the young child to feel physically safe and secure while at the same time aids respiration and digestion and reduces the possibility that the child will develop additional deformities.

Physical and occupational therapists (and parents) also help with ideas for adapting equipment and modifying materials for young children with physical impairments. For example, materials such as adapted scissors, adapted puzzles, and adapted eating utensils and cups need not be specially purchased. They are easily made from standard materials using Velcro, glue, and tape. Building up a spoon or fork handle with layers of tape may facilitate grasping so that a child can feed him- or herself. Velcro straps added to a musical instrument allow a child with an unsteady grasp to shake the tambourine as well as his or her peers without disabilities.

There is a wealth of creative ideas for adapting typical preschool activities for children with limited motor ability. Some special adaptations are described in Table 7.5. Teachers should keep the following considerations in mind for children with physical and health impairments:

- *Material and equipment modifications and adaptations should be kept as simple as possible:* The point is to change and modify only to the extent absolutely necessary to accomplish the desired purpose.

- *Procedures and planned experiences should be as similar as possible to those of peers without disabilities:* The rule is that the less intrusive the strategy, the higher preference it should be given. Avoid experiences that differ from those provided to peers without disabilities, interfere with daily routines, call undue attention to the child, or promote dependence. When alternative activity arrangements are necessary, the modifications should be as rich and varied as activities provided to peers without disabilities.

- *Optimal positioning for all activities is the goal:* Optimal positioning allows the child to relax, focus attention on the activity, and have sufficient controlled movement for independent functioning.

Table 7.5. Activity adaptations for children with limited motor abilities

Circle time
- Have the group sit in chairs rather than on the floor so that everyone is at eye level with the child in a wheelchair.
- If a child has communication difficulties, provide picture boards from which all the children choose a song or story or respond to calendar questions.
- Read stories that include children with disabilities.
- Increase peer interactions by modifying the words of songs to call for interaction: "If you're happy and you know it, hug a friend, or give five," and so forth.

Art activities
- Provide a variety of surfaces for painting; consider attaching paper to the wall, the refrigerator door, or the floor as alternatives to a table or easel.
- Cut off the legs of an easel; a child may find it easier to kneel or sit on a short stool.
- Use Velcro or yarn to fasten a paintbrush to the child's hand or wrist.
- Encourage the children to paint with their fingers, feet, and other body parts.
- Use edible paint (Jell-O and water, pudding, marshmallow whip) so that hand mouthing is not a problem.

Sensory play
- Provide a subset of sensory items on a tray on the floor or on a table that is wheelchair accessible.
- Place sensory items in a Ziploc bag and tape it to the table or wheelchair tray so that the items are easy to handle.
- Provide sponges, honey, peanut butter, marshmallow, fluff, mashed bananas, cotton candy, snow, whipped gelatin, and so forth for the children to experience the different textures.
- Blow bubbles, play with bubble wands, or use automatic blowers for children who may have difficulty blowing.

Books
- Be sure that bookshelves are at different levels so that the books are accessible to everyone.
- Provide headphones and tapes so that the children can listen to the stories.
- Provide a bookstand for children who are unable to hold a book.
- Include a variety of textured books (homemade or commercial).

Fine motor
- Adapt wood puzzles by adding large knobs on the pieces.
- Provide puzzles with auditory stimulation (music plays when a puzzle piece is fitted in the correct place).
- Provide large fine motor items—smaller items can be substituted as children with fine motor limitations become more proficient.
- Use Velcro to prevent materials from sliding on the table or tray.

Dramatic play
- Incorporate items that are large and easy to grasp and manipulate.
- Label shelves with pictures as well as words to facilitate easy cleanup.

Snacks
- Use bowls with suction to avoid sliding and "sippy" cups to avoid spills.
- Identify and assign (on a job board) suitable jobs to the child with limited motor abilities.
- Assemble all the children at the snack table, even if they are not all eating.

Gym and playground
- Provide a scooter board for the child with limited motor abilities: the child can push him- or herself around or be pulled by a peer.
- Provide a wading pool full of balls for the children to sit in and explore.
- Encourage wagon, blanket, and sheet pulls—a peer can pull the child.
- Ensure that sand tables and swings are accessible.

Computer center
- Encourage cooperative interactions with the battery-operated toys, switches, and computer games.
- Provide speech output devices that peers can program for a child with no speech.
- Provide alternative keyboards, touch-sensitive screens, and other appropriate peripherals.
- Place stickers on special keys for a particular program to help the children locate them more easily.
- Set a template or overlay over a keyboard so that only certain keys show.

Source: Sheldon (1996).

SUMMARY

This chapter has described four naturalistic instruction procedures—enhanced milieu teaching, activity-based intervention, embedded and distributed trials, and high-probability (high-*p*) procedures—that are intended to be implemented in the context of daily routines and activities (including play) in the natural environment. These procedures can promote children's development through access to and participation in the general curriculum in preschool and other center-based settings and daily routines in home and community settings. Moreover, they are as effective with toddlers as they are with preschoolers, and they can be implemented effectively by parents and other family members, therapists, paraeducators, and peers as well as teachers. In addition to naturalistic instruction procedures, this chapter described ways to 1) structure physical and social environments to influence behavior and learning and 2) modify instructional methods and activities to accommodate individual differences. Finally, the last section of the chapter has provided suggestions specifically focused on modifications and accommodations for children with sensory impairments, children with limited abilities, and children with health impairments.

•••••••••••••••••• **STUDY QUESTIONS** ••••••••••••••••••

1. Describe characteristics that are common to all *naturalistic intervention* procedures.

2. Describe and give examples of the six EMT procedures.

3. Compare and contrast EMT, ABI, and *embedded and distributed time delay procedures*.

4. Describe the rationale and procedures for *high-probability procedures*.

5. Identify and describe elements in the environment that influence children's access to activities and routines.

6. Discuss and give examples of ways to adapt instructional and play materials to facilitate participation of children with sensory impairment in routines and activities.

7. Discuss and give examples of ways to adapt instructional and play materials to facilitate participation of children with limited motor abilities and/or health impairments in routines and activities.

REFERENCES

Bates, E. (1976). *Language and context: The acquisition of pragmatics.* New York, NY: Academic Press.

Bricker, C., Pretti-Frontczak K., & McComas, N. (1998). *An activity-based approach to early intervention* (2nd ed.). Baltimore, MD: Paul H. Brookes Publishing Co.

Bricker, D.D., Cripe, J., & Norstad, S. (1990, October). *Activity-based intervention.* Paper presented at Post Conference Workshop, Council for Exceptional Children Conference. Albuquerque, New Mexico.

CAST. (2011). *Universal Design for Learning Guidelines version 2.0.* Wakefield, MA: Author.

Division for Early Childhood and the National Association for the Education of Young Children (DEC/AEYC). (2009). *Early childhood inclusion: A joint statement of the Division for Early Childhood (DEC) and the National Association for the Education of Young Children (NAEYC).* Chapel Hill, NC: The University of North Carolina at Chapel Hill, FPG Child Development Institute.

Halliday, M.A.K. (1977). How children learn language. In K.D. Watson & R.D. Eagleson (Eds.), *English in secondary schools: Today and tomorrow* (pp. 20–37). Ashfield, N.S.W.: English Teachers Association for New South Wales.

Hancock, T.B., & Kaiser, A.P. (2006). Enhanced milieu teaching. In R. McCauley & M. Fey (Eds.), *Treatment of language disorders in children* (pp. 203–233). Baltimore, MD: Paul H. Brookes Publishing Co.

Hart, B. (1982). So that teachers can teach: Assigning roles and responsibilities. *Topics in Early Childhood Special Education, 2*(1), 1–8.

Hart, B., & Risley, T.R. (1975). Incidental teaching of language in the preschool. *Journal of Applied Behavior Analysis, 8,* 411–420.

Hart, B., & Risley, T.R. (1995). *Meaningful differences in the everyday experience of young American children.* Baltimore, MD: Paul H. Brookes Publishing Co.

Kaiser, A.P. (2000). Teaching functional communication skills. In M.E. Snell & F. Brown (Eds.), *Instruction of students with severe disabilities* (5th ed., pp. 453–491). Columbus, OH: Merrill.

Kaiser, A.P., & Hancock T.B. (2003). Teaching parents new skills to support their young children's development. *Infants and Young Children, 16*, 9–21.

Kaiser, A.P., Ostrosky, M.M., & Alpert, K. (1993). Training teachers to use environmental arrangement and milieu teaching with nonvocal preschool children. *Journal of the Association of Persons with Severe Handicaps, 18*, 188–199.

Krantz, P.L., & Risley, T.R. (1977). Behavior ecology in the classroom. In K.D. O'Leary & S. O'Leary (Eds.), *Classroom management: The successful use of behavior management* (pp. 60–82). Elmsford, NY: Pergamon.

Macy, M.G., & Bricker, D. (2007). Embedding individualized social goals into routine activities in inclusive early childhood classrooms. *Early Childhood Development and Care, 177*, 107–120.

McCormick, L., & Feeney, S. (1995). Modifying and expanding activities for children with disabilities. *Young Children, 50*(4), 10–17.

McWilliam, R.A. (2010). *Routines-based early intervention: Supporting young children and their families.* Baltimore, MD: Paul H. Brookes Publishing Co.

National Lekotek Center. (n.d.). http://www.lekotek.org

National Professional Development Center on Inclusion. (2011. *Research synthesis points on quality inclusive practices.* Chapel Hill, NC: The University of North Carolina, FPG Child Development Institute, Author.

Pretti-Frontczak, K., & Bricker, D.D. (2004). *An activity-based approach to early intervention* (3rd ed.). Baltimore, MD: Paul H. Brookes Publishing Co.

Rosegrant, T., & Bredekamp, S. (1992). Planning and implementing transformational curriculum. In S. Bredekamp & T. Rosegrant (Eds.), *Reaching potentials: Appropriate curriculum and assessment for young children: Vol. 1* (pp. 66–91). Washington, DC: National Association for the Education of Young Children.

Rubin, K.H., & Howe, H. (1985). Toys and play behavior: An overview. *Topics in Early Childhood Special Education, 5*(3), 1–9.

Sadao, K.C., & Robinson, N.B. (2010). *Assistive technology for young children.* Baltimore, MD: Paul H. Brooks Publishing Co.

Sandall, S.R., & Schwartz, I.S. (2008). *Building blocks for teaching preschoolers with special needs* (2nd ed.). Baltimore, MD: Paul H. Brookes Publishing Co.

Santos, R.M., (2001). Using what children know to teach them something new: Applying high-probability procedures in the classroom and at home. In M. Ostrosky & S.R. Sandall (Eds.), *Teaching strategies: What to do to support young children's development* (Young Exceptional Children Monograph Series No. 3, pp. 71–80). Arlington, VA: Council for Exceptional Children, Division for Early Childhood.

Sheldon, K. (1996). "Can I play too?" Adapting common classroom activities for children with limited motor abilities. *Early Childhood Education Journal, 11*, 115–120.

Wolery, M. (1994). Implementing instruction for young children with special needs in early childhood classrooms. In M. Wolery & J.S. Wilbers (Eds.), *Including children with special needs in early childhood programs* (pp. 151–166). Washington, DC: National Association for the Education of Young Children.

Wolery, M. (2001). Embedding constant time delay procedures in classroom activities. In M. Ostrosky & S. Sandall (Eds.), *Teaching strategies: What to do to support young children's development* (Young Exceptional Children Monograph Series No. 3, pp. 81–90). Arlington, VA: Council for Exceptional Children, Division for Early Childhood.

Wolery, M., Ault, M.J., & Doyle, P.M. (1992). *Teaching students with moderate to severe disabilities: Use of response prompting strategies.* New York, NY: Longman.

Wolery, M., & Hemmeter, M.L. (2011). Classroom instruction: Background, assumptions and challenges. *Journal of Early Intervention, 33*, 371–380.

Zirpoli, S.B. (1995). Designing environments for optimal behavior. In T. Zirpoli (Ed.), *Understanding and affecting the behavior of young children* (pp. 123–149). Englewood Cliffs, NJ: Merrill.

8

Designing Culturally Relevant Instruction

Mary Jo Noonan

••••••••••••••• **FOCUS OF THIS CHAPTER** •••••••••••••••••

- Culturally compatible education
- Seven standards for culturally diverse classrooms
- The instructional conversation model
- Stages in learning English as a second language
- Recommendations to support English language learners
- Strategies for culturally and linguistically responsive intervention

Given the increasing cultural and linguistic diversity of the United States, it is critical that early childhood professionals be knowledgeable about procedures and strategies that are effective in meeting the needs of children from diverse backgrounds (Sandall, Hemmeter, Smith, & McLean, 2005). Some children and families of culturally and linguistically diverse backgrounds are Americans from sociocultural minority backgrounds (e.g., African Americans, Chinese Americans, Appalachians, Navajos). Others are relatively new to the United States and the American culture. Language experiences of children from culturally diverse families will vary from Standard American English to an English dialect or Creole; from bilingualism (or multilingualism) to little or no English. Proficiency in their home language, as well as in English, may be severely limited.

Culture has been defined as "shared ways of being, knowing, and doing" (Kana'iaupuni & Kawai'ae'a, 2008, p. 71). From an instructional point of view, the purpose of recognizing culture and its dynamics is to provide a basis for designing effective educational arrangements and practices. Addressing cultural considerations does not imply stereotyping. Instead, knowing a child's culture may offer insight into the norms or standards that influence behavior and thinking (Goodenough, 1981), and in turn, this information can be integrated into instruction to facilitate learning (Rueda & Stillman, 2012). Part of this insight involves identifying students' cultural knowledge, prior experiences, and performance styles that, if honored, will increase the effectiveness of instruction (Gay, 2010).

Cultural and linguistic variables must be addressed to provide an optimal educational experience; they are an inextricable part of learning, affecting all daily experiences and communications (Singh, 2011). Although it is nearly impossible to sort the effects of universally effective teaching practices from those of cultural accommodations, it is likely that both contribute to student learning (Goldenberg, 2004). Chapter 2 provides an introduction to cultural values from the fields of parenting and professional collaboration. This chapter focuses on how cultural differences—when a child's home culture and/or language are different from those of their school or early intervention services—impact environmental arrangements and instruction.

CULTURALLY COMPATIBLE EDUCATION

Children come to early childhood settings with social, communication, and behavioral competencies learned from experiences with their families and home communities. These experiences establish the expectation that behavior that was effective and acceptable for them in the past should be effective and acceptable in the present and future (Rogoff, 2003). A cultural mismatch occurs when the child's expectations are not realized in the early childhood setting. *Culturally compatible education* is an instructional approach characterized by modifications to the social, communication, and behavioral expectations of a learning environment to mirror the expectations of a child's home and community environment (Jordan & Tharp, 1979; Tharp & Dalton, 2007). The intent is to establish an educational environment that is familiar and consistent with children's competencies and expectations, thereby increasing participation and improving learning (Singh, 2011).

SEVEN STANDARDS FOR CULTURALLY DIVERSE CLASSROOMS

As early childhood programs become increasingly more culturally diverse (rather than characterized by a single cultural group), the goal of providing culturally compatible education becomes more challenging. To address this growing need, Tharp and Dalton (Tharp, 1997; Tharp & Dalton, 2007) studied and analyzed similarities associated with educational success across cultures. Merging earlier research on cultural differences in learning with cross-national research, they proposed that effective instruction for culturally diverse learners should address five standards. Recently, the standards were explored as they applied to early childhood programs (Wyatt, 2009; Yamauchi, Im, & Schonleber, 2012). These studies led to adaptations to the original five standards and added two standards. These are the seven standards for effective instruction with culturally diverse young children:

Standard 1: Teachers and students producing together (joint productive activity)
Facilitate learning through joint productive activity between teacher and students.

Standard 2: Developing language and literacy across the curriculum
Develop competence in the language(s) of instruction and of the disciplines throughout the day.

Standard 3: Making meaning—connecting school to students' lives (contextualization)
Embed curricular instruction in the interests, experiences, and skills of students' families and communities.

Standard 4: Teaching complex thinking
Challenge students toward cognitive complexity.

Standard 5: Teaching through instructional conversation (IC)
Engage students through dialogue.

Standard 6: Modeling
Promote children's observational learning.

Standard 7: Child- (student-) directed activity
Encourage learner decision making.

Applying the Standards

Standard 1: Teachers and students producing together (joint productive activity): Facilitate learning through joint productive activity between teacher and students. Requiring children to work jointly means that children participate in groups (small or large) in a single activity or create a single product. In contrast to many early childhood classrooms in which teachers prepare activities and learning centers in advance and monitor as children participate, joint productive activity requires that teachers join in as participants. The learning centers structure that characterizes many early childhood programs is easily adjusted to this standard when center activities are designed to require student collaboration toward a single product. As teachers and classroom staff monitor the children, they must also enter the activities and become collaborators (not group leaders) among the children. The teacher, for example, may enter a science learning center activity and collaborate in creating a "tornado bottle" (a water-filled bottle taped top-to-top with an identical empty bottle), or she may enter the home-living center, dress up, and play the role of a child in the family activity. Becoming a joint participant in the group allows the teacher to model participation in the activity, to assist children in learning to collaborate, and to be present as a communication partner for the children.

Standard 2: Developing language and literacy across the curriculum: Develop competence in the language(s) of instruction and of the disciplines throughout the day. Fitting well with the early learning standards/core standards (discussed in Chapter 4), the focus of the literacy standard is to embed literacy development—beginning with language development—throughout the entire early childhood curriculum, including self-management and social skill areas. Teachers are responsive to children's communication (verbal and nonverbal) by listening and observing intently and responding in ways that promote communication development (modeling, questioning, expanding; see enhanced milieu teaching in Chapter 7). Responsiveness is also evident when teachers respect children's interaction style, including their eye-contact, wait time (time between conversational turns), and comfort with spotlighting (calling attention to a single child with praise or a question rather than addressing the group). Early literacy development can be supported by activities that build new vocabulary, such as labeling items in the classroom, preteaching words associated with books and curricular activities, and modeling the use of new terms as they apply to familiar routines and activities. The literacy standard is also addressed by creating a classroom that is rich in literacy activities (speaking, listening, reading, and writing), allowing children to interact frequently with one another and classroom staff, and encouraging children's use of their first and second languages during instruction. Referring back to the joint productive activity example of making a tornado bottle in a new learning center, it can be introduced to the children during a large morning group activity. As the teacher describes the activity, he or she can highlight new vocabulary (*tornado, centripetal, liquid,* and *vortex*) by presenting word cards and raising questions with the children as he or she discusses each term. If the children start calling out answers and commenting as others are talking, the teacher respects the conversational style and restates or elaborates key ideas expressed by the children. The teacher groups the children for a short discussion of their own experiences with a tornado or stormy weather. He or she groups four children together who speak Vietnamese as their first language so that they may discuss their experiences in Vietnamese if they choose.

Standard 3: Making meaning—connecting school to students' lives (contextualization): Embed curricular instruction in the interests, experiences, and skills of students' families and communities. As illustrated above in the example of children discussing their experiences with a tornado or stormy weather, connecting the science activity to children's lives engages them in the activity. Evidence of engagement and making meaning out of the instruction is the children's descriptions of what the threatening weather looked like, what their families did when the warning sirens sounded, and how they felt during the storm. Contextualizing instruction creates a meaningful experience by linking new knowledge and skills with children's existing knowledge and skills. In addressing this standard, teachers learn about their students' homes and communities and provide opportunities for community-based learning (visiting the neighborhood library, helping out in a community garden). Parents are welcomed into the classroom to help build the home-school connection.

Standard 4: Teaching complex thinking: Challenge students toward cognitive complexity (CC). Too often, teachers of young children from culturally diverse backgrounds do not hold high expectations for the children. It is critically important that all children be provided with challenging instruction to motivate their learning and to teach complex thinking skills. Tharp (2006) operationalizes this standard by defining the concept of "challenging activities" in four ways:

1. Children are taught the *why*, not merely the *what* or the *how to*. In the tornado activity described above, the why is a bit of the physics behind the tornado. Even 3- and 4-year-olds can be introduced to the concepts of vortex and centripetal force, which explain the why of the tornado. This goes far beyond simply telling children what materials they need for an activity or how to put the materials together. Introducing cognitively complex concepts early can help children understand the concepts at greater depth in later grades when they encounter the topics (or related topics) again.

2. Children must not just acquire knowledge, they must use, apply, or generate new knowledge. Terms like *analyze, categorize, explore,* and *make judgments* are just a few of the characteristics associated with this type of cognitive complexity. Children engaged in the tornado activity can explore the properties of the minitornado by conducting experiments and reporting their findings.

3. Rather than relying on children to connect new information to existing information, teachers should illustrate connections to broader concepts or abstract ideas. The strength of centripetal force can be related to the concept of energy in all matter, for example.

4. Complex cognitive strategies, such as critical thinking, problem solving, or metacognitive strategies are taught. Again, teachers facilitate critical thinking by actively teaching such skills rather than hoping that the children acquire them. Critical thinking skills with the tornado activity, for example, could involve predicting what might happen with various types of water movements.

Standard 5: Teaching through instructional conversation: Engage students through dialogue. Questioning and sharing information and ideas through conversational dialogue develops basic thinking skills. In contrast to the more prevalent approach to instruction in which teachers provide information and assess the extent to which students can repeat or apply it, an instructional conversation model assumes that students can contribute knowledge, values, or experiences (students' cultures) to the learning activity (Vygotsky, 1978). Teachers listen to students and observe them carefully, assist them in expressing themselves (verbally and nonverbally), and then relate the instruction to the students' experiences and knowledge base. This approach contextualizes and individualizes learning and is discussed in more depth later in the chapter.

Standard 6: Modeling: Promote children's observational learning. To implement the modeling standard, the teacher must either present a completed sample of a product and/or demonstrate behaviors, thinking processes, or procedures that the children then practice. Continuing with the example of making the tornado bottle, the teacher demonstrates step-by-step how to construct the tornado bottle while verbally stating the key words of each step. In many early childhood activities, showing the children a completed model is counter to the value of honoring children's creativity, but might be used for inspiration (Yamauchi et al., 2012).

Standard 7: Child- (student-) directed activity: Encourage learner decision making. Child-directed activities are one of the hallmarks of developmentally appropriate practice. In child-directed activities, children make choices within assigned activities (choosing what color to dye the water for their tornado water) or choose among available activities (tornado bottle activity or bug activity in the science center). At more exemplary levels, child-directed activities include children generating their own ideas and constructions within an activity (suggesting adding glitter to the water in their tornado bottle) and generating their own topics and/or activities.

THE INSTRUCTIONAL CONVERSATION MODEL

Standard 5, teaching through instructional conversation (IC), is the central component of culturally compatible education and is an empirically tested model (Tharp, 1989; Tharp, 1997; Tharp & Dalton, 2007; Tharp & Gallimore, 1988; Tharp & Yamauchi, 1994). The IC model modifies the learning environment to address four cultural factors: 1) sociolinguistics, 2) cognition, 3) motivation, and 4) social organization.

Sociolinguistics

Sociolinguistics refers to the conventions or rules of conversational style. Studies have shown that when particular sociolinguistics of the classrooms are modified to more closely match those of children's home environments, student participation and learning improve (Kana'iaupuni, Ledward, & Jensen, 2010; Tharp & Dalton, 2007). Sociolinguistic variables that have been modified are wait time, discourse structures, and speech volume and eye gaze.

The time provided for individuals to speak and respond is known as *wait time* (Rowe, 1974). For a number of Native American Indian cultures, student participation is greater if wait time is extended (Greenbaum, 1983; Ingalls & Hammond, 2011; McCarthy & Benally, 2003; Phillips, 1983; Winterton, 1976). In contrast, children who are Native Hawaiians participate more in school when classroom discussions allow for negative wait times; that is, when children speak while someone else is speaking (*overlapping speech*) rather than waiting for the speaker to finish speaking (White & Tharp, 1988). To promote participation in an early childhood "circle time" with children of Hawaiian ancestry, for example, teachers should encourage children to speak out and overlap their responses with others as they would do in a conversation with family members at home. This is in contrast to giving children turns or requiring them to raise their hands and wait to be called on.

The second sociolinguistic variable, *discourse structures*, refers to verbal interactions during instruction. These include presentation of materials, voice inflections, and body movements. They occur somewhat rhythmically and may be established by the teacher or children (Tharp & Yamauchi, 1994). For example, a call-and-response rhythm characterizes the interactions of African American children and adults (Foster, 1998; Hale-Benson, 1986). This tempo and participation structure, similar to a negative wait time, is a form of active listening in which the listener calls out and verbally responds to the speaker. Its pace has been likened to a contest or rhythmical back and forth volley between speaker and listener (Hale-Benson, 1990). Esmailka and Barnhardt (1981) conducted a study of Athabascan Native American teachers in Alaska and their Athabascan students in a school in which the students were performing at or above national norms on standard measures of school success. They observed that the students set the rhythm during instruction and the teachers entered the activity later, following the tempo set by the students. These participation structures are in striking contrast to a *switchboard* structure that characterizes traditional Western classrooms in which the teacher regulates who speaks and when he or she speaks (Philips, 1976, 1983). In both examples described above, it appears that providing children with familiar participation structures seems to promote engagement. A number of varied participation structures have been identified across Native American groups (Erickson & Mohatt, 1982; Greenbaum, 1983; Ingalls & Hammond, 2011; McCarthy & Benally, 2003; Philips, 1976, 1983), African Americans (Hale-Benson, 1986, 1990), Latinos (Goldenberg & Gallimore, 1991), and Hawaiians (Au, 1980; Au & Mason, 1981).

In an early childhood setting, for example, a teacher should first watch children interacting in small groups, taking note of the rhythm of the children's activity and interactions to support their participation through discourse structures. Do the children take turns or work concurrently? Do they watch one another or work more independently? Does one child seem to direct the group? Does the pace of the activity or conversation seem slow or fast? As a group, are they quiet or talkative? When does a child initiate or enter a conversation? For how long does a child speak? What seems to cue a child to stop speaking? After careful observation of the groups, the teacher may enter the group, carefully following the existing rhythm of participation, pacing him- or herself to match the tempo of the group, adhering to apparent conversational rules (e.g., the group may allow children to speak for as long as they wish), and allowing the children to direct their activity as they were doing before he or she joined their group.

Speech volume is another sociolinguistic variable that differs across cultures and may affect children's participation in educational/intervention settings. Voice level ranges from soft to loud. Native Americans tend to speak at a soft volume (Darnell, 1979; Key, 1975). Because of their quiet tone, teachers who are not Native American may believe that the children are sullen or lack interest. And if non–Native American teachers speak in loud voices, the Native American children may judge their teachers to be mean.

The fourth and final sociolinguistic variable in the IC model is *eye contact*. As a sign of politeness and respect, children from African American and many

Native American cultures avoid or do not sustain eye contact with teachers. However, this may be perceived as rude or noncompliant by adults of other cultures (Darnell, 1979; Greenbaum, 1983; Johnson, 1971). To promote children's participation in early childhood settings, teachers should accept speech volume and eye-gaze patterns from children's home cultures. Teachers can identify family expectations for these behaviors by observing the children interact with their parents and other familiar adults or discussing the expectations with individuals who are knowledgeable about the practices of the pertinent culture.

Cognition

The second component of the IC model, *cognition*, refers to the thinking, problem-solving, and learning processes. Cross-cultural research suggests that culture has a significant influence on individuals' preference for instructional approaches and the conditions under which instruction is most effective (Joy & Kolb, 2009; Winzer & Mazurek, 1998). This component is sometimes referred to as *learning style* (Hilliard, 1989). Providing children with instructional situations that match their learning styles will increase their comfort level and understanding and thereby facilitate their participation. Cognitive or learning style variables that appear frequently in the literature include verbal thinking versus visual thinking, field dependence versus field independence, cognitive tempo, and cooperation versus competition (Joy & Kolb, 2009).

The dominant educational model in North America relies heavily on *verbal thinking* rather than *visual thinking* (Tharp, 1989; Tharp & Gallimore, 1988). In a verbal learning style, children are expected to learn information presented sequentially through oral explanations and written assignments. In contrast, the visual style presents learners with a context (perhaps a story) for linking the new information with previously acquired knowledge and experience. The actual presentation of new content may also include visual examples and opportunities for observation and participation. Cultures that tend to be characterized by verbal thinking include Euro-Americans, Japanese Americans, and Chinese Americans, and cultures that tend to prefer a visual learning style include Native Americans and Native Hawaiians. Other preferred learning modalities may include the kinesthetic (movement), tactile (touch), and multiple modalities (Shade, 1994; Shade, Kelly, & Oberg, 1997). In early childhood settings, verbal and visual thinking styles can be supported by presenting instructions, cues, and materials in both formats. For example, use charts with simple pictures to accompany verbal instructions, use visual activity schedules (a series of simple line drawings depicting each of the day's activities) concurrent with teacher directions to transition to the next activity, and provide audio-recorded instructional reminders to support paper and pencil or art activities.

Closely associated with the verbal versus visual thinking style is a cognitive style for processing information referred to as *field-dependent* or field-sensitive (Ramirez & Castenada, 1974) and *field-independent* (Witkin, Moore, Goodenough, & Cox, 1977). According to Witkin et al., learners who are field-dependent prefer a holistic style of instruction similar to the visual style presented above. They tend to be passive in receiving information, group-oriented, cooperative, and socially motivated. The field-dependent style is characteristic of collectivist cultures (the group is more valued than the individual) such as African Americans (Shade et al., 1997) and Mexican Americans (Ramirez & Castenada, 1974). Children who have a field-dependent learning style are sensitive to others' judgments and prefer close personal relationships (Correa & Tulbert, 1991). In contrast, children who have a field-independent style of learning are more likely to be from individualist cultures (the individual is more valued than the group), such as Euro-Americans and Asians (Shade et al., 1997). In general, these children prefer analytic, competitive, task-oriented, and experiential learning activities. They appear to be self-motivated and prefer to work independently. They are not strongly affected by others' judgments and favor formal relationships with teachers (Correa & Tulbert, 1991). Their learning style is similar to the verbal learning style described above. In an early childhood setting, for example, a reading comprehension activity for field-dependent learners might be a cooperative learning group in which small groups of children create a scene with building blocks depicting an event of the story. This would be in contrast to a field-independent activity in which the teacher asks the group questions about the story, expecting the children to raise their hands and respond individually.

Cognitive tempo refers to the tendency to be primarily impulsive or primarily reflective. The degree of impulsivity or reflectiveness is judged by the extent to which alternatives are considered when more than one solution is possible. When children are impulsive they tend to act quickly and without a course of action, make many errors, and have poor attention. On the other hand, reflective children respond more slowly, carefully, and systematically. They are persistent in their work, hold high standards for themselves, and make few errors. An impulsive learning style has been linked to reading and problem-solving difficulties (Epstein, Hallahan, & Kauffman, 1975). Some differences across ethnic groups have been reported for performance and cognitive tempo. Ayabe and Santos (1972) found that American second graders of Japanese and Chinese ancestry could perform at a fast tempo with significantly fewer errors than their Hawaiian, Filipino American, and Samoan American peers. Another study of young Asian Americans and Pacific Islander Americans indicated that cognitive tempo did relate to ethnicity (Kitano, 1983). Ordered according to the degree of reflectiveness, Chinese American children were the most reflective, followed by Hawaiians, Japanese Americans, Korean Americans, and Filipino Americans. Some gender differences were also noted: Chinese American boys were more reflective than the girls, and Japanese American and Hawaiian girls were more reflective than the boys in their respective ethnic groups. Recent research on cognitive tempo has explored the possibility of generational differences in cognitive tempo, hypothesizing that the current digital age of fast-moving images may contribute to more impulsive learning styles (Kenny, 2009).

In an early childhood setting, children with impulsive learning styles will be most successful working independently if tasks are simple. For more complex tasks, however, children with impulsive learning styles should be guided in strategies for analyzing and problem solving. For example, if 3-year-olds with an impulsive learning style are presented with a pouring task at a learning center, most will be able to participate independently following a single demonstration. For a learning center task of tanagrams (matching geometric blocks to a pattern), however, the children will be more successful if they are guided through a specific strategy for fitting the blocks to the pattern. The guidance should be repeated many times until the children can demonstrate the strategy independently.

Competitive classroom structures tend to be the norm in American schools. Children are encouraged and rewarded for high achievement, particularly when it is accomplished independently (Winzer & Mazurek, 1998). This style of schooling fits with capitalism and Euro-American values. Some cultures, however, value cooperation, sharing, and contribution to the group over competition, independence, and individual achievement. Children whose families place priority on cooperation and group efforts may be unwilling to compete, may look to peers for assistance, and may avoid excelling at tasks because they are reluctant to be singled out (spotlighted) and commended for their work. If educators are unaware of how a cultural value of cooperation may be affecting children's performance, they may incorrectly assume that some children are lazy, unmotivated, or of low ability (Grossman, 1995; Winzer & Mazurek, 1998). Furthermore, a competitive instructional setting does not optimize the educational achievement of children who are cooperatively oriented (Widaman & Kagan, 1987). Consistent with supporting children with a field-dependent learning style, cooperative learning groups are beneficial to children from cultures that place a high value on group contributions and collaboration. In the early childhood setting, a social skills lesson about "our neighborhood" could involve an outing exploring the community around the school. This is followed by a group activity in which children assemble a felt board picture representing what they learned about their neighborhood. The teacher facilitates conversation about the experience by questioning the children as they assemble their felt-board pictures. This would be in contrast to a more traditional approach in which the teacher stands in front of the group, describes the concept of neighborhood, and questions the children in a didactic format.

Motivation

The general attitude of a child toward learning has been referred to as *trait motivation*, whereas the child's desire to learn during a specific task is known as *state motivation* (Christophel, 1990). The distinction may be meaningful because culture can affect both differentially. For example, children who feel oppressed by the dominant Euro-American culture may approach their school experience with distrust and expectations for failure (Banks & Banks, 2009). Ogbu (1991) believes this is sometimes true for involuntary minorities (groups that did not become Americans by choice) such as Native Americans and African Americans. Tharp (1989) and Tharp and Gallimore (1988), however, have not found these characteristics in the Native American children they've studied. Nevertheless, being aware that some children may come to school mistrusting the education system and expecting failure highlights the importance of developing positive relationships with students and providing curricular supports that ensure success.

Trait motivation has also been shown to have positive effects on educational outcomes for children of culturally diverse backgrounds, including some who have experienced high degrees of linguistic barriers, prejudice, and teasing.

This has been the experience of recent Hmong, Vietnamese, and Korean immigrant children whose success has been attributed to trait motivation (Hirayama, 1985). These children approached schooling with strong parental, community, and cultural support for success.

State motivation, the drive to succeed at a specific task, has been shown to directly affect school participation and achievement of Hawaiian children and children from some Native American cultures (Tharp & Yamauchi, 1994). Classroom variables that seem to affect state motivation include relevance and interest level of materials, contingent reinforcement and punishment, and teacher-student relationships. For example, in one study Native American children in first through third grades told stories to their teachers, who transcribed them. The transcribed stories served as reading texts for the children. In a one-year posttest, the children using their transcribed stories as texts made greater oral language gains than the children in a control group. Parents also reported that more language-related activities occurred in the home because of the culturally relevant materials (Butterfield, 1983). Studies of verbal praise and punishment indicate that Hawaiian children participate more when clearly articulated school-based incentives are used (D'Amato, 1981). In contrast, Navajo children participate more in school when overt reinforcement and punishment are omitted. They engage more in educational activities when adults give them autonomy in their learning and allow them to take responsibility for organizing and completing their assigned work (Jordan, Tharp, & Vogt, 1985).

Social Organization

The fourth and final element of ICs, social organization, refers to the ways in which schools, classrooms, and teaching are structured. The traditional American classroom is teacher directed and relies primarily on whole class instruction and demonstration, followed by individual practice and testing. For some children of minority cultures, this social structure is associated with low attention to academic work and to the teacher, and greater attention to peers, often causing disruptions (Gallimore, Boggs, & Jordan, 1974). Instead, these children participate and learn more in classrooms organized around small-group instruction and cooperation that allow for peer interaction and support. The effectiveness of small-group social organization over the more traditional teacher-directed, individualized, and competitive classroom has been demonstrated for children who are Native Hawaiian (Tharp, 1989), Native American (Ingalls & Hammond, 2011; Leith & Slentz, 1984; Lipka, 1990; Philips, 1976), African American (Slavin, DeVies, & Edwards, 1983), and Mexican American (Castenada, 1976).

The IC model for teaching children of diverse cultural backgrounds provides an engaging learning environment that maximizes children's participation. Table 8.1 summarizes the IC variables, components of each, and recommendations for inclusive early childhood settings. Instruction is built around instructional exchanges that are sensitive to *sociolinguistic* variables, such as wait time and participation structures. *Cognition* variables are addressed by allowing children to use their preferred learning styles. Many children of culturally diverse backgrounds learn better visually than verbally. Content taught

Table 8.1. Instructional conversation model characteristics

Variable	Examples of components	Recommendations for promoting children's participation and learning
Sociolinguistics	Wait time	Observe groups of children and notice the wait time (time between conversational turns) during their interactions. Adhere to this observed wait time in classroom interactions. (Note that some wait times may be negative and characterized by overlapping speech.)
	Discourse structures	Observe groups of children and notice the tempo and style of the interactions (highly active, calling out, reserved, slowly taking turns, and so forth). Enter the group, taking care to follow the preestablished tempo. In didactic instruction, mirror the tempo observed in the children's groups and/or allow the children to set the rhythm of instruction.
	Speech volume and eye gaze	Accept the children's speech volume and eye gaze. Recognize that if a child's speech volume or eye gaze differs from your expectations, it may be a cultural variable rather than a sign of disrespect.
Cognition (learning style)	Verbal versus visual thinking (and other learning modalities)	Use visual and tactile prompts and materials to support verbal instruction. Notice if the children are moving a great deal while engaged in learning activities. If so, allow the movement if they remain on task.
	Field dependent versus field independent	Provide complete demonstrations or samples of tasks and activities, as well as step-by-step instructions. Teach in meaningful contexts (e.g., teach games on a playground or in the home setting in which they are likely to occur naturally). Schedule group work as well as individual work and notice which tends to be the more effective instructional arrangement. (When are children most successful?) Use the more effective instructional arrangement for most instruction.
	Cognitive tempo	Provide extra guidance and assistance for complex tasks to the children who appear to have an impulsive learning style. Teach the children methodical and systematic approaches (learning strategies) to use when confronted with complex tasks.
	Cooperation versus competition	Use group instruction and cooperative learning groups for children from cultures that are group oriented rather than individualistic and competitive. Provide group incentives and group rewards rather than individual ones. If calling on children to respond during an activity, allow peers to assist in a child's response.
Motivation	Trait motivation	Recognize that some children may not trust the educational system and may expect to fail. Provide a nurturing and accepting environment, rewarding the children for participating and attempting tasks. When instructional corrections are necessary, provide them privately and in a positive, constructive manner.
	State motivation	Become familiar with the cultures of the children you teach. Use materials and activities familiar to them (e.g., children's own stories, community settings, and events) as the context for instruction. Show caring and concern to the children to build rapport and a personal relationship. Provide immediate feedback for correct responding.

Variable	Examples of components	Recommendations for promoting children's participation and learning
Social organization	Small-group versus whole-group instruction	Use predominantly small-group instruction and cooperative learning groups for children from cultures that are group oriented.
	Teacher-directed versus child-directed activities	During small-group instruction, allow the children to follow their interests and direct the group.
	Peer-peer interaction versus peer-teacher interaction	For children from cultures that are group oriented, allow for extensive peer interaction (children helping one another and working collaboratively).

in the IC model is culturally relevant to enhance *motivation*. Furthermore, teachers are sensitive to how children respond to direct and structured behavioral consequences, realizing that some children learn well this way, while others learn better with a fair degree of autonomy. And finally, the overall *social organization* of the learning situation is dominated by small-group instruction and peer interaction.

Tharp refers to the standards as *universally potent features* of effective teaching for diverse children. As potent features, the practices have a great likelihood of engaging diverse learners (culturally heterogeneous groups of children) in their education and producing positive learning outcomes. Since these standards were proposed in the early 1990s, they have been validated through more than 40 studies (Tharp & Dalton, 2007), including studies involving preschool children (Tharp & Entz, 2003; Wyatt, 2009; Yamauchi et al., 2012).

STAGES IN LEARNING ENGLISH AS A SECOND LANGUAGE

Children of culturally diverse backgrounds may also be children who did not learn English as their first language. If they are not yet attending school, they may be totally immersed in their family's native language and have little exposure to English. Others who attend early intervention settings, child care, preschool, or school programs may be in the process of acquiring English as a second language (ESL). In either situation, these children, known as English language learners (ELLs), have unique needs associated with their cultural and linguistic diversity that must be addressed in providing effective education.

Salend (2001) proposed that school-age children progress through six stages in ESL learning:

1. *Preproduction or silent period:* Initially, children are quiet and focus on comprehension. They rely on contextual and other clues (e.g., peer modeling) to derive meaning and to express themselves nonverbally. Nonverbal response modes are an appropriate expectation during this phase.

2. *Telegraphic or early production period:* When children acquiring a second language begin speaking, they do so with short two- and three-word

sentences. It is apparent that their comprehension is limited. Simple language activities, such as naming and responding to easy questions, may be helpful.

3. *Interlanguage and intermediate fluency period:* Longer phrases and complex sentences emerge during this period, sometimes mixing first and second languages. This is an appropriate time to focus on vocabulary development and encourage children to test their expanding abilities with their new language.

4. *Extension and expansion period:* Comprehension has clearly improved and children produce complex sentences during this period. Specific instruction in grammar and vocabulary is helpful.

5. *Enrichment period:* In this period, children can benefit from learning strategies to help them with specific language needs (e.g., a particular rule of grammar).

6. *Independent learning period:* Children can participate and learn effectively across a range of instructional activities and in heterogeneous peer groups.

Although the six stages of second language learning proposed by Salend were formulated with reference to school-age children, in all likelihood younger children follow the same progression once they are exposed to a second language for extended periods of time (e.g., when they enter a center-based or school-based program). Being familiar with these stages of second language learning will help professionals understand and set appropriate expectations for children learning English. A professional familiar with these stages, for instance, will not assume that a toddler—a recent immigrant to the United States and an ELL—who has never spoken in a playgroup conducted in English is delayed in language development without first observing the child in his home in which his native language is spoken. Instead, the professional will recognize that it is common for ELLs to go through the *preproduction or silent* stage. Second language learning expectations for young children and those with language delays or differences need to reflect children's current level of language development in their native language. For example, if a child has not yet begun to use single words or point to pictures to label objects in his or her native language, labeling objects with English words would probably not be an appropriate expectation.

RECOMMENDATIONS TO SUPPORT ENGLISH LANGUAGE LEARNERS

The IC model has been evaluated extensively with ELL children and found to be highly effective in promoting early literacy skills. In a review of 73 studies of ELLs, the U.S. Department of Education What Works Clearinghouse ranked the IC Model as the most effective intervention approach for improving reading skills and as the second most effective approach for increasing English literacy skills (Institute of Educational Sciences, 2006). Note that literacy skills are generally taught concurrently with English language skills while children are acquiring the language. Early childhood services for young children who are ELLs should address the five standards for diverse learners discussed at the beginning of this chapter (Tharp, 1997; Tharp & Entz, 2003), with the IC model embedded throughout all activities (Yamauchi et al., 2012).

Professionals should assume that all children, even those with communication delays and/or cognitive disabilities, can learn a second language to the same extent that they have acquired a first language; there is no evidence to the contrary (Barrera, 1993). In addition to implementing the IC model, there are six approaches to instruction that are helpful to young children in acquiring ESL (Barrera, 1993; Bunce, 2003; Laturnau, 2001; Salend & Salinas, 2003): 1) capitalize on *all* communication skills, 2) focus on content, 3) teach in context, 4) provide relaxed environments and comprehensible input, 5) use cooperative learning methods, and 6) teach coping strategies.

Capitalize on All Communication Skills

In providing services to young children with special needs who do not have English as their first language, a primary concern is that they have an effective way to communicate. Effective communication allows children to understand their experiences and the expectations of others, to have their needs met, and to continue developing their communication skills. Remember that all communication is not verbal: Prelinguistic and nonverbal communication skills must also be supported. To support children's present communication skills and concurrently address their academic goals, instruction should continue in their native language (including the use of academic materials in the native language) if possible. For infants and young children who are not in school, this may mean that a family member or friend who is fluent in the child's native language plays a central role in the delivery of early intervention services if the teacher does not speak the native language. When children who are ELLs begin school, they may receive bilingual instruction so that their communication, language arts, and other academic skills may be addressed concurrently. If instruction in a child's native language is not possible, verbal communication should be supplemented with visual cues, gestures, facial expressions, modeling, and other concrete prompts to assist the child in understanding.

Focus on Content

While teaching and interacting with children who are ELLs, teachers and others should respond to the *intent or meaning* of a child's communication rather than the form or grammar. In other words, children's grammar should not be corrected, but rather the adult should respond appropriately to the child's message. (If the child requests "me wants up," pick him or her up rather than correct her grammar!) Responding to a child's communicative intent will foster a climate that welcomes and encourages communication; frequently correcting a child's communication or requiring more sophisticated use of grammar may inadvertently punish attempts to use the new language. Responding to meaning rather than form is based on observations of how parents naturally facilitate language acquisition with typically developing children and is the same strategy recommended for children who are delayed in learning language (but are not ELLs).

Teach in Context

Although a primary recommendation is to focus on the content of a child's communication, this does not imply that English is not taught. English is taught in context—that is, in the course of a child's typical schedule of activities—when the vocabulary and communication are needed. Teaching in context not only provides natural reinforcers for communication, it links communication to meaningful events. For example, in preparation for lunch during preschool, teachers can emphasize key vocabulary and sing self-help and mealtime songs ("This is the way we wash our hands, wash our hands, wash our hands"). Repeating words and phrases about hand washing while actually doing it is more meaningful than taking a child aside and asking him to imitate the words or phrases associated with picture cards. Songs are an effective instructional approach because they generally include repetition: Repetition helps to teach children the rhythm, pitch, volume, and tone of their new language.

During the course of daily activities in the home, child care center, or school, the naturalistic language teaching strategies of *expansion* and *elaboration* should be implemented (see also Chapter 7). An adult expands on a child's utterance by repeating a slightly lengthier version of what the child says. For example, if the child is building with blocks and says, "Block fall," the adult can reply with an expansion, "The block fell down." An elaboration also expands on what the child says, but differs from an expansion because it adds more information: "The red blocks fell and made a loud noise!"

Other strategies for teaching language in context include 1) teaching literacy through whole language, 2) using focused contrasts to illustrate grammatical forms, and 3) recording instructions on audiotape. The first strategy, whole language, is *teaching in context*. Rather than (or in addition to) an instructional time designated for literacy activities, literacy instruction is embedded throughout the day in various subjects and activities. In a child care setting, familiarizing children with books may occur as part of creative movement and cooking activities (rather than only during reading time). And in a kindergarten class, learning phonetic sounds can be embedded in community walks that are a part of social studies (identifying initial sounds as objects are named during the walk), calendar time during morning circle (identifying initial sounds of the days of the week, the weather, and so forth), and art activities (identifying initial sounds of shapes and colors). Conducting prereading, reading, and other language arts in a variety of activities takes advantage of natural teaching opportunities and maintains an emphasis on language learning throughout the day. *Focused contrasts*, the second strategy for teaching in context, are comments made by an adult to illustrate two closely related grammatical forms. Bunce (2003, p. 393) provided the following focused contrast example of what an adult might say as a child is playing with dolls: "The mommy *is* walk*ing* to the house. Look! She walk*ed* in." Frequent experience with the two closely related grammatical forms will help the child understand the differences in meaning. And *recording instructions on audio devices*, the third strategy for teaching in context, may help a child improve receptive language skills by giving her the opportunity to review instructions for an activity as many times as she feels is necessary to understand them.

Provide Relaxed Environments and Comprehensible Input

Comprehensible input means that the child is provided with communication that is understandable given his or her present language abilities (Krashen, 1982; Krashen & Terrell, 1983). A relaxed environment is usually one with comprehensible input and a situation in which the child feels free to use his or her developing language skills (adults accept all communication attempts and respond to meaning). In the early stages of second language learning, the goal is to help the child learn the new language; later the goal will be for the child to use the new language to obtain new knowledge or skills.

The distinction between learning a new language and using a language to learn refers to two kinds of language proficiency: basic interpersonal communicative skills (BICS) and cognitive/academic language proficiency (CALP) (Cummins, 1984). Daily conversation is associated with BICS. It takes place in context-embedded situations that are rich in paralinguistic and situational cues. In contrast, CALP is associated with more decontextualized academic situations. One cannot assume that a child's BICS and CALP are equivalent. In other words, for a child who is learning ESL, it cannot be assumed that because she uses English well in oral conversation that she has adequate proficiency for learning academics in English (Bunce, 2003). While focused on decoding and learning a language, a child cannot also be expected to learn *through* that language—the processes are too different (Westby, 1985).

For many young children who are ELLs and receiving early childhood special education, the emphasis on second language learning will be focused on BICS. As these children acquire the basic communication skills in English, it is critical that they be provided with a relaxed environment and comprehensible (meaningful) input. The following are recommendations for providing comprehensible input:

- *Adjust speech:* Speak in simple, short sentences using vocabulary in the child's repertoire. Simple sentences are those with a straightforward grammatical structure, such as subject-verb ("Anisa eats"), verb-object ("Bring cup"), and subject-verb-object ("Dog has your shoe!"). In simplifying sentences, avoid using idioms, slang words or phrases, and pronouns.

- *Provide descriptions:* Talk about what the child is doing or observing while the activity is in progress. ("You found the teddy bear card. You matched the cards. You have another turn.") Providing descriptions of ongoing events links language to context. Because the intent is to provide meaningful input in a relaxed situation rather than to elicit conversation, use comments rather than questions.

- *Use concrete and contextual cues:* Concrete cues are prompts that are clear and obvious, rather than subtle or abstract. Examples include visuals (pictures, charts), modeling, gestures, facial expressions, voice changes, and pantomimes. Contextual cues are prompts provided in a specific place or time to take advantage of additional information in the environment. Placing a picture on a classroom cubby of a child holding her lunch bag and sweater is an example of a concrete cue indicating where the child should place her sweater and lunch bag. It is also a contextual cue because the picture is placed on the cubby, providing additional information about the place where her belongings are to be stored. Placing the cubbies close to the classroom door would be an additional contextual clue because the children would be likely to see them the moment they walk into the classroom.

- *Use familiar and holistic experiences:* Familiar experiences may assist a child in comprehending language because the materials, setting, and expectations are already understood by the child. For example, providing rules for using playground equipment, such as a slide ("Climb up the ladder, not up the slide"), will be easier for a child to understand if she has experience with a slide. A child who has experience with a slide may know that she may fall if she attempts to climb up the slide (rather than the ladder) or that another child may bump into her or knock her down if she is climbing up the slide when the other child is coming down. The child's experience provides a context that aids in understanding the language. Using familiar adults in providing intervention may also add to the familiarity of the experience. Holistic experiences provide a more meaningful context for understanding language compared with discrete or isolated ones. For example, providing step-by-step directions for a task (such as an art activity) may be helpful, but the directions will be more understandable if the child can see the finished product concurrent with the step-by-step guidance.

- *Teach new vocabulary:* In preparation for an activity, review a few new vocabulary words that are central to talking about the activity. If visiting an animal shelter, for example, reviewing the names of the animals ("cat," "dog," "rabbit," "guinea pig") and relevant verbs ("pet," "hold," "carry," "lock") might help the child in understanding language during the visit. Key words may be highlighted through repetition, increased volume, or exaggeration.

Use Cooperative Learning Methods

Cooperative learning methods are described in detail in Chapter 11. They are advantageous to children who are ELLs for a number of reasons. First, they may minimize stress by allowing for observing and nonresponding. Lowering stress may help the child attend to the activity and may provide safe opportunities for speaking. More linguistically capable peers serve as models, providing descriptions, directions, and questions in a meaningful context. The relaxed group setting is an opportunity for building peer support networks. This can be done informally (some children initiate assisting others) or formally (through strategies such as a buddy system—assigning a peer to provide assistance), or by peer tutoring (peer assigned to teach a specific task).

Teach Coping Strategies

Some children who are ELLs may be shy or hesitant to ask for help or clarification. Others may be from cultures in which it is inappropriate to ask for help directly. When adults observe that a child needs help or clarification, they can model "Help, please" with a calm expression and a smile to teach that asking for assistance is permissible. For a child who is not yet using speech, the child may be guided to take another's hand as a request for assistance. The child can be taught that it is permissible to ask peers for assistance. Providing children who are learning English with coping strategies may alleviate stress and frustration when they do not understand what to do or what is expected. Similarly, other learning strategies may be beneficial for ELLs, particularly in early childhood education settings. For example, a child may be taught to ask "Say it differently, please" if he doesn't understand a direction, or he may be taught to "look and follow" what a peer is doing if he doesn't understand what is expected.

STRATEGIES FOR CULTURALLY AND LINGUISTICALLY RESPONSIVE INTERVENTION

In many cases, the cultural and linguistic considerations discussed above will need to be interwoven to create an appropriate and responsive intervention program for a young child with disabilities, whether the child is receiving services at home, at a community child care setting, or in school. Which strategies are used will be individualized to each child, family, and setting. Table 8.2 summarizes strategies to support ELLs. The following are examples for an infant, toddler, and kindergarten student:

Example: Mei Mei—an Infant Receiving Home-Based Services

Mei Mei is 13 months old. She and her parents and 5-year-old brother are recent immigrants from Hong Kong. Mei Mei has low muscle tone and is learning to sit during playtime, eat snacks and meals, get dressed, and take a bath. She communicates mostly with gestures (pointing to what she wants) and facial expressions (pouting or crying when she is unhappy). She is very attached to her mother. One of Mei Mei's goals is to request more of an activity. This will be taught in the context of a repetitious turn-taking game while seated on her mother's lap. Examples of cultural and linguistic accommodations to this activity are as follows:

Cultural Accommodations Mei Mei's mother and brother will first model the game (holding hands, facing each other, singing, rocking back and forth, and stopping; brother says, "more" and the game begins again). Modeling the complete activity may assist Mei Mei in understanding the expectation if she is a field-dependent learner. While the brother and mother model, the interventionist will note if the wait time for turn taking appears to be very short (or overlapping) or long. When it is Mei Mei's turn with mother, the interventionist will prompt Mei Mei's mother (if necessary) to match the wait time observed when the brother modeled the activity. The interventionist will also encourage Mei Mei's brother to play the game with her. Although he is only 5 years old, he regularly helps care for Mei Mei (a *social organizational variable*).

Linguistic Accommodations Mei Mei's brother and mother will sing to her in Cantonese—the language they use in their home—during the turn-taking game as a strategy to *provide a relaxed environment and comprehensible input*. When the repetitious game stops, any gesture or verbalization will be accepted to indicate "more." Accepting any communication form *capitalizes*

Table 8.2. Recommendations and strategies for a supportive language-learning environment in inclusive early childhood settings

Capitalize on all communication skills
- Respond to nonverbal communication (facial expressions, gestures, and so forth) as well as verbal communication.
- Provide instruction in child's strongest language.
- Use visual cues, gestures, facial expressions, and other concrete cues when teaching in English.

Focus on content
- Respond to meaning (the intent of the child's communication).
- Do not correct grammar.

Teach in context
- Teach during ongoing activities (e.g., label objects during activity).
- Use expansion and elaboration.
- Use focused contrasts to illustrate grammatical forms.
- Provide audio-recorded instructions.

Provide a relaxed environment and comprehensible input
- Recognize that a child's conversational skills (basic interpersonal communicative skills, BICS) are probably not equivalent to the child's ability to learn through the language (cognitive/academic language proficiency, CALP).
- Adjust speech (simplify).
- Provide descriptions.
- Use concrete and contextual cues.
- Use familiar and holistic experiences.
- Teach new vocabulary.

Use cooperative learning methods
- Use small group activities.
- Assign children to assist one another.
- Assign peer tutors.

Teach coping strategies
- Model requests for assistance from adults or peers.
- Teach child to ask for clarification.
- Teach child to observe and imitate peers.

on all communication skills. Mei Mei's mother or brother will respond by restarting the game (*responding to meaning*) and saying something similar to "Play again!" alternately in Cantonese and English. Saying "Play again!" *expands* on Mei Mei's response, *teaches during an ongoing activity,* and provides comprehensible input by using both languages (*using simple speech, a familiar experience,* and *contextual cues*).

Example: Toa—a Toddler in Early Head Start

Toa and his family are originally from American Samoa. They moved to the United States 2 years ago when Toa was 12 months old to have greater access to family health care. Toa is now 3 years old and attends Early Head Start five mornings a week. He speaks softly in English, using single words or two-word sentences, and often avoids eye contact with adults. Toa has spina bifida and is unable to move around the classroom independently. One of his goals is to request assistance as needed to do an activity (e.g., imitate movements, retrieve an object that is out of reach).

Cultural Accommodations   Two of Toa's aunties are classroom volunteers. His aunties will be asked to assist in conducting free-play activities similar to those that their children play at home (*addressing state motivation by using familiar activities*). An example is a body-part song ("Where is your _____?") that Samoan adults frequently play with children ("O fea o iai lou _____?" [ulu, isu, gutu, taliga, mata, lima]). Classroom staff will pay close attention to Toa and will model "Help, please" when he appears to need assistance in imitating the song motions or obtaining a material or toy that is out of reach. Staff will respond and provide assistance immediately to any verbalization or gesture, accepting low speech volume and eye gaze (even if Toa doesn't make eye contact). If Toa does not say "Help, please," staff will model the request a second time while providing assistance.

Linguistic Accommodations   Responding to any verbalization that Toa makes as a request for assistance will *capitalize on all communication skills* and is a response to *meaning rather than grammar*. Repeating the model when Toa does not imitate provides *expansion*. And finally, teaching Toa to request assistance is a *coping strategy* that Toa may be able to use in situations when he lacks comprehension.

Maile—a Kindergarten Student

Maile is a 5-year-old of Hawaiian descent who lives with her grandparents and three siblings in a rural coastal area. She attends a developmentally appropriate, fully inclusive kindergarten. Maile has developmental delays and is working on preacademic skills similar to those of her classmates.

Cultural Accommodations   Use small-group activities for practicing preacademic skills, allowing children to help one another, model for one another, and converse while they work. (The Hawaiian culture tends to be *group-oriented and values peer interaction*). Ask the class as a whole to talk about their activity to summarize the lesson. Allow more than one child to talk at a time (*negative wait time*) and to call out answers (Hawaiian *discourse structure*).

Linguistic Accommodations   Accept *pidgin* (Hawaiian *Creole* English) grammar when Maile responds (*capitalize on all communication skills; focus on content*). In addition to accommodating her group-oriented cultural style, using the small-group activities will provide a linguistic accommodation that will promote more language use. Use peer tutors within the small-group situation when Maile needs assistance with assigned tasks.

SUMMARY

Supporting children of diverse backgrounds to participate and learn in early intervention and early childhood special education requires that cultural and linguistic variables be addressed. The seven standards for effective instruction with diverse young children and the IC model describe approaches and modifications to sociolinguistic, cognition, motivation, and social organization variables that have been shown to improve children's participation and learning in educational situations. The modifications are designed to align a child's experiences and expectations in educational environments with those of home environments. Children of diverse cultures may also benefit from linguistic accommodations: Some children will have languages other than English as their first language, and others may have learned a cultural variation of Standard American English. The IC model promotes reading and English literacy skills among ELLs. Additionally, six approaches can assist children in acquiring English: 1) capitalize on all communication skills, 2) focus on content, 3) teach in context, 4) provide relaxed environments and comprehensible input, 5) use cooperative learning methods, and 6) teach coping strategies. Instructional strategies for diverse learners should include cultural and linguistic accommodations and be designed on an individualized basis.

STUDY QUESTIONS

1. Referencing the definition of *culture*, discuss several ways in which culture may influence a child's educational experiences.

2. Identify and describe the three components of *culturally compatible education*.

3. Define the four cultural factors associated with the *instructional conversation* (IC) model: sociolinguistics, cognition, motivation, and social organization.

4. Choose one sociolinguistic variable associated with the IC model and provide an example of how it may be modified to support a child's learning in a home-based early intervention setting and in an inclusive preschool setting.

5. Discuss various ways that *cooperative learning groups* can be modified to create culturally compatible education.

6. List and describe Salend's (2001) six stages that school-age children progress through when learning English as a second language.

7. Describe a rationale for bilingual instruction for children who are ELLs.

8. What does it mean to "teach in context" for children who are ELLs? Provide an example for a preschool setting.

9. Define and contrast the terms *basic interpersonal communication skills (BICS)* and *cognitive/academic language proficiency (CALP)*. What is the implication of the concepts for addressing the needs of young children who are ELLs?

10. Identify and describe three strategies for providing children who are ELLs with *comprehensible input*.

References

Au, K. (1980). Participation structures in a reading lesson with Hawaiian children: Finding a culturally appropriate instructional event. *Anthropology and Education Quarterly, 11,* 91–115.

Au, K., & Mason, J. (1981). Social organizational factors in learning to read: The balance of rights hypothesis. *Reading Research Quarterly, 17,* 115–152.

Ayabe, H.I., & Santos, S. (1972). Conceptual tempo and the Oriental American. *Journal of Psychology, 81,* 121–123.

Banks, J.A., & Banks, C.A.M. (2009). *Multicultural education: Issues and perspectives.* New York, NY: John Wiley & Sons.

Barrera, I. (1993). Effective and appropriate instruction for all children: The challenge of cultural/linguistic diversity and young children with special needs. *Topics in Early Childhood Special Education, 13,* 461–487.

Bunce, B. (2003). Children with culturally diverse backgrounds. In L. McCormick, D.F. Loeb, & R.L. Schiefelbusch (Eds.), *Supporting children with communication difficulties in inclusive settings: School-based language intervention* (pp. 367–407). Boston, MA: Allyn & Bacon.

Butterfield, R.A. (1983). The development and use of culturally appropriate curriculum for American Indian students. *Peabody Journal of Education, 61,* 50–66.

Castenada, A. (1976). Cultural democracy and the educational needs of Mexican American children. In R.L. Jones (Ed.), *Mainstreaming and the minority child* (pp. 181–194). Reston, VA: Council for Exceptional Children.

Christophel, D. (1990). The relationships among teacher immediacy behaviors, student motivation, and learning. *Communication Education, 39,* 335–345.

Correa, V., & Tulbert, B. (1991). Teaching culturally diverse students. *Preventing School Failure, 35*(3), 20–25.

Cummins, J. (1984). *Bilingualism and special education: Issues in assessment and pedagogy.* Clevedon Avon, UK: Multilingual Matters.

D'Amato, J. (1981). *Power in the classroom.* Paper presented at the annual meeting of the American Anthropological Association, Los Angeles.

Darnell, R. (1979). *Reflections on Cree interactional etiquette: Educational implications* (Working Papers in Sociolinguistics No. 57). Austin, TX: Southwestern Educational Development Laboratory.

Epstein, M.H., Hallahan, D.P., & Kauffman, J.M. (1975). Implications of the reflectivity-impulsivity dimension for special education. *Journal of Special Education, 9,* 11–25.

Erickson, F., & Mohatt, G. (1982). Cultural organization of participation structures in two classrooms of Indian students. In G. Spindler (Ed.), *Doing the ethnography of schooling: Educational anthropology in action* (pp. 132–174). New York, NY: Holt, Rinehart & Winston.

Esmailka, W., & Barnhardt, C. (1981). *The social organization of participation in three Athabaskan cross-cultural classrooms.* Fairbanks, AK: University of Alaska Center for Cross Cultural Studies. Retrieved from Education Resource Information Center web site: http://www.eric.ed.gov/ERICWebPortal/detail?accno=ED231571

Foster, M. (1998). *Black teachers on teaching.* New York, NY: Norton.

Gallimore, R., Boggs, J.W., & Jordan, C. (1974). *Culture, behavior, and education: A study of Hawaiian-Americans.* Beverly Hills, CA: Sage.

Gay, G. (2010). *Culturally responsive teaching: Theory, research, and practice.* New York, NY: Teachers College Press.

Goldenberg, C. (2004). Literacy for all children in the increasingly diverse schools of the United States. In N. Unrau & R. Ruddell (Eds.), *Theoretical models and processes of reading* (5th ed., pp. 1636–1666). Newark, DE: International Reading Association.

Goldenberg, C., & Gallimore, R. (1991). Local knowledge, research knowledge, and educational change: A case study of first-grade Spanish reading improvement. *Educational Researcher, 20*(8), 2–14.

Goodenough, W.H. (1981). *Culture, language, and society* (2nd ed.). Menlo Park, CA: Benjamin/Cummings.

Greenbaum, P. (1983). *Nonverbal communications between American Indian children and their teachers.* Lawrence, KS: Native American Research Associates. Retrieved from Education Resource Information Center website: http://www.eric.ed.gov/ERICWebPortal/detail?accno=ED239804

Grossman, H. (1995). *Special education in a diverse society.* Boston, MA: Allyn & Bacon.

Hale-Benson, J.E. (1986). *Black children: Their roots, culture and learning styles* (Rev. ed.). Baltimore, MD: Johns Hopkins University Press.

Hale-Benson, J.E. (1990). Visions for children: African-American early childhood education programs. *Early Childhood Research Quarterly, 5,* 199–213.
Hilliard, A.S. (1989). Teachers and cultural styles in a pluralistic society. *NEA Today, 7*(6), 65–69.
Hirayama, K.K. (1985). Asian children's adaptation to public schools. *Social Work in Education, 7,* 213–230.
Institute of Educational Sciences. (2006). *What Works Clearinghouse: Instructional conversations and literature logs.* Retrieved from http://ies.ed.gov/ncee/wwc/interventionreport.aspx?sid=236
Ingalls, L., & Hammond, H. (2011). The match between Apache Indians' culture and educational practices used in our schools: From problems to solutions. *College Teaching Methods & Styles Journal, 3*(1), 9–18.
Johnson, D. (1971). Black kinesics: Some nonverbal communication patterns in black culture. *Florida Reporter, 9,* 1–2.
Jordan, C., & Tharp, R.G. (1979). Culture and education. In A.J. Marsella, R.G. Tharp, & T. Ciborowski (Eds.), *Perspectives in cross-cultural psychology* (pp. 265–285). New York, NY: Academic Press.
Jordan, C., Tharp, R.G., & Vogt, L. (1985). *Compatibility of classroom and culture: General principles with Navajo and Hawaiian instances* (Working paper). Honolulu, HI: Kamehameha Schools/Bishop Estate, Center for the Development of Early Education.
Joy, S., & Kolb, D.A. (2009). Are there cultural differences in learning style? *International Journal of Intercultural Relations, 33*(1), 69–85.
Kana'iaupuni, S.M., & Kawai'ae'a, K.K.C. (2008). *E lauhoe mai na wa'a: Toward a Hawaiian indigenous education teaching framework.* Retrieved from Education Resource Information Center web site: http://www.eric.ed.gov/ERICWebPortal/recordDetail?accno=ED523184
Kana'iaupuni, S., Ledward, B., & Jensen, U. (2010). *Culture-based education and its relationship to student outcomes.* Honolulu, HI: Kamehameha Schools, Research and Evaluation.
Kenny, R. (2009). Evaluating cognitive tempo in the digital age. *Educational Technology Research and Development, 57*(1), 45–60.
Key, M.R. (1975). *Paralanguage and kinesics: Nonverbal communication.* Metuchen, NJ: Scarecrow.
Kitano, M. (1983). Early education for Asian-American children. In O.N. Saracho & B. Spodek (Eds.), *Understanding the multicultural experience in early childhood education* (pp. 45–66). Washington, DC: National Association for the Education of Young Children.
Krashen, S.D. (1982). *Principles and practices in second language acquisition.* Elmsford, NY: Pergamon.
Krashen, S.D., & Terrell, T.D. (1983). *The natural approach: Language acquisition in the classroom.* Elmsford, NY: Pergamon.
Laturnau, J. (2001). *Standards-based instruction for English language learners.* Honolulu, HI: Pacific Resources for Education and Learning.
Leith, S., & Slentz, K. (1984). Successful teaching strategies in selected Northern Manitoba schools. *Canadian Journal of Native Education, 12,* 24–30.
Lipka, J. (1990). Integrating cultural form and content in one Yup'ik Eskimo classroom: A case study. *Canadian Journal of Native Education, 17,* 18–32.
McCarthy, J., & Benally, J. (2003). Classroom management in a Navajo middle school. *Theory Into Practice, 42*(4), 296–304.
Ogbu, J.U. (1991). Immigrant and involuntary minorities in comparative perspective. In M. Gibson & J.U. Ogbu (Eds.), *Minority status and schooling: A comparative study of immigrant and involuntary minorities* (pp. 3–33). New York, NY: Garland.
Philips, S.U. (1976). Some sources of cultural variability in the regulation of talk. *Language in Society, 5,* 81–95.
Philips, S.U. (1983). *The invisible culture.* New York, NY: Longman.
Ramirez, M., & Castenada, A. (1974). *Cultural democracy, bicognitive development and education.* New York, NY: Academic Press.

Rogoff, B. (2003). *The cultural nature of human development.* New York, NY: Oxford University Press.

Rowe, M.B. (1974). Wait time and rewards as instructional variables: Their influence on language, logic, and gate control: Part 1. Wait time. *Journal of Research in Science Teaching, 11,* 81–97.

Rueda, R., & Stillman, J. (2012). The 21st century teacher: A cultural perspective. *Journal of Teacher Education, 20*(10), 1–9.

Salend, S.J. (2001). *Creating inclusive classrooms: Effective and reflective practices* (4th ed.). Columbus, OH: Merrill/Prentice Hall.

Salend, S.J., & Salinas, A. (2003). Language differences or learning difficulties: The work of the multidisciplinary team. *Teaching Exceptional Children, 35*(4), 36–43.

Sandall, S., Hemmeter, M.L., Smith, B.J., & McLean, M.E. (2005). *DEC recommended practices: A comprehensive guide for practical application in early intervention/early childhood special education.* Longmont, CO: Sopris West.

Shade, B.J. (1994). Understanding the African-American learner. In E.R. Hollins, J.E. King, & W.C. Hayman (Eds.), *Teaching diverse populations: Formulating a new knowledge base* (pp. 175–189). Albany, NY: State University of New York Press.

Shade, B.J., Kelly, C., & Oberg, M. (1997). *Creating culturally responsive classrooms.* Washington, DC: American Psychological Association.

Singh, N.K. (2011). Culturally appropriate education: Theoretical and practical implications. In J. Reyhner, W.S. Gilbert, & G.S. Lockard (Eds.), *Honoring our heritage: Culturally appropriate approaches for teaching indigenous students* (pp. 11–42). Flagstaff, AZ: University of Arizona. Retrieved from Northern Arizona University web site: http://jan.ucc.nau.edu/jar/HOH/Honoring.pdf#page=23

Slavin, R., DeVies, D., & Edwards, K. (1983). *Cooperative learning.* New York, NY: Longman.

Tharp, R.G. (1989). Psychocultural variables and constants: Effects on teaching and learning in schools. *American Psychologist, 44,* 349–359.

Tharp, R. G. (1997). *From at-risk to excellence: Research, theory, and principles for practice; Research report 1.* Santa Cruz, CA: Center for Research on Education, Diversity & Excellence. Retrieved from eScholarship University of California web site: http://escholarship.org/uc/item/8nc0979r.pdf

Tharp, R.G. (2006). Four hundred years of evidence: Culture, pedagogy, and Native America. *Journal of American Indian Education, 45*(2), 6–25.

Tharp, R.G., & Dalton, S.S. (2007). Orthodoxy, cultural compatibility, and universals in education. *Comparative Education, 43*(1), 53–70.

Tharp, R.G., & Entz, S. (2003). From high chair to high school: Research-based principles for teaching complex thinking. *Young Children, 58*(5), 38–44.

Tharp, R.G., & Gallimore, R. (1988). *Rousing minds to life: Teaching, learning, and schooling in social context.* New York, NY: Cambridge University Press.

Tharp, R.G., & Yamauchi, L.A. (1994). *Effective instructional conversation in Native American classrooms.* (Educational Practice Report No. 10). Santa Cruz, CA: National Center for Research on Cultural Diversity and Second Language Learning.

Vygotsky, L.S. (1978). *Mind and society: The development of higher mental processes.* Cambridge, MA: Harvard University Press.

Westby, C.E. (1985). Learning to talk—talking to learn. In C.S. Simon (Ed.), *Communication skills and classroom success* (pp. 181–218). San Diego, CA: College-Hill.

White, S., & Tharp, R.G. (1988, April 5–9). *Questioning and wait time: A cross-cultural analysis.* Paper presented at the annual meeting of the American Educational Research Association, New Orleans, LA.

Widaman, K.F., & Kagan, S. (1987). Cooperativeness and achievement: Interaction of student cooperativeness with cooperation versus competitive classroom organization. *Journal of School Psychology, 25,* 355–365.

Winterton, W.A. (1976). *The effect of extended wait-time on selected verbal response characteristics of some Pueblo Indian children* (Unpublished doctoral dissertation). University of New Mexico, Albuquerque.

Winzer, M., & Mazurek, K. (1998). *Special education in multicultural contexts* (2nd ed.). Upper Saddle River, NJ: Prentice Hall.

Witkin, H.A., Moore, C.A., Goodenough, D.R., & Cox, P.W. (1977). Field-dependent and field-independent cognitive styles and their educational implications. *Review of Educational Research, 47*, 1–64.

Wyatt, T.R. (2009). The role of culture in culturally compatible education. *Journal of American Indian Education, 48*(3), 47–63.

Yamauchi, L.A., Im, S., & Schonleber, N.S. (2012). Adapting strategies of effective instruction for culturally diverse preschoolers. *Journal of Early Childhood Teacher Education, 33*(1), 54–72.

9

Teaching Children with Autism

Mary Jo Noonan

FOCUS OF THIS CHAPTER

- Learning characteristics of children with autism
- Instructional procedures effective for most children, including those with autism
- Specialized procedures focused on children with autism
- Model programs for children with autism

Children with autism spectrum disorder (usually referred to simply as autism) include children who vary widely in their abilities and educational needs. Autism was first defined as a disorder in 1943 by the psychologist Leo Kanner. He had encountered a number of children who had behavioral characteristics and needs that were strikingly different from children with intellectual disabilities and developmental delay. In particular, the children with autism had typical physical growth and development, but they also had social relationship difficulties, speech-language delays and differences, and obsessions with environmental sameness and/or stereotypies (repetitive movements such as finger flicking) and self-stimulations. Since that time, definitions and diagnostic criteria have been promulgated by a number of organizations and policies (e.g., Individuals with Disabilities Education Improvement Act [2004], Autism Society of America [n.d.], *Diagnostic and Statistical Manual of Mental Disorders* [American Psychiatric Association, 2013], but the central defining characteristics of the disorder have not changed. Diagnostic criteria have been distinguished among individuals with few or mild characteristics (Asperger syndrome) and those with more or pronounced characteristics (pervasive developmental disorder [PDD], including autistic disorder). In this chapter, the term *autism* will be used to refer to all labels and disorders on the autism spectrum, but keep in mind that the characteristics and needs will vary in number and degree (from mild to severe).

LEARNING CHARACTERISTICS OF CHILDREN WITH AUTISM

Many of the distinguishing characteristics of autism have important implications for instruction. Specifically, they suggest that certain content, instructional approaches, and environmental arrangements will be more effective than others. The following characteristics of children with autism should be considered in designing specialized instruction.

Communication and Social Needs

One of the most noticeable concerns of children with autism is that they have significant communication and social delays or differences. These delays and differences are often noticeable before the children are 1 year of age. One of the earliest apparent differences is that many infants and young children with autism do not engage in *joint attention* (Wetherby, Prizant, & Schuler, 2000). Joint attention is a social-communication skill whereby the child follows the gaze of an adult (that is, the child looks in the same direction and at the same thing or event that the adult is looking at). It is an important skill because it establishes a context for communication: The communication partners (in this case, the young child and adult) focus their communications and interactions on what they are looking at together. As children with autism become toddlers, their communication needs become more marked. For example, a mother may be worried when her 18-month-old child is not attempting to communicate or socialize (e.g., not pointing or otherwise indicating that she wants desired objects, not gesturing or vocalizing to be picked up or to get attention, not playing typical baby games such as peekaboo, crying when tired or frustrated but not looking to an adult for comfort). Frequently, children with autism make little or no eye contact. They appear isolated and unaware of people and events in their environment. Some have socialization and communication behaviors that are markedly different from their age peers. For example, a child with autism may talk using only phrases and sentences imitated from cartoons. Or the child may play with toys in a repetitive and/or ritualistic manner (e.g., sorting and lining up plastic dishes) rather than in more object-specific or socially influenced ways (e.g., playing "tea party" with the cups and dishes) as age peers would do.

Related to their apparent isolation, children with autism have difficulty taking the perspective of others (Baron-Cohen, Leslie, & Frith, 1985)—a psychological ability referred to as *theory of mind* (Premack & Woodruff, 1978). In their landmark 1985 study, Baron-Cohen et al. studied a group of young children with autism matched on intelligence measures with children who had Down syndrome and children without a disability. They found that the children with autism were unable to impute mental states or beliefs to others (understand what others might be feeling or thinking), whereas their peers were able to do so. This finding suggested a unique social deficit, rather than an intellectual deficit, that distinguished children with autism from other children with and without disabilities. Theory of mind deficits or delays are apparent in young children with autism when they fail to show even the most basic language and social skills: They behave toward other people as though they are objects without feelings or communication abilities. For example, the child with autism takes a parent's hand to the sink when wanting a drink of water, or the child does not look or attend when another child cries.

Generalization Needs

The behavior of children with autism is often characterized as rigid. The children tend not to transfer skills learned in one situation to another, and they have difficulty in adapting or modifying skills to fit new situations. For example, a child with autism may learn to pop open the toothpaste lid but not generalize the skill to the pop-up top on the shampoo bottle; or she may learn to say "please" when she wants something to drink, but she may not transfer the use of the word to dinnertime when she wants something to eat, or to play activities to request a particular toy.

Preoccupation with Sameness

Many children with autism are most content and capable when expectations, materials, and other environmental variables remain constant or unchanged. For example, the child who sorts and lines up plastic dishes may be content while organizing the materials, but if asked to stop and put the materials away, he may become upset, even to the point of having a tantrum. Similarly, if he completes the task and someone disturbs the orderliness of his work (moves the toys aside or puts them away), he may react very strongly. When children with autism have a strong preference for consistency or order, it is not uncommon for families to be extremely cautious to avoid disturbing the materials or environmental arrangements on which the children focus.

Challenging Behavior

Children with autism frequently have numerous behavioral challenges: They may isolate themselves (hide under furniture), act aggressively toward others (hit, kick, push), injure themselves (bite, pinch, head bang), and/or demonstrate other socially inappropriate behaviors. As discussed in detail in Chapter 10, challenging behavior usually serves a communication purpose. Because children with autism have significant communication needs, it is not surprising that challenging behaviors are present.

Dawson and Osterling (1997) have suggested that effective programs for children with autism, given the children's unique characteristics and concerns, should include the following:

1. *Curriculum content emphasizing attending skills, imitation (gestural and verbal), language comprehension and use, appropriate toy play (functional and symbolic), and social interaction (with adults and with peers):* Attending and imitative skills are emphasized because they are *tool skills* that facilitate subsequent learning (and are often lacking in children with autism). Language comprehension and use and social interaction skills are included because they are high-need areas for children with autism. Appropriate toy play is a cognitive skill area that is included because children with autism often have difficulty understanding the social purpose of objects and the use of symbols (language learning relies on the use of symbols).

2. *A highly supportive teaching environment and generalization strategies:* The term *highly supportive* implies that instruction is carefully planned and executed based on the unique needs and strengths of the child. Supportive teaching often includes instructional objectives that are just slightly beyond the child's current performance level, direct instruction methods (see Chapter 6), and a consistent schedule (see Chapter 13). Because generalization difficulties are prevalent among children with autism, generalization strategies should be included in all instructional plans (see Chapter 6).

3. *Learning environments that are predictable and routine:* As discussed fully in Chapter 13, predictability and routines teach children what to expect. In turn, knowing what to expect supports children in demonstrating appropriate behavior and promotes independence. It's important to note that predictability and routines add order to what would otherwise seem a chaotic world. Children with autism commonly show a high preference for orderliness. Establishing predictable and routine learning environments capitalizes on a preferred learning style, creates a familiar and comfortable situation, and thereby facilitates learning.

4. *A functional, positive approach to problem behaviors:* A functional approach to problem behaviors focuses on teaching socially appropriate alternative responses to replace the problem behavior. In other words, children are taught socially acceptable ways (usually a communication skill) to get what they want (reinforcement), thereby eliminating the need for problem behavior. In addition, a number of positive strategies should be employed to prevent problem behavior, and the use of punishment should

be avoided. Chapter 10 describes functional and positive assessment and intervention procedures for challenging behavior.

5. *Carefully planned transitions to next setting:* Transitions are often difficult times for children with autism because changing from one activity to the next has the effect of ending an ongoing routine. As already discussed, children with autism prefer sameness and orderliness; ending a routine is viewed as disruptive. Therefore, transitions need to be planned, and related skills (identifying next activities, putting away materials) should be taught.

6. *Family involvement:* As emphasized throughout this text, family support is a critical component of early childhood special education. Because the extensive communication, social, and behavioral needs of children with autism may affect all aspects of family life, supports might include involving family members in planning and implementing interventions. For example, family members can participate in developing and conducting an intervention to teach a child to make eye contact and to point to a desired object (a social-communication objective).

These six items describe components of effective programs (also known as *comprehensive treatment models*) for children with autism. The recommendations of Dawson and Osterling (1997) are echoed in a more recent report from the National Research Council (2001). Additionally, the National Research Council recommends that young children with autism receive group instruction as well as individual instruction and opportunities for supported interaction with their peers who do not have disabilities.

Reviews of programs for young children with autism indicate that intensive, behaviorally based practices have the strongest evidence of effectiveness, while other models show promise (Howlin, Magiati, & Charman, 2009; Odom, Boyd, Hall, & Hume, 2010; Reichow & Wolery, 2009). While most behaviorally based programs begin with intensive individualized instruction in segregated settings (Lovaas, 1987; McEachin, Smith, & Lovaas, 1993), evidence for the effectiveness of inclusive behavioral programs is accumulating (Boulware, Schwartz, Sandall, & McBride, 2006; McGee, Morrier, & Daly, 2000; Stahmer & Ingersoll, 2004; Strain & Bovey, 2011). Most behaviorally based programs (inclusive and segregated), however, include naturalistic and parent-implementation components (Boyd, Odom, Humphreys, & Sam, 2010). Given that comprehensive intervention programs are not uniformly effective for all children, decisions on matching programs to children ultimately must be individualized and based on child outcome data (Howlin et al., 2009; Sandall et al., 2011; Simpson, 2005).

Just as reviews of comprehensive program models for children with autism have found that behaviorally based models have the most positive effectiveness data, recent reviews of evidence-based practices for young children with autism—focused on specific interventions and/or instructional approaches—concluded that behaviorally based interventions are currently the only interventions that are solidly supported by research and considered well established (Matson & Smith, 2008; Odom et al., 2003; Simpson, 2005). Other procedures (peer-mediated interventions, visual supports, self-monitoring, and involving parents) have been shown to be emerging and effective and probably efficacious

(Odom et al., 2003). The next two sections of this chapter focus on behaviorally based instructional procedures: 1) those for early childhood intervention that are effective for young children with disabilities and also applicable to children who have autism, and 2) those designed specifically for children with autism. This chapter concludes with a description of seven comprehensive model programs for children with autism.

INSTRUCTIONAL PROCEDURES EFFECTIVE FOR MOST CHILDREN, INCLUDING THOSE WITH AUTISM

The following eight instructional approaches have been shown to be effective for many children with autism, presumably because they fit with the children's learning styles and address critical developmental needs: 1) direct instruction, 2) naturalistic instruction, 3) general case instruction, 4) cues (versus general prompts), 5) prompt and cue fading, 6) group instruction, 7) augmentative communication, and 8) positive behavior support. Although these procedures are discussed in detail elsewhere in this text, this discussion focuses on special considerations in applying the procedures with children who have autism.

Direct Instruction

Chapter 6 fully describes *direct instruction,* which is defined as the consistent use of one or more prompts, a correction procedure, and a reinforcement strategy to teach an operationally defined behavior. For example, a child may be taught to ask her sibling to play with her by handing the sibling a toy. There may be a three-step prompting and correction procedure: 1) The adult points to the toy and waits 4 seconds; 2) if there is no response or an incorrect response the adult hands the child the toy, points to the sibling, and waits 4 seconds; and 3) if there is no response the adult guides the child to the sibling, guides the child to hand the sibling the toy, and says, "Jamie, please play with me." When the child hands the sibling the toy, the adult plays the child's favorite music softly as the reinforcer. Using a precise and consistent direct instruction procedure fits with the preferences for sameness and predictability that characterize the learning styles of many children with autism. And, indeed, research indicates that children with autism learn relatively quickly with systematic instruction (Dawson & Osterling, 1997; Lovaas, 1987; Matson & Smith, 2008).

As with any application of direct instruction, it is important to individualize the prompts and correction procedures for each child (Barton, Lawrence, & Deurloo, 2012). Children with autism tend to respond better to visual prompts compared with auditory prompts. However, teachers must be responsive to each child's performance data for each instructional plan. In other words, view each instructional plan as a "worksheet" to be modified based on its effectiveness. If the data for an instructional plan indicate that a child doesn't use a prompt (i.e., rarely or never responds correctly to a prompt), eliminate that prompt from the plan and use ones that are effective in eliciting correct responses.

Attentional Issues In addition to ensuring that prompts are individualized, it may be necessary to include an attentional prompt in the direct instruction plan. Many children with autism attend predominantly to objects and the physical world and seem to ignore the social world. For some children, a prompt eliciting attention to the teacher (or adult) prior to the prompt associated with the instructional objective will improve instructional effectiveness. Returning to the example above of teaching a child to ask a sibling to play, the teacher might call the child by name and make eye-to-eye contact prior to delivering each prompt.

Although eye contact is a typical way that children demonstrate attention, there may be other valid indicators of attention for children who rarely make eye contact. Some children may stop their play and become still. Others may turn their attention from one set of materials to another. And still others may orient their body and/or face toward the speaker even though they don't make direct eye contact. If direct eye-to-eye contact is difficult to achieve, look for other indicators (such as the three presented here) that the child is attending, implement the direct instruction, and monitor learning. If the child shows progress, direct eye contact may not be a requisite to effective instruction. Attentional prompts may still be included in instruction, but attention may be operationalized as a behavior other than eye contact.

Reinforcement Issues Because of significant social delays and needs, children with autism may not be reinforced by verbal praise or affection—reinforcers commonly used with young children with special needs. It may seem difficult to identify potential reinforcers for children with autism because they do not show the same interests as their peers without disabilities. The following are three examples of approaches that may be used to identify instructional reinforcers: 1) test the effectiveness of verbal praise and social reinforcement, 2) conduct a reinforcer survey, and 3) assess the use of high-probability (high-*p*) activities, including stereotyped behaviors.

The first approach, *testing the effectiveness of verbal praise and social reinforcement*, is suggested for pragmatic reasons: Before assuming that verbal praise or social reinforcement will not be effective (even when a child has significant social needs and/or does not make eye contact), test it as part of a direct instruction plan. If the instructional plan is effective, then a very natural and highly generalizable reinforcement strategy has been identified and is available for instruction.

The second approach includes two procedures that may be used to identify a set of highly preferred items (which could include food) that are likely to function effectively as reinforcers. One procedure is to conduct a *reinforcer survey*, either by asking a child to name favorite items or presenting numerous items to a child (often two at a time) and noting the child's most frequent choices. Observing a child's choices is often used for children who do not speak or cannot name their preferences. Studies have indicated that choice assessments evaluating a number of potential reinforcers is a valid method for identifying effective reinforcers and should be used periodically because children's preferences may change frequently (Carr, Nicolson, & Higbee, 2000; Love, Carr, Almason, & Petursdottir, 2009). Research on children's self-report of potential reinforcers, however, suggests that self-report is not always an accurate method for identifying effective reinforcers (Northup, 2000; Northup, George, Jones, Broussard, & Vollmer, 1996).

Another procedure for assessing potentially effective reinforcers is to measure the time a child spends engaged (interacting) with items that appear to be highly preferred. Items are presented to the child one at a time and then are ranked according to the duration of engagement. The longer a child interacts with an object, the more likely it is that the object will be an effective reinforcer. This procedure has been shown to be valid and easy to administer (Hagopian, Rush, Lewin, & Long, 2001; Pace, Ivancic, Edwards, Iwata, & Page, 1985).

Applying the Premack principle, *using high-probability (high-p) activities as reinforcers*, is a third approach that may be used for assessing reinforcer effectiveness. High-*p* activities are identified by noting which activities a child most frequently chooses in free-play situations with access to a variety of materials. The child is then given access to a high-*p* activity as a reinforcer for a correct response. Instructional progress can be used to confirm or disconfirm whether the activity is an effective reinforcer. Although children may enjoy engaging in some activities for extended periods of time, access to an activity reinforcer can be brief (10 or 15 seconds). Some teachers prompt the child by saying "My turn!," signaling that the child should hand the teacher the play item (or turn away from the activity) and return to the instructional activity. Stereotypy (repetitive movements with or without objects) can also be used as a high-*p* activity reinforcer and may be especially effective if its availability is restricted to when it is provided as a reinforcer (Hanley, Iwata, Thompson, & Lindberg, 2000).

Direct instruction is an effective and valuable component of a comprehensive program for children with autism (Steege, Mace, Perry, & Longenecker, 2007). For direct instruction to be maximally effective, instructional prompts should be individualized, attentional prompts may need to be added, and reinforcement assessments may be used to improve reinforcer effectiveness.

Naturalistic Instruction

As described in Chapter 7, a hallmark of naturalistic instruction (or *milieu teaching*) is providing instruction at times determined by the child's interest (e.g., when the child points to something out of reach, when the child attempts to gain a peer's attention). A premise is that child-determined occasions for instruction are motivating because the child is actively engaged and goal oriented. If the child is highly motivated, naturally occurring reinforcement may be effective. Given that many children with autism are socially isolated and favor consistency, naturalistic instruction is a good fit. Rather than attempting to draw the child's focus to the adult's interest and searching for effective artificial reinforcers, attend to the child's focus and conduct instruction when the child indicates a high level of motivation.

Another advantage of naturalistic instruction for children with autism is that it promotes generalization (Steege et al., 2007). As noted in the introduction to this chapter, children with autism tend to be rigid in their behaviors and routines and have difficulty with generalization. Naturalistic instruction promotes generalization because teaching situations vary considerably: Incidental teaching occasions throughout the day involve different people (children and adults), different activities, different materials, different responses, and different reinforcers. The variety of stimulus conditions promotes generalization (Stokes & Baer, 1977). In addition, reinforcers associated with naturalistic instruction are likely to be naturally occurring, and thus promote generalization because they are available in noninstructional situations.

Instructional plans for incidental teaching are identical in format to other direct instruction plans, except that *child-determined occasions for instruction* are specified. To implement the plans, teachers or family members follow their typical routines and maintain a watchful eye for the occasions for instruction (e.g., when the child expresses frustration—bangs the toy or whines—after a wind-up toy stops moving). When an occasion for instruction is observed, the adult approaches the child and follows the prompting procedure specified in the instructional plan. The prompt may be to make eye contact with the child and wait 5 seconds (a time delay to encourage communication), it may be to model the expected response ("Help, please"), or it may be another type of prompt (e.g., verbal direction, physical guidance). Correction and reinforcement procedures are also implemented as stated in the instructional plan.

General Case Instruction

As previously discussed, direct instruction is effective with children who have autism because of its consistency and predictability. Although consistency of instruction promotes learning new skills, it may impede generalization, particularly among children who like sameness and orderliness. As noted in Chapter 6, it is critical to develop direct instruction plans that include strategies to promote generalization. Incidental or milieu teaching is one way to promote generalization (discussed above). Another strategy is general case instruction (Kleeberger & Mirenda, 2010). In general case instruction (discussed in Chapter 6), the behavioral objective is stated as a generalized skill; instead of an objective to request a drink of water, for example, the objective is to request a desired item (drink, food, toy, clothing). The skill variations are carefully selected to represent the range of items represented by the general case objective (*request a desired item*) and are taught concurrently rather than sequentially. Other generalization strategies (e.g., teaching across people, places, materials, times; using mediation strategies) may also be included to increase the likelihood of generalization.

Cues

Chapter 6 defined prompting strategies, including cues. *Cues are prompts (anything that helps a child make a correct response) that direct a child's attention to salient characteristics of a stimulus.* For example, an identifying characteristic of an alphabet letter is its shape (salient characteristic) rather than its color (nonsalient characteristic). For a child learning to discriminate a lowercase *b* from a *p*, *d*, and *q*, salient characteristics include the direction and location of the straight line relative to the circle. A cue that would direct a child's attention to the location and direction of the straight line may be to make the line portion of the *b* bold and to draw it as an arrow pointing up (↑). Cues are a particularly effective type of prompt for children with autism because some children with autism have difficulty attending to multiple and relevant stimulus characteristics. This is known as *stimulus overselectivity* (Lovaas, Koegel, &

Schreibman, 1979; Lovaas & Schreibman, 1971). Providing cues rather than other types of prompts highlights the discriminative characteristics of stimuli that children with autism might otherwise not notice.

Prompt and Cue Fading

Because children with autism prefer consistency, they may become prompt dependent. In other words, they may rely on instructional prompts or cues (and the adults who provide the prompts and cues) even after they have acquired a new skill. Prompt dependency limits independence and generalization. To counteract this tendency, a direct instruction plan should specify steps for fading instructional prompts so that children respond to naturally occurring prompts. Fading is the gradual removal of a prompt by decreasing its saliency (a verbal prompt gradually gets quieter; a pictorial or visual prompt successively gets smaller or lighter), physical proximity (a prompt is gradually moved away from the stimulus), or temporal proximity (the time between a natural prompt and an instructional one is gradually lengthened). If fading is conducted too quickly, errors result or the child does not respond. Therefore it is important that fading be conducted slowly with careful monitoring for errors. If errors occur, the saliency of a prompt should be increased to reestablish correct responding, and a more gradual fading procedure should be conducted.

Group Instruction

Early intervention and early childhood special education services provided to young children with autism tend to emphasize individualized instruction. Often the children are assisted by skills trainers who provide extensive one-to-one instruction for several hours per day in a child's home and sometimes in a child's classroom. Although intense (predominantly one-to-one instruction) intervention has been associated with greater developmental gains for many children with autism compared with less intense programs (Lovaas, 1987; McClannahan & Krantz, 1993; National Research Council, 2001), there is recent evidence that other less intensive interventions focused on communication and joint attention can have significant positive effects (Howlin et al., 2009). Additionally, there is no indication that one-to-one instruction is superior in quality to larger child-to-staff ratios (Strain, Wolery, & Izeman, 1998). Instead, the quality of instruction and the competence of the teachers may be the more important variables.

In addition to one-to-one instruction, all children with autism should receive group instruction. Group instruction is important for children with autism because the diagnosis of autism is based on extensive communication and social needs. The group arrangement provides the necessary context for teaching communication and social skills with peers—a context that is otherwise not available (Leaf, Dotson, Oppeneheim, Sheldon, & Sherman, 2010). Chapter 11 describes several additional benefits of group instruction (e.g., opportunity for observational learning, peer modeling, turn taking) as well as group instructional procedures.

It is important that group instructional arrangements be age appropriate: Infants and toddlers may be in groups for child care and recreation programs (especially parent–toddler programs), and their groups tend to be small (two to six children or parent–child dyads). Children age 3 and older are frequently in large groups of 20 or more children for child care, preschool, kindergarten, and recreational programs. They may also receive instruction in small groups (three to six children) within the large-group setting.

As noted in Chapter 11, children may need to be taught how to participate in groups and eased into group situations (Carnahan, Musti-Rao, & Bailey, 2009; Collins, Gast, Ault, & Wolery, 1991; Koegel & Rincover, 1974). A child may begin group instruction with just one other child. When she demonstrates progress on her instructional goals and learns basic group-participation skills, such as responding to a peer and sitting quietly while the other child takes a turn, a third child may be added to the group. Additional children may be added to the group, in turn, as the child with autism demonstrates success in the small-group arrangement.

Augmentative Communication

Although augmentative communication is not an instructional procedure per se, it is a support/adaptation that may facilitate speech and language acquisition and reduce problem behaviors (Ganz et al., 2012; Lal, 2010; Schlosser & Wendt, 2008). As noted in the introduction to this chapter, significant communication needs is a defining characteristic of children with autism. Many young children with autism have little or no spoken language and therefore may have a difficult time communicating their desires and needs. Chapter 10 notes that challenging behavior most often serves a communicative function. This implies that problem behavior is occurring because appropriate communication skills are lacking.

Augmentative communication provides an alternative means for children who do not speak to express their wants and needs. As reviewed in Chapter 13, there are a number of augmentative communication systems and modes from which to select, including gestures, sign language, and visual systems (symbols, pictures, and/or photographs) that may be arranged in books, on boards, or on key rings. Electronic devices, including ones that "speak," are also available. Although visual systems in books or on key rings are popular because they are portable and can be understood by a wide audience, one system is not inherently better than another. Indeed, some children will use a combination of systems. The important thing is that all children have an effective means to express themselves. If children are not talking by age 2, they should be taught some form of augmentative communication. Research indicates that augmentative systems do not interfere with the development of speech and may actually facilitate speech (Ganz et al., 2012; Schlosser & Wendt, 2008).

Speech pathologists are important members of the intervention team for children with autism and may be instrumental in developing and teaching a child to use an augmentative communication system. Once a communication mode and system have been selected, instructional considerations mentioned previously in this chapter (direct instruction, naturalistic instruction, general case instruction, cues, and prompt and cue fading) should be incorporated into the instructional plan to teach the child to use the augmentative system. The

Picture Exchange Communication System (PECS) is a pictorial augmentative communication system developed specifically for children with autism. It is described in detail later in this chapter.

Positive Behavior Support

As previously mentioned, children with autism commonly have severe behavioral challenges associated with their communication needs. Chapter 10 describes the positive behavior support model designed to identify the function of problem behavior, prevent the need for problem behavior, teach alternative replacement behaviors (usually communication skills), and eliminate the reinforcement that maintains the challenging behavior. Because it is a communication-based approach (Carr et al., 1994), positive behavior support is particularly well suited to children with autism who often have significant communication needs (Vismara & Rogers, 2010). Positive behavior support strategies should be incorporated throughout a child's day and across the adults and settings the child frequents.

Summary of Instructional Procedures

The eight instructional approaches addressed in this chapter (direct instruction, naturalistic instruction, general case instruction, cues, fading prompts and cues, group instruction, augmentative communication, and positive behavior support) are addressed in detail in other chapters in this text. They are highlighted here because they address one or more of the unique learning characteristics and needs of children with autism. Direct instruction is an effective teaching strategy because children with autism have a learning preference that appreciates consistency. On the other hand, the strong preference for sameness that children with autism tend to have mitigates against generalization. Naturalistic instruction and general case instruction are proven approaches that facilitate generalization during the initial acquisition stage of learning. A preference for sameness also means that prompt fading must be planned and implemented very carefully to ensure independent responding and prevent prompt dependence. Group instruction addresses the social needs of children with autism to develop peer relationships and associated communication skills. And finally, augmentative communication and positive behavior support address the considerable needs that most children with autism have relative to communication and social skills.

SPECIALIZED PROCEDURES FOCUSED ON CHILDREN WITH AUTISM

In addition to the instructional procedures described above and in other chapters, this text presents instructional procedures that have been developed specifically for children with autism. Some are variations of the procedures just described; others are unique. The special procedures described in this section are not exhaustive, but they are ones used extensively with children who have autism. There are five special procedures: 1) discrete trial training, 2) floortime, 3) PECS, 4) visual supports, and 5) peer-mediated intervention.

Discrete Trial Training

Discrete trial training (DTT) is a direct instruction method. It is typically conducted in a one-to-one teaching arrangement in which an interventionist implements a direct instructional plan repeatedly. The repeated trials format is contrary to the earlier recommendations in this chapter that direct instruction be implemented throughout the day at times when a skill is needed, often using naturalistic (milieu) teaching strategies. Although the repeated trials format is associated with generalization concerns, DTT is the foundation of the Lovaas Institute developed and directed by Ivar Lovaas, a leading researcher in the field of autism. The name Lovaas has come to be almost synonymous with DTT. Lovaas has held firm to his belief that DTT should be central to intervention for young children with autism and points to program evaluation data as support for his position (Lovaas, 1987; McEachin et al., 1993). Note that DTT is *not* a comprehensive behavioral intervention program for young children with autism; it is an instructional component of a broader intervention program (Steege et al., 2007).

As indicated, DTT is a repeated trials arrangement of direct instruction. Skills are taught with a consistent delivery of a prompt, correction(s), and reinforcement. When one trial is completed, the next trial begins. It is common to present 10 to 20 trials of DTT per skill. If a child is being taught to recognize his printed name, for example, two cards are placed on a table in front of him, one with his printed name and one with another name. The child is prompted, "Timmy, point to your name." When Timmy points to his name (with or without additional prompts), he is reinforced as indicated in the instructional plan. The two cards are then rearranged in front of Timmy and the instructional plan is implemented again. This process is repeated until the specified number of trials has been conducted.

Although recommended practices for children with severe disabilities include more naturalistic trial arrangements with instruction occurring throughout the day and embedded in meaningful activities (Barton et al., 2012), there may be situations when the repeated trials format of DTT would be more effective than the distributed trial arrangement. Bambara and Warren (1993) suggested that repeated trials are well suited to shaping new behaviors. Over successive repeated trials, the adult or teacher can gradually modify and reduce prompts, requiring that the child perform the skill with increasing independence. It is also easier to ensure that a sufficient number of trials are conducted each day and that instruction is implemented consistently when a repeated trials format is used. Another advantage of repeated trials for children with autism is that they fit with learning styles that are characterized by orderliness and consistency.

DTT may be a primary method of instruction for some children with autism. However, it is essential that strategies for generalization be implemented for all instructional objectives. The highly systematized and consistent nature of DTT may facilitate initial skill acquisition, but it will also hinder generalization. Strategies such as naturalistic instruction (milieu teaching), general case instruction, and other generalization techniques (e.g., mediate generalization, use of naturally occurring reinforcers; see Chapter 6) must be implemented concurrently with DTT.

Floortime

Floortime is the cornerstone of the Developmental, Individual-Difference-Based (DIR) intervention model for young children with autism (Greenspan & Wieder, 2006). The DIR model and floortime procedures emphasize following a child's lead to establish communicative interactions, building social relationships, supporting affective development, and facilitating sensory development. This approach is in clear contrast to the DTT model, which is highly directive and controlled by the teacher. In floortime, the parent or teacher attempts to enter the child's world by joining the play or activity initiated by the child. In contrast, the objective of DTT is to shift the child's focus from her own world to the world beyond herself by attending to the adult or teacher, following directions, and participating in activities initiated by the adult or teacher.

Parents are often the primary interventionists in conducting floortime because the strategy is designed to build or strengthen a child–adult relationship—a relationship that is often weak or severely lacking when the child has autism. Floortime sessions are typically conducted for 20 to 30 minutes, 8 to 10 times per day, with the overall amount of intervention varying from 10 to 25 hours per week (Schertz & Odom, 2004). Floortime is conducted by first observing the child and deciding how to approach and enter the play. In observing the play, the child's emotions and temperament are noted. Next, the adult approaches by acknowledging the child's emotional states and interests ("You are excited about collecting your dinosaurs and putting them all in the same place"). The adult may then enter the child's play by assisting with the activity, being careful to let the child direct the course of events and set the emotional tone. The adult can also extend and expand the child's play, making supportive comments and being careful not to be intrusive. Supportive comments may be descriptive of the activity ("I think you've found all the dinosaurs") or tone ("You are so happy to have the dinosaurs all together!") and may include statements or questions that clarify and support creativity ("The dinosaurs seem happy to be together. Can other animals join them? Which ones? Now that they are all together, what are the dinosaurs going to do next?"). When the child responds by building on the adult's comments, he closes the *circle of communication*. The child's responses may be verbal ("The dinosaurs are family. They live together.") or nonverbal (the child picks up a dinosaur, looks at its face, smiles, and makes the dinosaur dance). It is up to the adult to follow the child's lead, enter the play again, and open a new circle of communication. The floortime strategy can be used with functional and/or socially influenced play, as well as perseverative, stereotypic play. In addition, floortime can be conducted even if a child says "no" by commenting and building on the child's mood and response ("You don't want anyone else to touch your dinosaur." "Should I put it back?" "Where should I put it?").

In addition to following a child's lead and expanding on her play, floortime can include adult responses that 1) obstruct the child's play and create problems to be solved; 2) introduce symbolism (pretend play with objects, dress-up, puppetry); 3) develop abstract thinking by talking about feelings, alternative outcomes to problem situations, a wide range of real and pretend topics, and asking questions ("why" questions, opinions); and 4) develop motor planning skills by helping children learn to "undo" situations (uncover a hidden toy, fix a mistake with a puzzle) and engage in multiple-step activities. Typically, the adult challenges the child gently with attempts to open communication circles and responds empathically and supportively to the child's mood and reactions.

Picture Exchange Communication System

For many children with autism, understanding the meaning and use of language is a primary communication concern. Language meaning, or *semantics*, requires a cognitive understanding of objects, actions, and how the environment "works." Language use (or *pragmatics*) involves social knowledge and includes skills such as conversational turn taking and using words and a voice tone appropriate for the social rules of the situation. Pragmatics also includes an understanding that language is a communication tool used to accomplish objectives. For example, if we are thirsty we use language to ask for a drink of water, or if we don't understand something, we ask for clarification. Some children with autism have speech that is limited to *echolalia*, repeating what others say to them apparently without understanding the communication. In other situations, children with autism memorize phrases and sentences from observation of others or DVDs, television, and other media. Some of these children use the memorized phrases and sentences appropriately to comment while playing or to respond to others' comments and questions. Sometimes only the adults most familiar with the child (parent or skills trainer) recognize the origins of the language. Although these children have difficulty generating novel communications (and this ultimately restricts their communication abilities), they demonstrate functional levels of semantic and pragmatic skills because they can use the phrases and sentences effectively.

PECS is an augmentative communication approach designed to address the semantic and pragmatic communication needs of children with autism (Frost & Bondy, 1994). PECS uses photographs or simple line drawings to create communication books and schedules. Children use the pictures and symbols to communicate by removing them from the book or schedule and handing them to an adult. For example, a child may take a "breakfast" picture (line drawing showing bowl and cup) off the daily schedule and hand it to her mother as they walk to the table for breakfast. When breakfast is finished and the child needs to wash up for school, she returns to the schedule, places the breakfast picture on it, removes the bathroom picture, and hands it to her parent. By using the communication pictures and symbols in a schedule, a child learns that symbols have meaning. Concurrently, the PECS schedule helps the child learn daily routines and expectations. This creates meaning and expectations in the child's life and establishes a context for communication. Although the child may not initially comprehend the word "breakfast," following repeated use of the PECS breakfast symbol she may come to understand that the symbol means it's time for the morning meal.

The PECS program is detailed in a training manual and uses basic behavioral intervention techniques, such as shaping and reinforcement, for instruction (Frost & Bondy, 1994). Children are first taught to use individual pictures to initiate a request. To avoid prompt dependency and promote initiations, verbal prompts are not used. The program then builds vocabulary and sentence structure, beginning with the simple grammatical form "I want _____." Children are also taught to comment and respond to questions. PECS is used widely and regarded as an effective and worthwhile program (Boyd et al., 2010; Siegel, 2000; Vismara & Rogers, 2010; Yamall, 2000). Although there are a number of published reports describing its effectiveness (Bondy & Frost, 1993, 1994; Peterson, Bondy, Vincent, & Finnegan, 1995; Schwartz, Garfinkle, & Bauer, 1998), experimental data supporting its use are just beginning to emerge in the literature (Charlop-Christy, Carpenter, Le, LeBlanc, & Kellet, 2002; Yoder & Stone, 2006a, 2006b).

Visual Supports

As noted, many children with autism respond better to visual than to auditory stimuli. Recognizing this characteristic, picture schedules have been used to teach children with autism to transition from one activity to the next (Boyd et al., 2010). Picture schedules may be created as a list of the day's activities noted in both words and photos or line drawings. The adult reviews the list with the child before beginning the set of activities and then draws the child's attention to the list again as one activity ends and the next is to begin. Sometimes, as described earlier in this chapter, a picture schedule is used in conjunction with PECS. In using a PECS picture schedule, a child removes the corresponding PECS symbol at the beginning of the activity and then returns it to the schedule at the conclusion of the activity. The remaining PECS symbols are removed and returned to the schedule successively as the child proceeds through the day's activities. Visual cues have also been successfully used to teach children symbolic play and social-communication skills.

Peer-Mediated Intervention

Teaching peers without disabilities to promote communication and social skill use among children with disabilities is referred to as peer-mediated intervention. The effectiveness of these procedures has been demonstrated in inclusive early childhood settings since the late 1970s (Ragland, Kerr, & Strain, 1978; Sperry, Neitzel, & Engelhardt-Wells, 2010) and are discussed in detail in Chapter 12. The procedure is to teach young children without disabilities to initiate interactions with their peers with autism ("Sherry, I have the blocks. Please play with me.") or to be responsive to interaction attempts (responding with "Hi Sherry! Do you want to share my snack?"). For children with autism who rarely initiate or respond to their peers, peer-mediated interventions support the reciprocal nature of social interactions and are, therefore, a crucial component of inclusive programs serving young children with autism (Odom & Strain, 1986).

MODEL PROGRAMS FOR CHILDREN WITH AUTISM

While research-supported instructional techniques are a critical component of early childhood education for young children with autism, many have significant needs that are best addressed through a comprehensive intervention program. Seven exemplary programs for children with autism are described here. These programs were selected because they represent a growing number of well-established interventions, are supported with program evaluation data and/or experimental data, and represent comprehensive approaches to addressing the needs of children with autism (Odom et al., 2010). Note, however, that no single program is universally effective for all children with autism (Howlin et al., 2009; Reichow & Wolery, 2009). Three of the seven programs are inclusive early childhood programs.

1. Learning Experiences and Alternative Program for Preschoolers and their Parents: LEAP

2. Developmental, Individual-Difference, Relationship-Based Approach: DIR

3. Developmentally Appropriate Treatment for Autism: Project DATA

4. Treatment and Education of Autistic and Related Communication Handicapped Children: Project TEACCH

5. Lovaas Institute

6. Pivotal Response Training

7. Denver Model

LEAP, Project DATA, and a part of the Denver Model called Early Start are inclusive early education models. Project TEACCH is a model that can be implemented in segregated or inclusive settings. Lovaas Institute, Pivotal Response Training, and DIR are usually conducted in segregated settings (at least initially).

There is consensus that intervention for children with autism needs to start early (often before a child is 2 years old) and must be fairly intense (sometimes 30 to 40 hours per week) (Strain et al., 1998). A key difference among the model programs is the extent to which the intervention approaches are intrusive or nonintrusive. An intrusive program is one requiring that the child attend and follow the instructions of the adult or teacher. Nonintrusive approaches attempt to enter the child's world and capture his attention without interference or upset. Two behavioral models, the Lovaas Institute and Pivotal Response Training, are fairly intrusive models. Project TEACCH is less intrusive, and the DIR model is perhaps the least intrusive approach.

Learning Experiences and Alternative Program for Preschoolers and Their Parents: LEAP

LEAP, an inclusive early childhood education model, was developed in 1981 by Strain et al. at the University of Pittsburgh and implemented in public school settings (Strain, Barton, & Dunlap, 2012). It was the first inclusive public-school-based model for young children with autism. LEAP includes intensive behavioral, data-based interventions and develops strategies to promote child engagement in activities and with peers. The peer-mediated interventions described in the previous section of this chapter and in detail in Chapter 12 were developed through LEAP. The model is now well established and has been replicated numerous times (Strain & Bovey, 2011). Replications begin in typical preschools by first establishing high-quality preschool instruction for typically developing children (several different early childhood curricula have been used in the replication sites). In addition to peer-mediated intervention, key features of the model include incidental instruction on individual education program objectives embedded into daily routines and activities and extensive family training focused on the behavioral needs of the children with autism in home and community settings. Recent research indicates that LEAP has strong empirical support and meets the stringent criteria of being an evidence-based practice (National Research Council, 2001; Odom et al., 2010; Strain & Bovey, 2011; Vismara & Rogers, 2010).

Developmental, Individual-Difference, Relationship-Based Approach

The floortime procedures reviewed earlier in this chapter were developed through the DIR model, designed by Stanley Greenspan at the George Washington University Medical School in the District of Columbia (Greenspan & Wieder, 2006). The DIR model focuses on broad developmental areas of need—such as emotional development—rather than on specific skill needs or skill areas, as in the Lovaas Institute program and Pivotal Response Training. Greenspan views autism as a multisystem regulatory disorder affecting sensory processing, reactions to stimuli, and the forming of relationships.

The focus of DIR is on nurturing the child's development of self and self-expression. Individualized intervention plans are designed based on an assessment that produces a functional developmental profile. The profile indicates a child's strengths and needs related to emotional development; sensory, modulation, processing, and motor planning; and relationships and interactions. An individualized plan for a child is comprehensive and includes floortime (following the child's lead; problem-solving activities; motor and sensory activities); speech therapy; sensory integration therapy (occupational and/or physical therapy); a daily educational program (inclusive program when possible); perhaps biomedical intervention (e.g., medications that might help a child's attending); and a consideration of nutrition, diet, and other programs designed to improve sensory motor skills.

Developmentally Appropriate Treatment for Autism: Project DATA

Developed by Ilene Schwartz and her colleagues at the University of Washington, Project DATA is a model program designed to merge recommended practices in early childhood education with those in early childhood special education and autism (Boulware et al., 2006). Unlike the other model programs, the central feature of Project DATA is a high-quality, inclusive early childhood program designed in accordance with developmentally appropriate practice (see Chapter 1). Children with autism attend the early childhood program for approximately 12.5 hours per week. Individualized instruction is provided by embedding the instruction in the ongoing classroom activities and routines. Strategies that promote generalization and maintenance are also implemented in regular classroom activities. The other components of Project DATA were developed to support the success of each child with autism in the inclusive early childhood program. These support components include

1) extended instructional time, 2) technical and social support for families, 3) collaboration and coordination across services, and 4) transition support. Extended instructional time provides approximately 8 additional hours per week of individualized intensive services focused on each child's individual needs. Intensive services may include a range of effective approaches such as DTT, naturalistic instruction (milieu teaching), and embedded instruction. Technical and social support for families consists of monthly home visits, resource coordination (e.g., child care, parent support groups, community services), parent support and networking get-togethers, and a father's evening. Collaboration and coordination across services helps facilitate communication among professionals who provide services to the family and/or child but are not a part of Project DATA (e.g., a family may hire a speech therapist for their child). And finally, transition support involves strategies to assist the family and child as the child exits Project DATA and enters a new school (often a public school).

Treatment and Education of Autistic and Related Communication-Handicapped Children: Project TEACCH

Project TEACCH was developed in the early 1970s by Eric Schopler at the University of North Carolina at Chapel Hill (Mesibov, 2005). TEACCH is a statewide program serving infants through adults with autism and their families in North Carolina. The model utilizes a combination of approaches to design an individualized program based on a child's skills, interests, and needs. Intervention approaches are selected to fit with the culture of autism or the learning preferences of many individuals with autism; for example, a preference for sameness and consistency or a preference for visual prompts rather than verbal ones. Individual programs designed through Project TEACCH emphasize altering the environment to accommodate the characteristics of a child (e.g., allowing a child to maintain orderly arrangements of items), using visual organizers (e.g., picture schedules), implementing work systems (e.g., daily work organized in baskets), and providing direct instruction. More so than the model programs discussed thus far, TEACCH includes a family support component and considers aspects of an individual's life beyond independent work skills (e.g., communication, social, leisure areas). As noted above, TEACCH can be implemented in segregated or inclusive settings (Carnahan, Harte, Schumacher, Hume, & Borders, 2011).

Lovaas Institute

Developed by Ivar Lovaas in the 1960s at the University of California–Los Angeles, the Lovaas Institute (also known as the Young Autism Project) has the longest history of the programs described here. Without question, it is the program with the largest database. As noted earlier, DTT is the central feature of the program. DTT procedures, data collection strategies, scheduling and implementation recommendations, and programs (i.e., lessons) are fully described in a published manual (Lovaas, 2002). Instruction covers 15 areas, all of which are addressed within a year's time. Program areas focus on self-help, early academics, and communication skills and include the following: establishing cooperation with simple requests; matching and sorting;

early receptive language; nonverbal imitation; play skills; verbal imitation; receptive labels; arts and crafts; self-help skills; expressive labels; reading and writing; color, shape, and size; "I want, I see, I have"; prepositions; and emotions. Most of the intervention is conducted in a one-to-one situation, with the child and the interventionist seated across from each other. Following 6 to 12 months of intensive one-to-one intervention, Lovaas recommends that children gradually be moved into nursery or preschool programs with an individual assistant.

Lovaas has reported that nearly half of the children with autism who participated in the Lovaas Institute have "recovered" (Lovaas, 1987; McEachin et al., 1993). He defined recovery as having an adequate IQ and the ability to participate in mainstream education. There has been much controversy in response to the Lovaas data and the claims of recovery (Mesibov, 1993; Schopler, Short, & Mesibov, 1989), with most of the criticisms and questions focused on the manner in which participants were selected (i.e., were they representative of most children with autism, or were they primarily children with mild autistic characteristics?) and the outcome measures (i.e., do the assessment tools adequately measure the most important behavioral concerns of children with autism?). A recent evaluation of the Lovaas Institute program across 12 samples of children yielded mixed results, including the failure of some children to benefit from the program (Howlin et al., 2009; Reichow & Wolery, 2009). Despite the controversy and limitations, there is widespread agreement that children who participate in the program frequently make substantial skill gains (Eldevik et al., 2009).

Pivotal Response Treatment

The pivotal response treatment model (Koegel & Koegel, 2012) developed by Lynn and Robert Koegel and their colleagues at the University of California–Santa Barbara is an outgrowth of the Lovaas Institute. The Koegels worked with Lovaas in the 1970s and developed their model to address what they believed were some of the shortcomings of the Lovaas Institute, primarily the artificial nature of the intervention situation, the appearance that children were unhappy during DTT, and issues with generalization. The Koegels believed that children with autism could be self-motivated. Their model uses behavioral procedures (direct instruction) and provides intervention in the context of play and functional activities. Child choice is incorporated throughout the model. They have also built a theoretical framework that defines and provides a rationale for identifying *pivotal responses,* key skill areas that can greatly enhance the overall development of children with autism. Pivotal response areas are the core of their approach.

Pivotal responses refer to skill areas that, when acquired, produce "large, collateral improvements in other areas" (Koegel, Koegel, Harrower, & Carter, 1999). The model is described as an efficient intervention approach because it targets skills that affect wide areas of functioning and does not simply teach a series of isolated skills. Pivotal response areas were identified as key areas for intervention because they are typically high-need areas for children with autism. There are four pivotal response areas: 1) responsivity to multiple cues, 2) motivation, 3) self-management, and 4) self-initiations.

Responsivity to multiple cues, the first pivotal response area, addresses stimulus overselectivity, a characteristic of many children with autism. Stimulus overselectivity means that a child has difficulty attending to multiple cues and instead focuses on a limited number of stimulus features or characteristics, often irrelevant ones. While a teacher is providing instructions for a new activity, for example, a child with stimulus overselectivity is focused on the buzzing of a fluorescent light. Stimulus overselectivity results in serious difficulties in acquiring social and language skills and a failure to generalize, because the children do not attend consistently to their social world. In pivotal response training, direct instruction is used to highlight relevant stimulus characteristics and requires that a child respond to multiple cues.

Motivation, the second pivotal response area, is evident when a child responds often and quickly to instruction and shows indications of positive affect, such as interest, enthusiasm, and happiness. Increases in motivation have been associated with decreases in disruptive behaviors. Motivational strategies include providing choices throughout the day, using natural and functional reinforcers (rather than artificial ones), interspersing maintenance trials (practice with previously acquired skills) with acquisition trials, and reinforcing attempts.

The third pivotal response area is *self-management*. It is considered a critical skill for success in inclusive environments. Self-management includes the child setting goals and selecting reinforcers, self-monitoring progress, and requesting reinforcement when appropriate. The self-monitoring strategy used to teach children to be aware of their own behavior is gradually faded, and the generalization of self-monitoring to natural environments is assessed.

The fourth pivotal response area is the communication skill of *self-initiation*. It refers to spontaneously asking questions, seeking information, and initiating conversations. Such skills are often lacking in children with autism but are critical for learning in natural environments without adult intervention.

Denver Model

The Denver Model and the Early Start Denver Model—a counterpart for toddlers—are inclusive intervention models that adhere to a framework that integrates applied behavior analysis, the developmental model, and a relationship-based approach (Dawson et al., 2010; Rogers & Dawson, 2009). Intervention is intensive and applies ABA principles to teaching skills of joint attention and engagement, interpersonal interaction, and verbal and nonverbal communication. There is also a strong parent-training component. The model follows an interdisciplinary approach, including speech, occupational, and physical therapists, to address children's needs across the range of developmental areas. Intervention occurs in natural environments, such as the home and inclusive preschool settings. A recent controlled experimental study of Early Start was conducted with children beginning the program before age 2.5 years. Compared to children with autism in existing community programs, children in the experimental group made significant improvements on measures of intelligence, adaptive behavior, and language, and children in the experimental group were significantly more likely to have an improved status on measures associated with the severity of their autism diagnosis (Dawson et al., 2010).

SUMMARY

Autism is a diagnosis based on social and communication difficulties, an obsession with sameness and/or stereotypy, and self-stimulation. These unique characteristics have implications for instruction. This chapter reviewed several instructional approaches described elsewhere in this text that have been shown to be effective with children who have autism. These strategies include 1) direct instruction, 2) naturalistic instruction, 3) general case instruction, 4) cues (versus general prompts), 5) prompt and cue fading, 6) group instruction, 7) augmentative communication, and 8) positive behavior support. They are highlighted here because they address the unique educational needs of children with autism and are well suited to the learning styles of most children with autism. In addition, DTT, floortime, PECS, visual supports, and peer-mediated intervention were described—five instructional approaches developed specifically for children with autism. The chapter concluded with descriptions of seven model programs: LEAP, DIR, Project DATA, Project TEACCH, Lovaas Institute, Pivotal Response Treatment, and the Denver Model.

STUDY QUESTIONS

1. Describe the learning characteristics of children with autism. For each characteristic you identify, discuss the ways (positive and negative) that it might affect learning.

2. Briefly describe the eight general instructional procedures (direct instruction, naturalistic instruction, general case instruction, cues, prompt and cue fading, group instruction, augmentative communication, positive behavior support) reviewed in this chapter. Describe why each of these procedures may be important to providing effective instruction for children with autism.

3. Define *discrete trial training (DTT)*. Discuss the pros and cons of using this procedure.

4. What is *floortime*? Compare and contrast it to DTT.

5. Describe how you might use PECS to help a 4-year-old child with autism who doesn't speak to participate in an inclusive preschool classroom.

6. Define and describe the four pivotal response areas of the *pivotal response treatment program*. Propose an intervention strategy to teach a skill in each of the four areas.

7. Discuss several ways that Project DATA merges recommended practices for children with autism.

8. Drawing from previous chapters that have discussed culture and learning, discuss cultural issues that might affect parents' receptivity to each of the model programs for children with autism.

REFERENCES

American Psychiatric Association. (2013). *Diagnostic and statistical manual of mental disorders: DSM-V*. Arlington, VA: American Psychiatric Publishing, Inc..

Autism Society of America. (n.d.). *Diagnosis*. Retrieved from http://www.autism-society.org/about-autism/diagnosis

Bambara, L.M., & Warren, S.F. (1993). Massed trials revisited: Appropriate applications in functional skill training. In R.A. Gable & S.F. Warren (Eds.), *Strategies for teaching students with mild to severe mental retardation* (pp. 165–190). Baltimore, MD: Paul H. Brookes Publishing Co.

Bambara, L.M., Warren, S.F., & Komisar, S. (1988). The individualized curriculum sequencing model: Effects on skill acquisition and generalization. *Journal of the Association for Persons with Severe Handicaps, 13*, 8–19.

Baron-Cohen, S., Leslie, A.M., & Frith, U. (1985). Does the autistic child have a "theory of mind"? *Cognition, 21*(1), 37–46.

Barton, E., Lawrence, K., & Deurloo, F. (2012). Individualizing interventions for young children with autism in preschool. *Journal of Autism and Developmental Disorders, 42*(6), 1205–1217.

Bondy, A.S., & Frost, L.A. (1993). Mands across the water: A report on the application of the picture exchange communication system in Peru. *The Behavior Analyst, 16*, 123–128.

Bondy, A., & Frost, L. (1994). The picture exchange communication system. *Focus on Autistic Behavior 9*, 1–19.

Boulware, G.L., Schwartz, I.S., Sandall, S.R., & McBride, B.J. (2006). Project DATA for toddlers: An inclusive approach to very young children with autism spectrum disorder. *Topics in Early Childhood Special Education, 26*(2), 94–105.

Boyd, B.A., Odom, S.L., Humphreys, B.P., & Sam, A.M. (2010). Infants and toddlers with autism spectrum disorder: Early identification and early intervention. *Journal of Early Intervention, 32*(2), 75–98.

Carnahan, C., Musti-Rao, S., & Bailey, J. (2009). Promoting active engagement in small group learning experiences for students with autism and significant learning needs. *Education and Treatment of Children, 32*(1), 37.

Carnahan, C., Harte, H., Schumacher, K., Hume, K., & Borders, C. (2011). Structured work systems: Supporting meaningful engagement in preschool settings for children with autism spectrum disorders. *Young Exceptional Children, 14*(1), 2–16.

Carr, E.G., Levin, L., McConnachie, G., Carlson, J.L., Kemp, D.C., & Smith, C.E. (1994). *Communication-based intervention for problem behavior: A user's guide for producing positive change.* Baltimore, MD: Paul H. Brookes Publishing Co.

Carr, J.E., Nicolson, A.C., & Higbee, T.S. (2000). Evaluation of a brief multiple-stimulus preference assessment in a naturalistic context. *Journal of Applied Behavior Analysis, 33*(3), 353–357.

Charlop-Christy, M.H., Carpenter, M., Le, L., LeBlanc, L.A., & Kellet, K. (2002). Using the Picture Exchange Communication System (PECS) with children with autism: Assessment of PECS acquisition, speech, social-communication behavior, and problem behavior. *Journal of Applied Behavior Analysis, 35*, 213–231.

Collins, B.C., Gast, D.L., Ault, M.J., & Wolery, M. (1991). Small group instruction: Guidelines for teachers of students with moderate to severe handicaps. *Education and Training in Mental Retardation, 26*, 18–32.

Dawson, G., & Osterling, J. (1997). Early intervention in autism. In M.J. Guralnick (Ed.), *The effectiveness of early intervention* (pp. 307–326). Baltimore, MD: Paul H. Brookes Publishing Co.

Dawson, G., Rogers, S., Munson, J., Smith, M., Winter, J., Greenson, J., Donaldson, A., & Varley, J. (2010). Randomized, controlled trial of an intervention for toddlers with autism: The Early Start Denver Model. *Pediatrics, 125*(1), e17–e23.

Eldevik, S., Hastings, R.P., Hughes, J.C., Jahr, E., Eikeseth, S., & Cross, S. (2009). Meta-analysis of early intensive behavioral intervention for children with autism. *Journal of Clinical Child & Adolescent Psychology, 38*(3), 439–450.

Frost, L.A., & Bondy, A.S. (1994). *The picture exchange communication system training manual.* Cherry Hill, NJ: Pyramid Educational Consultants.

Ganz, J.B., Earles-Vollrath, T.L., Heath, A.K., Parker, R.I., Rispoli, M.J., & Duran, J.B. (2012). A meta-analysis of single case research studies on aided augmentative and alternative communication systems with individuals with autism spectrum disorders. *Journal of Autism and Developmental Disorders, 42*(1), 60–74.

Greenspan, S.I., & Wieder, S. (2006). *Engaging autism: Using the floortime approach to help children relate, communicate, and think.* Boston, MA: Da Capo Press.

Hagopian, L.P., Rush, K.S., Lewin, A.B., & Long, E.S. (2001). Evaluating the predictive validity of a single stimulus engagement preference assessment. *Journal of Applied Behavior Analysis, 34*, 475–485.

Hanley, G.P., Iwata, B.A., Thompson, R.H., & Lindberg, J.S. (2000). A component analysis of "stereotypy as reinforcement" for alternative behavior. *Journal of Applied Behavior Analysis, 33*, 285–297.

Howlin, P., Magiati, I., & Charman, T. (2009). Systematic review of early intensive behavioral interventions for children with autism. *Journal on Intellectual and Developmental Disabilities, 114*(1), 23–41.

Individuals with Disabilities Education Improvement Act (IDEA) of 2004, PL 108-446, 20 U.S.C. §§ 1400 *et seq.*

Kanner, L. (1943). Autistic disturbances of affective contact. *Nervous Child, 2,* 217–250.

Kleeberger, V., & Mirenda, P. (2010). Teaching generalized imitation skills to a preschooler with autism using video modeling. *Journal of Positive Behavior Interventions, 12*(2), 116–127.

Koegel, R.L., & Koegel, L.K. (2012). *The PRT Pocket Guide: Pivotal Response Treatment for Autism Spectrum Disorders.* Retrieved from Education Resource Information Center website: http://www.eric.ed.gov/ERICWebPortal/recordDetail?accno=ED531708

Koegel, L.K., Koegel, R.L., Harrower, J.K., & Carter, C.M. (1999). Pivotal response intervention: I. Overview of approach. *Journal of the Association for Persons with Severe Handicaps, 24,* 174–185.

Koegel, R.L., & Rincover, A. (1974). Treatment of psychotic children in a classroom environment: I. Learning in a large group. *Journal of Applied Behavior Analysis, 7,* 45–49.

Lal, R. (2010). Effect of alternative and augmentative communication on language and social behavior of children with autism. *Educational Research and Reviews, 5*(3), 119–125.

Leaf, J.B., Dotson, W.H., Oppeneheim, M.L., Sheldon, J.B., & Sherman, J.A. (2010). The effectiveness of a group teaching interaction procedure for teaching social skills to young children with a pervasive developmental disorder. *Research in Autism Spectrum Disorders, 4*(2), 186–198.

Lovaas, O.I. (1987). Behavioral treatment and normal educational and intellectual functioning in young autistic children. *Journal of Consulting and Clinical Psychology, 55,* 3–9.

Lovaas, O.I. (2002). *Teaching individuals with developmental delays: Basic intervention techniques.* Austin, TX: PRO-ED.

Lovaas, O.I., Koegel, R.L., & Schreibman, L. (1979). Stimulus overselectivity in autism: A review of research. *Psychological Bulletin, 86,* 1236–1254.

Lovaas, O.I., & Schreibman, L. (1971). Stimulus overselectivity of autistic children in a two stimulus situation. *Behaviour Research and Therapy, 9,* 305–310.

Love, J.R., Carr, J.E., Almason, S.M., & Petursdottir, A.I. (2009). Early and intensive behavioral intervention for autism: A survey of clinical practices. *Research in Autism Spectrum Disorders, 3*(2), 421–428.

Matson, J.L., & Smith, K.R.M. (2008). Current status of intensive behavioral interventions for young children with autism and PDD-NOS. *Research in Autism Spectrum Disorders, 2*(1), 60–74.

McClannahan, L.E., & Krantz, P.J. (1993). The Princeton Child Development Institute. In S.L. Harris & J.S. Handleman (Eds.), *Preschool education programs for children with autism* (pp. 107–126). Austin, TX: Pro-Ed.

McEachin, J.J., Smith, T., & Lovaas, O.I. (1993). Long-term outcome for children with autism who received early intensive behavioral treatment. *American Journal of Mental Retardation, 97*(4), 359–372.

McGee, G.G., Morrier, M.J., & Daly, T. (2000). The Walden early childhood programs. In *Preschool Education Programs for Children with Autism* (pp. 157–190). Austin, TX: PRO-ED.

Mesibov, G.B. (1993). Treatment outcome is encouraging. *American Journal of Mental Retardation, 97,* 379–380.

Mesibov, G.B. (2005). *What is TEACCH?* Retrieved May 23, 2005, from University of North Carolina at Chapel Hill, TEACCH website: http://www.teacch.com

National Research Council. (2001). *Educating children with autism.* Washington, DC: National Academies Press.

Northup, J. (2000). Further evaluation of the accuracy of reinforcer surveys: A systematic replication. *Journal of Applied Behavior Analysis, 33,* 335–338.

Northup, J., George, T., Jones, K., Broussard, C., & Vollmer, T. (1996). A comparison of reinforcer assessment methods: The utility of verbal and pictorial choice procedures. *Journal of Applied Behavior Analysis, 29,* 201–212.

Odom, S.L., Boyd, B.A., Hall, L.J., & Hume, K. (2010). Evaluation of comprehensive treatment models for individuals with autism spectrum disorders. *Journal of Autism and Developmental Disorders, 40*(4), 425–436.

Odom, S.L., Brown, W.H., Frey, T., Karasu, N., Smith-Canter, L.L., & Strain, P.S. (2003). Evidence-based practices for young children with autism: Contributions from single-subject design research. *Focus on Autism and Other Developmental Disabilities, 18*(3), 166–175.

Odom, S.L., & Strain, P.S. (1986). A comparison of peer-initiation and teacher-antecedent interventions for promoting reciprocal social interaction of autistic preschoolers. *Journal of Applied Behavior Analysis, 19*(1), 19–59.

Pace, G.M., Ivancic, M.T., Edwards, G.L., Iwata, B.A., & Page, T.J. (1985). Assessment of stimulus preference and reinforcer value with profoundly retarded individuals. *Journal of Applied Behavior Analysis, 18*, 249–255.

Peterson, S.L., Bondy, A.S., Vincent, Y., & Finnegan, C.S. (1995). Effects of altering communicative input for students with autism and no speech: Two case studies. *Augmentative and Alternative Communication, 11*, 93–100.

Premack, D., & Woodruff, G. (1978). Does the chimpanzee have a theory of mind? *Behavioral and Brain Sciences, 1*(4), 515–526.

Ragland, E.U., Kerr, M.M., & Strain, P.S. (1978). Behavior of withdrawn autistic children: Effects of peer social initiations. *Behavior Modification, 2*(4), 565–578.

Reichow, B., & Wolery, M. (2009). Comprehensive synthesis of early intensive behavioral interventions for young children with autism based on the UCLA young autism project model. *Journal of Autism and Developmental Disorders, 39*(1), 23–41.

Rogers, S.J., & Dawson, G. (2009). *Early Start Denver Model for young children with autism: Promoting language, learning, and engagement.* New York, NY: Guilford Press.

Sandall, S.R., Ashmun, J.W., Schwartz, I.S., Davis, C.A., Williams, P., Leon-Guerrero, R.M., Boulware, G.L., & McBride, B.J. (2011). Differential response to a school-based program for young children with ASD. *Topics in Early Childhood Special Education, 31*(3), 166–177.

Schertz, H.H., & Odom, S.L. (2004). Joint attention and early intervention with autism: A conceptual framework and promising approaches. *Journal of Early Intervention, 27*, 42–54.

Schlosser, R.W., & Wendt, O. (2008). Effects of augmentative and alternative communication intervention on speech production in children with autism: A systematic review. *American Journal of Speech-Language Pathology, 17*(3), 212–230.

Schopler, E., Short A., & Mesibov, G. (1989). Relation of behavioral treatment to normal educational functioning: Comment on Lovaas. *Journal of Consulting and Clinical Psychology, 57*, 162–164.

Schwartz, I.S., Garfinkle, A.N., & Bauer, J. (1998). The picture exchange communication system: Communicative outcomes for young children with disabilities. *Topics in Early Childhood Special Education, 18*, 144–159.

Siegel, B. (2000). Behavioral and educational treatments for autism spectrum disorders. *The Advocate, 33*, 22–25.

Simpson, R.L. (2005). Evidence-based practices and students with autism spectrum disorders. *Focus on Autism and Other Developmental Disabilities, 20*(3), 140–149.

Sperry, L., Neitzel, J., & Engelhardt-Wells, K. (2010). Peer-mediated instruction and intervention strategies for students with autism spectrum disorders. *Preventing School Failure: Alternative Education for Children and Youth, 54*(4), 256–264.

Stahmer, A.C., & Ingersoll, B. (2004). Inclusive programming for toddlers with autism spectrum disorders: Outcomes from the children's toddler school. *Journal of Positive Behavior Interventions, 6*(2), 67–82.

Steege, M.W., Mace, F.C., Perry, L., & Longenecker, H. (2007). Applied behavior analysis: Beyond discrete trial teaching. *Psychology in the Schools, 44*(1), 91–99.

Stokes, T.F., & Baer, D.M. (1977). An implicit technology of generalization. *Journal of Applied Behavior Analysis, 10*, 349–367.

Strain, P.S., Barton, E.E., & Dunlap, G. (2012). Lessons learned about the utility of social validity. *Education and Treatment of Children, 35*(2), 183–200.

Strain, P.S., & Bovey, E.H. (2011). Randomized, controlled trial of the LEAP model of early intervention for young children with autism spectrum disorders. *Topics in Early Childhood Special Education, 31*(3), 133–154.

Strain, P.S., Wolery, M., & Izeman, S. (1998). Considerations for administrators in the design of service options for young children with autism and their families. *Young Exceptional Children, 1*(2), 8–16.

Vismara, L.A., & Rogers, S.J. (2010). Behavioral treatments in autism spectrum disorder: What do we know? *Annual Review of Clinical Psychology, 6,* 447–468.

Wetherby, A.M., Prizant, B.M., & Schuler, A.L. (2000). Understanding the nature of communication and language impairments. In B.M. Prizant & A.M. Wetherby (Eds.), *Autism spectrum disorders: A transactional developmental perspective* (Vol. 9, pp. 109–141). Overland Park, KS: AAPC.

Yamall, P. (2000). Current interventions in autism: A brief analysis. *The Advocate, 33,* 25–27.

Yoder, P., & Stone, W.L. (2006a). Randomized comparison of two communication interventions for preschoolers with autism spectrum disorders. *Journal of Consulting and Clinical Psychology, 74*(3), 426–435.

Yoder, P., & Stone, W.L. (2006b). A randomized comparison of the effect of two prelinguistic communication interventions on the acquisition of spoken communication in preschoolers with ASD. *Journal of Speech, Language, and Hearing Research, 49*(4), 698–711.

10
Challenging Behavior

Mary Jo Noonan

FOCUS OF THIS CHAPTER

- Levels of intervention for challenging behavior
- Positive behavior support at the tertiary level
- Functional assessment: why, with whom, and when does challenging behavior occur?
- Hypothesis development and verification
- Design of positive behavior support plans

Most challenging behavior of young children is within the bounds of developmental expectations. It is resolved through maturation, general parenting, and developmentally appropriate practices in early childhood education. For example, a toddler may cry when corrected or frustrated, a preschooler may hit a peer to obtain a toy, and a kindergarten child may talk back to a parent. Without specialized assessments and intervention, the toddler who screams will probably learn to use words to express her feelings, the preschooler will develop patience and learn the rules about sharing and turn taking, and the kindergarten child will come to understand that he must listen and be polite when corrected for misbehavior. Although these behaviors can be frustrating to professionals and parents, they are typical behaviors of the early childhood years and not cause for alarm. Professionals who work with young children must remember that on a daily basis children are confronted with the complex task of learning socially appropriate behavior. Rather than focusing attention on managing misbehavior, a proactive approach to helping children learn appropriate behavior should be emphasized.

LEVELS OF INTERVENTION FOR CHALLENGING BEHAVIOR

For approximately 10% of preschool-age children, however, challenging behaviors may be extreme and require specialized intervention (Kupersmidt, Bryant, & Willoughby, 2000). Addressing behavioral challenges in the preschool years is vitally important, as there is research suggesting that preschoolers with behavior problems are expelled at three times the rate of students in kindergarten through grade 12 (Gilliam, 2005). Furthermore, longitudinal studies indicate that early behavior problems are strong predictors of ongoing behavior problems into the elementary and secondary school years (Brennan, Shaw, Dishion, & Wilson, 2012).

Current intervention models for addressing problem behavior during the early childhood years follow a programwide approach (Benedict, Horner, & Squires, 2007; Hemmeter, Fox, Jack, & Broyles, 2007; Lewis, Beckner, & Stormont, 2009; Muscott, Pomerleau, & Szczesiul, 2009). These models draw from approaches to positive behavior support (PBS) for elementary- and secondary-age students (c.f. Sugai et al., 2000) and generally include three levels of intervention. They have been demonstrated to be effective in home and inclusive community preschool settings. As described by Benedict et al. (2007), the levels become increasingly more focused on individual child needs and increasingly more intense:

- The primary level is the classroom, school, or program level that addresses all children, staff, and settings. The focus is on establishing and maintaining a safe and predictable environment for young children and promoting positive relationships. This level of behavior support includes strategies such as explicit classroom rules and clearly marked activity areas. The primary level of PBS is sufficient for preventing and intervening with the behavioral challenges of approximately 80% of the children.

- The secondary level may be necessary for approximately 15% of the children. These are children with at-risk behaviors, such as more marked social skill and behavioral needs (children who have difficulty following directions or children who grab and yell rather than ask to join a playgroup).

Secondary-level positive supports are targeted interventions conducted with the entire class or small groups of children. These interventions may involve commercially available social skill curricula or teacher-constructed strategies, such as teaching cooperation and friendship skills (Powell, Dunlap, & Fox, 2006).

- The tertiary level is the most intense level of PBS. This level of intervention is individualized and is required for only about 5% of the children in early childhood settings. These are the children who do not respond to the primary and secondary levels of the model and have chronic and/or severe challenging behavior. Programs that implement a schoolwide PBS model have a leadership team that helps guide the planning, assessment, implementation, and data-based monitoring of tertiary-level interventions.

This chapter is concerned with interventions for chronic and serious challenging behaviors that require tertiary-level interventions.

POSITIVE BEHAVIOR SUPPORT AT THE TERTIARY LEVEL

At the tertiary level, PBS is a multicomponent intervention model that 1) includes families as team members in assessment, planning, intervention, and monitoring; 2) assesses when, where, with whom, and why challenging behavior occurs; 3) restructures environments, lifestyles, and activities to prevent further occurrences of challenging behavior; and 4) teaches appropriate social-communication behaviors that serve the same purpose as challenging behavior. The PBS model emphasizes the use of proactive, educational, and reinforcement-based methods (Powell et al., 2006). A basic premise of PBS is that challenging behavior is a method of communication for the child. Thus, it is important to identify what the child is communicating with the challenging behavior so that a socially appropriate replacement behavior may be identified and taught.

PBS differs from more traditional behavioral approaches in several important ways (see Table 10.1):

- Traditional behavioral approaches are narrowly focused on the child and on reducing or eliminating the child's challenging behavior. In contrast, PBS emphasizes that behavior occurs in context. It focuses not only on the child and the challenging behavior but also on understanding and modifying broad and specific environmental variables, including the physical setting, overall lifestyle, activities, schedules, persons present, nature of social interactions, and events preceding and following the challenging behavior (Luiselli & Cameron, 1998).

- Traditional behavioral assessment focuses on the topography (physical characteristics and appearance) and quantification of the challenging behavior: What does it look like and how often does it occur? In contrast, PBS emphasizes a two-part functional assessment. The first part is identifying variables that predict the occurrence of the challenging behavior and, alternatively, the occurrence of appropriate behavior in the same types of situations. The second part is identifying the function of the challenging behavior (usually a communication function). The function of a problem behavior is its purpose or the reason *why* the behavior occurs.

Table 10.1. Comparison of traditional behavioral approaches and positive behavior support

Elements of approach	Traditional behavioral approach	Positive behavior support
Focus	Challenging behavior	Environment, child, challenging behavior, communication need (replacement behavior)
Assessment	Description and quantification of challenging behavior (what, when, where, with whom, frequency, rate, duration, intensity)	Function (purpose) of challenging behavior and conditions associated with occurrence/nonoccurrence of challenging behavior, and alternative appropriate behavior
Intervention	Punishment or other aversive techniques	Environmental preventive arrangements and reinforcement-based instruction

- Traditional behavior modification approaches rely on punishment or other aversive interventions to decrease or stop the challenging behavior. In contrast, PBS uses positive interventions that address the function of the challenging behavior. These interventions include arranging the environment to prevent or eliminate the need for challenging behaviors and teaching socially appropriate replacement behaviors (behaviors that serve the same purpose as challenging behaviors).

The PBS model evolved to address efficacy and ethical issues associated with traditional behavioral approaches that relied on punishment and aversive techniques. First, behavior reductions obtained through punishment and aversive interventions were frequently not maintained and were often accompanied by increases in new challenging behaviors. PBS addresses these concerns by teaching new socially appropriate behaviors that serve the same purpose as the challenging behaviors. Such new behaviors receive the same reinforcers and thus are maintained (e.g., if crying and calling for a parent both serve the same purpose of getting parental attention, parental attention is the reinforcer for both behaviors). Second, many professionals are uncomfortable with the use of punishment or aversive interventions for ethical reasons: Physical punishments (e.g., water mist, forced exercise, electric shock) and restraints that would not be considered appropriate for individuals without disabilities should not be used with children who have disabilities. An additional ethical concern is that undesirable side effects, such as aggression or withdrawal, frequently occur with punishment. A final issue is that punishment or aversive procedures are insufficient interventions because they do not result in the child learning appropriate behavior. PBS addresses this issue because it is an educational approach that always includes an instructional component to teach a socially acceptable replacement behavior.

Major Components of the Positive Behavior Support Model

The PBS model has three major components: a crisis plan, functional assessment, and a support plan. The crisis plan is an emergency plan focused on stopping the behavior and maintaining safety should the challenging behavior occur prior to developing and implementing the support plan or should

Table 10.2. Tertiary level of the positive behavior support model

Components

Functional assessment
- Purpose/function of challenging behavior
- Contextual antecedent variables and triggers

Support plan
- Crisis management procedures
- Supports to prevent challenging behavior
- Supports to encourage appropriate behavior
- Supports to teach effective replacement behaviors
- Supports to maintain and generalize behavior changes
- Data-based monitoring

the challenging behavior occur despite having the support plan in place. It is not an intervention (Carr et al., 1994). Functional assessment includes various evaluation methods directed at determining the purpose (i.e., *function*—and there may be more than one) of the challenging behavior as well as identifying environmental and antecedent situations associated with the occurrence and nonoccurrence of the challenging behavior (Powell et al., 2006). A hypothesis of the function of the challenging behavior provides direction for selecting a socially appropriate replacement behavior. Understanding situations and variables associated with the occurrence and nonoccurrence of challenging behavior is important for designing environmental arrangements that prevent challenging behavior and support socially appropriate replacement behaviors. The support plan is a multicomponent strategy built on the information obtained in the functional assessment. A support plan includes preventive strategies and supports for appropriate behavior, replacement behaviors, and maintenance and generalization (Carr et al., 1994; Janney & Snell, 2000). Table 10.2 summarizes the components of the PBS model. Each of these components will be discussed in detail in the remainder of the chapter.

Influences on Appropriate and Challenging Behavior

Before turning attention to the details of implementing the PBS model, it is important to consider the variables that influence whether challenging behavior occurs or not. Four influences are social judgment, maintaining variables, variables that trigger challenging behaviors, and contextual influences.

Social Judgment Whether a behavior is considered a problem or not is a matter of opinion, or social judgment. Behavior is essentially "neutral" and is considered a problem only when someone decides that it is inappropriate. In early intervention and early childhood special education, that person might be a parent, a close family friend, or a professional who is involved with the child. Because it is a subjective decision, it is possible that all members of a child's team might not agree that the behavior is a problem. Furthermore, each individual's judgment of whether the behavior is a problem has a number of influences, including culture, education, experiences, relationships and history with the child, child development philosophies and perspectives, expectations for children, and so forth. For example, if a toddler yells out after she eats each bite of food, her mother may find this very upsetting and even embarrassing because she is concerned that it means her child is not well behaved or dislikes mealtime. In contrast, a speech-language pathologist might be delighted, assuming that the child is attempting to communicate a request for more food. Who is correct about whether or not challenging behavior exists in these situations? This is a question that can only be answered by the entire team. However, as noted earlier, family concerns should always be viewed as important and valid and should usually carry more weight than professional opinion in decision making.

Variables that Maintain Behavior A basic principle of behavior is that if it is being maintained or is increasing, it is being reinforced. A corollary is that if the behavior is being reinforced, it is serving a purpose or function for the child. Thus, to effectively decrease or eliminate challenging behavior, it is necessary to conduct assessments that will identify the reinforcer. This tells us why a child is engaging in the behavior. It answers the question, "What does the child *get* for the behavior?" With a hypothesis of what the reinforcer is, supports can be designed to eliminate reinforcement of the challenging behavior, thus rendering it ineffective (O'Neill et al., 1997), and to provide reinforcement for socially acceptable replacement behavior.

The reasons or purposes for challenging behavior are referred to as *functions*. There are four possible functions for challenging behavior: gaining attention; obtaining something tangible; escaping, terminating, or avoiding something; or self-regulation (self- or sensory-reinforcement) (Carr et al., 1994; Janney & Snell, 2000, Neilsen & McEvoy, 2004). If someone consistently and immediately approaches a child or talks to her when she engages in challenging behavior, *gaining attention* is a plausible hypothesis. The response may appear to be positive, such as redirecting the child to do something else or complimenting an appropriate behavior that occurred just prior to the challenging behavior. The response may be sympathetic, such as holding the child and preventing the challenging behavior, or it may be a reprimand ("Stop that! Throwing things is not okay."). Regardless of the nature or tone of the response, if an individual usually responds to a behavior, attention may be the purpose.

The second function of challenging behavior is to obtain something tangible, such as a toy or food. It might be that the child requests something and is initially denied. When the request is not granted, challenging behavior occurs (e.g., a tantrum) and continues until finally the adult gives in and provides the desired item. In some situations, challenging behavior will serve to stop, escape, or avoid an undesirable situation or activity. This is the third function. For example, a child may repeatedly and forcibly kick the crib when placed in it for bedtime. If the typical result is removal from the crib, the child may be escaping the undesirable situation of having to go to bed. Finally, performing challenging behavior may be reinforcing to the child in that it provides sensory stimulation. For example, head banging may mask the pain of an ear infection, eye poking may provide interesting visual stimulation for a child who is blind, and continuous rocking may be soothing to a child. Challenging behaviors that function as self-reinforcement are particularly difficult to decrease or eliminate because the variables that maintain the behavior reside within the child (internal stimulation) rather than as part of the social context that is more easily altered. Fortunately, most challenging behavior is not maintained by self-reinforcement.

Variables that Trigger Behavior Although reinforcers are a powerful variable in maintaining and increasing behavior, specific events that precede a behavior can significantly affect whether or not it occurs. These *triggers* are called discriminative stimuli, or S^Ds (Carr, Carlson, Langdon, Magito-McLaughlin, & Yarbrough, 1998). They are specific events that prompt or cue behavior. For example, saying "No. That's not the way to do that!" may trigger a tantrum. Although knowing the trigger for a behavior does not tell us the purpose or function of the behavior, this information is important for assessment and planning because triggers can be highly predictive of appropriate and inappropriate behavior. If we can identify the trigger for a particular challenging behavior, we can eliminate or avoid that trigger and instead include triggers associated with appropriate behavior.

Contextual Influences The context of challenging behavior refers to the physical, temporal, social, and physiological situation associated with the challenging behavior (Carr, Reeve, & Magito-McLaughlin, 1996). All elements of the context have the potential to increase or decrease the likelihood that challenging behavior will occur. For example, a child might be more likely to refuse to do schoolwork if it is a warm day (physical context), if it is late in the day (temporal context), if the classroom is crowded and bustling with activity (social context), or if she slept poorly the night before (physiological context). Variations in contextual influences may result in differing opinions among team members regarding the occurrence or seriousness of the challenging behavior. However, contextual influences are critical assessment data that may suggest situations when challenging behavior is most likely to occur and when interventions are most needed.

These four major influences on behavior—social judgment, maintaining variables, variables that trigger challenging behavior, and contextual influences—are addressed throughout the remainder of this chapter. They determine whether professionals and parents judge that challenging behavior exists and are critical assessment data for constructing effective PBS plans.

FUNCTIONAL ASSESSMENT: WHY, WITH WHOM, AND WHEN DOES CHALLENGING BEHAVIOR OCCUR?

As discussed in Chapter 3, assessment includes a broad array of approaches to evaluate a child's strengths and needs in the home and other environments. Assessment for the purpose of developing a PBS plan examines the physical and social context in which challenging behavior occurs. Examining the context of challenging behavior produces information about why it occurs (function), with whom it occurs (social context), and when it occurs (physical and/or social context). It may also illuminate similar contexts in which challenging behavior does not occur. Information about the function and context of challenging behavior is best obtained using multiple assessment strategies, such as interviews and observational assessment (Neilsen & McEvoy, 2004).

Interviews

Interviews provide assessment data gathered from persons who are well acquainted with the young child exhibiting the challenging behavior. It is common to interview one or both parents and sometimes other family members, babysitters, early intervention personnel, early childhood educators, and others who see the child regularly. The interview questions are designed to elicit specific information about the behavior, the child's current communication and social skills, and the context in which the behavior occurs (Neilsen & McEvoy, 2004). Observational assessment is also conducted to validate the interview data, provide quantifiable data, and examine data in situations not covered by the interview. Sample questions included in a functional assessment interview are listed in Table 10.3.

Table 10.3. Questions frequently asked in a functional assessment interview

Challenging behavior

1. What are the behaviors that concern you?
2. What do they look like?
3. How often do they occur (per hour, day, or week)?
4. How intense are they? How do you judge how intense they are?

Communication and social skills

1. How does the child communicate basic needs such as hunger, thirst, or discomfort (wet diaper, not feeling well)?
2. How does the child communicate a desire for attention or to be held?
3. How does the child reject something, indicate "no," and express a preference?
4. For which adults or children does the child show a clear preference?
5. Does the child play simple turn-taking games (e.g., peekaboo)? Please describe.
6. How does the child respond to new social situations (e.g., going to a playground for the first time, having visitors)?
7. How does the child interact when other children are present?

Physiological context

1. Are there concerns related to eating?
2. Are there concerns related to sleeping?
3. What is the child's typical sleep schedule?
4. Does the child have allergies?
5. Does the child have frequent ear infections or other respiratory illnesses?
6. Does the child have any chronic health concerns?
7. Does there seem to be any relationship between challenging behavior(s) and eating, sleeping, and/or other health concerns?

Social context

1. Is there a particular person who is usually present when challenging behavior(s) occurs?
2. Are there particular social situations that seem to be associated with challenging behavior(s)?

Environmental and activity context

1. What is the child's typical daily schedule?
2. Is there a particular place or activity that seems to be associated with challenging behavior(s)?
3. Is there a particular place or activity that is likely to be free of challenging behavior(s)?
4. What are the child's favorite places and activities?

Cultural Considerations When the professional conducting a functional assessment interview is of a culture different from that of the child's family, the interviewer must use effective cross-cultural communication skills. The interviewer must be aware of how culture affects values, judgments, and attitudes concerning challenging behavior, assessment, and intervention. In their model of cross-cultural competence, Kalyanpur and Harry (1999) suggested that the professional must first be aware of the influences of culture on personal beliefs and values concerning disabilities, families, and the issues being addressed. These are one's own cultural biases. If a professional is aware of personal biases, he or she can recognize that such beliefs and values are subjective and neither right nor wrong. Next, Kalyanpur and Harry recommend that the professional adopt a stance of *cultural reciprocity,* sharing personal values and beliefs with families. Personal disclosure invites families to respond likewise by sharing their own values and beliefs. As professionals and parents get to know one another through cultural reciprocity, they may develop a relationship built on mutual understanding and trust.

As noted earlier, cultural differences among professionals and families may account for disparities in judgments as to the extent to which a behavior is or is not considered a challenge or problem. Culture may affect a family's participation in assessment and intervention as well as their comfort level associated with implementing recommendations from professionals. Throughout the assessment and intervention process, it is critical that professionals respect and honor family perspectives while continuing to build cultural reciprocity in their relationship.

Observational Assessment

Information obtained through interviews will indicate times and situations associated with the challenging behavior. It may also suggest probable hypotheses about the purpose that the challenging behavior is serving. This preliminary information is useful for planning times to conduct observational assessment. The purposes of observational assessment are to 1) confirm that the challenging behavior exists, 2) document occurrences of the challenging behavior, 3) provide information on the contexts of the challenging behavior and variables associated with it, and 4) formulate hypotheses about the function (purpose) of the behavior. Recognizing that challenging behavior usually serves a communicative purpose ("I want attention," "I don't want to do this," "I want that _____"), each observation of the challenging behavior may be recorded on a notecard describing its social context. Carr et al. (1994) suggested that notecards include the following contextual information: interpersonal situation (who is present), behavior, and social consequence (what someone says or does when the challenging behavior occurs). Figure 10.1 is a sample of an observation recorded in this manner.

Another format for recording observations of challenging behavior is an A-B-C record (Bijou, Peterson, & Ault, 1968). *A* represents the *antecedents* (conditions or events) that precede the challenging behavior, *B* represents the *behavior* (the challenging behavior and any other child behaviors), and *C* is the *consequence.* An A-B-C record is typically written on a piece of paper divided into three columns labeled A, B, and C. As in the example shown in Figure 10.1,

Observation of challenging behavior		
Child: Chelsea	**Observer:** Toni	**Date:** 5/22/13
Challenging behavior: Hits her head with her fist		**Activity:** Sandbox
Interpersonal context: Two girls (toddlers) and one boy (4 years old) in sandbox; Chelsea's mom and two other moms are watching from a park bench at the edge of the sandbox. **Behavior:** Chelsea takes shovel from one of the girls. The girl takes it back. Chelsea hits herself in the head six times. **Social consequence:** Chelsea's mom goes to the sandbox, tells Chelsea not to do that, and hands Chelsea her own shovel.		

Figure 10.1. Sample notecard: Observed social context of challenging behavior.

it is important that the social situation (interpersonal context and social consequence) be recorded, given the assumption that challenging behavior usually serves a communicative function. In addition, the observer may write a continuous description of the situation(s) and child behaviors. This provides a rich description of the context of the child's behavior. It may also provide information about several events preceding the challenging behavior and may uncover behavior chains associated with challenging behavior. For example, Figure 10.2 is an A-B-C record of the same events noted on the observation card in Figure 10.1. The A-B-C record reveals that Chelsea asked for the shovel twice before she took it from the toddler. Knowing that taking the toy was not Chelsea's first attempt to obtain it suggests that it might be possible to intervene before Chelsea's behavior escalates to challenging behavior.

Observational assessment should be conducted across several activities, settings, and days to obtain sufficient information about the contexts and variables associated with challenging behavior. In reviewing A-B-C records or behavioral observation cards, the consequences suggest the purpose or function of the behavior. In the example illustrated in Figure 10.1 and 10.2, the consequences are attention from the child's mother and receipt of the requested item. The A-B-C record also reveals a behavioral chain of two ineffective (but socially appropriate) verbal requests preceding the challenging behavior. In this instance, the challenging behavior occurred only after the peer took the shovel back from Chelsea. This suggests that Chelsea's challenging behavior was triggered by the physical action of the toddler taking the toy rather than the verbal refusals that preceded the physical action. The antecedent situation of young children at play may also be associated with challenging behavior. It is plausible that Chelsea's challenging behavior occurs mostly with younger children who have not yet learned sharing or turn taking. Additional observations and A-B-C recordings will indicate whether these are plausible interpretations and predictable variables. Observations should be conducted until the information obtained indicates consistent patterns of consequences, behavioral chains, antecedent situations, and triggers. Sometimes observational assessment may be completed in a few hours, at other times, a few days.

HYPOTHESIS DEVELOPMENT AND VERIFICATION

Once the interview and observational assessment information yield a clear picture of the child's challenging behavior and associated variables, hypotheses

A-B-C assessment		
Child: Chelsea	**Observer:** Toni	**Date:** 5/22/13
Challenging behavior: Hits her head with her fist		**Activity:** Sandbox play
Antecedent	Behavior	Consequence
Two toddlers (girls) and one 4-year-old boy are playing in the sandbox when Chelsea arrives. Chelsea's mom sits down on a park bench at the edge of the sandbox; two mothers are sitting on another nearby bench.	Chelsea stands by her mom and watches the children play.	The children remain focused on their play. None of the children look at Chelsea.
Chelsea's mom: "It's O.K., Chelsea. You can play, too."	Chelsea looks at her mom and says "Pail, Mom."	Chelsea's mother hands her a pail and some other sand toys.
	Chelsea slowly enters the sandbox, and squats off to the side. She watches the other children.	The other children continue with their play and do not look at Chelsea.
	Chelsea moves close to the girls and watches them dig in the sand with their shovels.	One of the girls looks at Chelsea and then moves, turning her back to Chelsea.
	Chelsea reaches toward a shovel and says, "Please. Me play."	One girl looks at Chelsea. Both girls move away from Chelsea a bit.
	Chelsea reaches again and says, "Please."	One girl turns to her and shouts, "No!"
	Chelsea takes the shovel from the girl who shouted at her.	The girl takes the shovel back and says, "Mine."
	Chelsea backs away, hits herself on the head six times, and begins crying.	Chelsea's mom goes to the sandbox, tells her not to do that, and hands Chelsea her own shovel.
	Chelsea cries softly and begins digging in the sand with her shovel.	Chelsea's mom rubs her back and softly repeats, "It's O.K. It's O.K."

Figures 10.2. A-B-C record of challenging behavior (same situation as Figure 10.1)

about the function (purpose) of the behavior and when it is likely to occur (context and triggers) must be developed. These hypotheses will be used to guide the development of the PBS plan.

Hypotheses About Function

Knowing why a behavior occurs (its purpose) is essential information for identifying a socially appropriate communication behavior that will be taught as an alternative response to the challenging behavior. Hypotheses about function will indicate why a challenging behavior occurs. The effect produced by a behavior indicates its function. In other words, the consequence of a behavior reveals its purpose. Referring again to the scenario described in Figures 10.1 and 10.2: Why did Chelsea hit herself in the head? To develop a hypothesis to this question, look to the effect or consequence of the behavior: Chelsea hit herself to obtain adult attention and a desired object (her mother went to her and gave her a shovel). Observing and recording many observations of the challenging behaviors across a number of situations and times will help to determine if both functions (attention and obtaining a desired object) are typical or if one function occurs more frequently than the other.

As noted earlier, there are four possible functions of challenging behavior: gaining attention, obtaining something, escaping/terminating something, or providing self-reinforcement. Escaping/terminating something would be the hypothesis when the child does not have to do an activity or is removed from a situation as a result of challenging behavior. For example, if Chelsea's mother removed Chelsea from the sandbox when she hit herself on the head, the hypothesis would be that Chelsea hit herself to escape/terminate playtime in the sandbox. Escape is a fairly common function of challenging behaviors and is often accomplished through tantrums and aggression.

Self-reinforcement is the hypothesis when challenging behavior is not consistently associated with one of the other three functions (gaining attention, obtaining something, escaping/terminating something), all of which are *socially mediated*, that is, requiring another person to accomplish his or her purpose (Carr et al., 1994). When challenging behavior serves the function of self-reinforcement, the child is being reinforced by the behavior itself. Self-reinforcement is sometimes referred to as *self-regulation*. The function of self-regulation is to adjust the child's sensory experiences and internal state of stimulation: that is, feeling calm or being alert (Janney & Snell, 2000). For example, eye poking may produce sensations of light that the child finds very appealing; children who hit or bite themselves may experience a reduction or masking of another pain (like an earache or headache) or may feel a "high" sensation as chemical endorphins are released by the central nervous system to soothe their pain. Behaviors such as hand flapping may be self-stimulating and serve as entertainment or play. Numerous studies have shown that providing alternative sensory stimulation (headphones with music, decorative lights, handheld electronic games, and so forth) may result in a reduction in self-reinforcing challenging behavior (Kennedy & Souza, 1995).

Hypotheses About Context and Triggers

Although the effect or consequence of challenging behavior indicates why it occurs, the social situation and other antecedents suggest when it is likely to occur. Contextual variables may be physical, temporal, social, or physiological. Continuing to analyze the situation of Chelsea in the sandbox, contextual variables that might increase the likelihood of her engaging in challenging behavior include the physical variable of being in the sandbox (perhaps the texture of sand is unpleasant and makes her irritable), the temporal variable of having been away from home for 2 hours while her mother ran errands, the social variable of toddlers (who don't share!) or crowding (four children in a small sandbox), or the physiological variables of hunger (lunchtime is approaching) and fatigue (nap follows lunchtime). As in developing hypotheses about the function of challenging behavior, it is necessary to look at many instances of challenging behavior to develop reasonable hypotheses. Reviewing many observational records of challenging behavior may yield this example of a hypothesis about the context of a challenging behavior: Chelsea is most likely to engage in challenging behavior when she is playing near several young children in a crowded area.

As stated, *triggers* to challenging behavior are specific events or S^Ds (discriminative stimuli) that significantly affect whether a behavior occurs or not. In the example of Chelsea's self-injury, Chelsea hit her head immediately after the toddler took the shovel from her. Additional observational records should be reviewed to determine whether there are similar discrete events that immediately precede Chelsea's self-injury. A hypothesis about a trigger for her challenging behavior may be that Chelsea is likely to hit herself when an object is taken away from her.

It is tempting to look to the antecedents to hypothesize why a challenging behavior occurs (e.g., Chelsea wants the shovel back), but the context, conditions, or triggers do not reinforce (i.e., maintain or increase) challenging behavior. Similarly, the toddler taking the shovel from Chelsea isn't why Chelsea hit herself. The toddler taking the shovel from Chelsea was the trigger for Chelsea's self-injury. Parental attention or actually obtaining the desired object was the reinforcing consequence (the effect/purpose) of Chelsea's challenging behavior.

As evident in the above examples, it is possible to develop hypotheses about the function, antecedents, and triggers of challenging behavior for each observation, but more valid hypotheses are likely if numerous observations are reviewed. In many cases, challenging behavior will serve more than one function and have multiple antecedent conditions and triggers associated with it. A list of hypotheses should be developed following a thorough review of all interviews and observational records. The family should be an integral part of the assessment and interpretation process.

Functional Analysis

The only valid way to verify hypotheses about challenging behavior is to test each one through a brief experiment called *functional analysis* (Carr, 1977; Iwata, Dorsey, Slifer, Bauman, & Richman, 1982). This often requires the support of a behavior specialist who has expertise in functional analysis and is not a part of the social situations associated with challenging behavior. If a behavior specialist is available, it is advantageous to conduct the functional analyses before developing the PBS plan. The results of the functional analyses will increase the likelihood that the PBS plan addresses the true antecedents, triggers, and functions of challenging behavior. Often, however, the precision and rigor of functional analyses are not necessary when ample functional assessment information has been obtained (Horner, Albin, Todd, & Sprague, 2006). For this reason, full details of how to conduct functional analyses are not presented here. Instead, it is recommended that functional analyses be conducted only when a behavior specialist is available to provide the necessary assistance.

DESIGN OF POSITIVE BEHAVIOR SUPPORT PLANS

PBS plans are designed assuming that the hypotheses are correct. They also informally test the hypotheses. Hypotheses about antecedent conditions and triggers are used to develop strategies to prevent challenging behavior from occurring and to promote appropriate behavior. Hypotheses about the function(s) of challenging behavior are used to select socially appropriate behaviors that will be taught to the child as alternatives or replacement behaviors so that the challenging behavior is not necessary. Components of a comprehensive PBS plan are as follows:

1. Crisis management plan
2. Supports to prevent challenging behavior
   - Modify or eliminate contextual variables
   - Modify or eliminate triggers
   - Interrupt escalating chain of behavior
3. Supports to encourage appropriate behavior
   - Provide choice and high-preference situations
   - Embed cues
   - Present positive social comments
   - Create meaningful, interesting, and predictable routines and activities
   - Use supported routines, task simplification, and preteaching
4. Supports to teach effective replacement behaviors
   - Teach proactively
   - Teach functionally equivalent communication responses
   - Teach behaviors that are more effective than challenging behavior
5. Supports to maintain and generalize behavior changes
   - Teach *effective* replacement behaviors
   - Introduce delayed and intermittent reinforcement
   - Teach across people, places, and activities
   - Address all functions of challenging behavior concurrently
   - Teach in controlled situations first; then in less controlled situations
6. Data-based monitoring
   - Monitor challenging behavior
   - Monitor replacement behavior

Appendix 10.1 includes a sample PBS plan. The remainder of the chapter describes how to construct each component of a comprehensive PBS plan.

Cultural Considerations

As described earlier, culture will affect judgment concerning whether challenging behavior exists, interpretation of assessment information, and acceptability of intervention procedures. Professionals can facilitate family participation in designing intervention procedures by discussing the interpretation of assessment information and resultant hypotheses. Reviewing each instance of challenging behavior recorded during the observational assessment process can do this. First, discuss whether or not there is agreement that challenging behavior occurred during the observation. This will contribute to a continuing process of clarifying what is and is not challenging behavior (an issue that is highly influenced by culture). If there is agreement that challenging behavior occurred, come to consensus on the antecedents of and consequences to the challenging behavior during that specific observation. If the family was not present for that observation, describe the observed antecedents and consequences to the family. Finally, discuss a hypothesis about the function or *why* the challenging behavior occurred (referring to the consequences) and note if a contextual variable or trigger that might increase the likelihood of the challenging behavior was present (referring to the antecedents). The hypotheses are probably the most subjective and culturally influenced part of this process, but with continuous reference to the antecedents and consequences, it should be possible to reach consensus.

Crisis Management Plan

During the assessment and intervention phases of PBS, challenging behavior may sometimes occur. It is necessary to have a plan for responding when this happens. Sometimes the occurrence of challenging behavior will seem minor. At other times it may create a serious situation in which the behavior is intense or extreme, potentially placing the child or others in danger of harm. Whenever challenging behavior occurs—whether it is minor or severe—the family and professionals who support the child should respond following a preestablished crisis management plan. Note that this is not an intervention; it is an agreed upon strategy for minimizing the immediate effects of challenging behavior and keeping the child and others safe until the PBS plan begins to take effect.

Carr et al. (1994) provided five recommendations for a crisis management plan. First, occurrences of nonharmful challenging behavior may be ignored. The parent or professional who observes the occurrence can casually turn away and pretend that the behavior did not occur. Second, if it's not believable to pretend that the challenging behavior did not occur, calmly redirect the child's attention by introducing a cue for appropriate behavior. For example, if the child is angry and throws a toy, a parent might approach the child with a favorite book and say, "Let's read a story together." Third, if the behavior is intense or severe, furniture or other objects may have to be moved to prevent the child from becoming injured. Fourth, it may be prudent to request children who are nearby to move to another location. Fifth, it may be necessary to momentarily restrain the child. If the team developing the crisis management plan believes that restraint might sometimes be necessary, parents and professionals who may have to apply the restraint should receive training in the safe use of restraint. In reviewing these five suggestions, it should be apparent that they don't teach appropriate behavior; they only serve to stop the challenging behavior and protect the child and others. Remember, a crisis management plan is a short-term plan only and is not likely to eliminate challenging behavior or the need for a multicomponent PBS plan.

Supports to Prevent Challenging Behavior

The hypotheses developed from the assessment information may include one or more contextual variables (antecedent conditions or situations) or triggers that seem to predict when challenging behavior is likely to occur. The PBS plan modifies or eliminates these variables when reasonable to do so (Neilsen & McEvoy, 2004). For example, if Chelsea is most likely to engage in self-injury at the playground when she is in a small area crowded with other children, that situation can be eliminated. There are activity areas at the playground other than the sandbox. If the sandbox is crowded, her parent can take her to a less crowded area for play. When the entire playground is crowded, her parents can make note of such times and change their schedule for visiting the playground. Similarly, if taking an object from Chelsea is a trigger for self-injury, her play environments can be arranged to include more than one of each type of toy so that others will be less likely to take a toy from Chelsea. Play in proximity to very young children (1- through 3-year-olds) might also be avoided in favor of 4- and 5-year-olds, because the younger children are the ones who are most likely to take toys from others.

It is important to consider whether contextual variables and triggers associated with challenging behavior are necessary elements of a child's routines and activities. If, for example, Chelsea was going to start preschool in a few months, the PBS plan might initially include avoiding areas crowded with young children. The plan might also include a strategy to help Chelsea become accustomed to playing appropriately with an increasing number of young children in close proximity. If Chelsea has a younger sibling and/or is frequently with younger cousins, then it might not be feasible to remove the trigger of a child taking a toy from her. Other strategies that encourage appropriate behavior and teach socially appropriate replacement behaviors will have to be implemented, especially when the trigger is likely to be present.

In some situations, assessment information will have indicated that challenging behavior is associated with an escalating chain of behavior. For example, Chelsea made two verbal requests for the shovel that were unsuccessful (she was not given the shovel). Only then did she engage in self-injury. Additional assessment information might confirm whether Chelsea's challenging behavior typically follows multiple failed communication attempts. If this is confirmed as a behavior chain leading to self-injury, one preventive strategy to include in a PBS plan is to interrupt the escalating behavior chain (Kazdin, 2001). When Chelsea's communicative requests are unsuccessful, the parent or professional can interrupt the situation by restating the request and encouraging the other child or adult to fulfill the request, or the parent or professional can fulfill the request. If it's not appropriate or possible to satisfy Chelsea's request, she can be removed from the situation and redirected to another task that she enjoys.

Supports to Encourage Appropriate Behavior

In addition to strategies that prevent challenging behavior, a PBS plan should include contextual variables and triggers associated with appropriate behavior. Generally, high-preference, child-selected, and predictable situations, routines, and activities are associated with little or no challenging behavior

(Janney & Snell, 2000; Park & Scott, 2009). These antecedent/contextual variables provide the child with a sense of control.

Choice and High-Preference Situations, Routines, and Activities   Many children—and particularly those with disabilities—are given very little choice in their daily lives. Instead, adults orchestrate their routines and activities, generally so that the daily schedule is convenient for the adults. This doesn't mean the adults don't give any consideration to the children's preferences and interests, but the daily schedule is often far from what the children would choose if they had the opportunity to create their own schedules. Honoring a child's preferences not only gives the child some control over his or her daily life but communicates respect for the child.

For most children, the adult-constructed schedule is not a problem and includes many things that children enjoy. However, when children have severe challenging behavior they are often communicating a desire to control at least some of their world. As noted earlier, the purpose of most challenging behavior is to communicate "I want something" (attention, an object, or something to end/stop). Therefore, one way to decrease challenging behavior is to create a schedule reflecting child choice (Park & Scott, 2009). Such a schedule would include situations, routines, and activities that are highly preferred by the child. For an infant or young child with limited communication, this means that parents and professionals must carefully observe to determine what preferences and choices the child is expressing. For example, an infant may be extremely fussy and demonstrate challenging behavior in the early morning because she wants to get out of her crib immediately on wakening and eat, in contrast to staying in the crib until both parents finish showering and dressing. Parents might be willing to adjust their morning schedules and alternate one getting up and feeding the infant while the other showers. Allowing the child to choose her wake-up and feeding time may be all that is necessary to eliminate challenging behavior in the early mornings.

Embedded Routines and Cues for Appropriate Behaviors   Another strategy for encouraging appropriate behavior in situations in which challenging behavior frequently occurs is to introduce or embed routines or cues that prompt appropriate behavior (Carr et al., 1998). For example, Chelsea and her father may have a favorite routine in which Dad sings "Itsy Bitsy Spider" while walking his fingers up her leg, arm, neck, and face to the top of her head. Chelsea giggles with anticipation of the ticklish feeling whenever he does this. The song and the walking motion of Chelsea's father's fingers are routines and cues for appropriate behavior. The PBS plan can use this routine by embedding it at times they know Chelsea is likely to engage in self-injury. For example, when Chelsea is waiting her turn in a game with neighborhood children, her dad might unobtrusively sit behind her and sing softly in her ear and occasionally walk his fingers along her back or shoulders. Because this routine is associated with appropriate behavior, it may serve as a prompt for Chelsea to continue demonstrating appropriate behavior. Similarly, if Chelsea has learned to take turns when prompted by a timer, the cues of turning the timer to 5 minutes and stating, "O.K. Let's share this toy by taking turns every 5 minutes," could be introduced in the preschool setting.

Two strategies to encourage appropriate behavior related to embedding are *interspersed requests* (Horner, Day, Sprague, O'Brien, & Heathfield, 1991)—also known as *high probability requests* (Davis, Brady, Williams, & Hamilton, 1992)—and *positive social comments* (Kennedy, Itkonen, & Lindquist, 1995). The interspersed-requests strategy can encourage appropriate behavior for children who demonstrate challenging behavior when asked to follow directions. The procedure is to make a few short requests that are not associated with challenging behavior. Once the child has responded appropriately to easy requests, a more difficult request is made (difficult meaning that the request typically results in challenging behavior). An example would be asking a kindergarten child to take out his favorite pencil, point to a word that begins with the letter *b* (two easy requests), and copy the letter *b* (difficult request). The interspersed request strategy may be considered when a child has demonstrated the ability to respond to a request (i.e., the response has already been acquired) yet engages in challenging behavior when the request is presented. As discussed earlier, it is essential to consider whether demands being placed on a child are necessary and appropriate.

The *positive social comments* strategy is similar to interspersed requests, but rather than make requests, the adult makes several comments that are likely to put the child in a good mood prior to the difficult request. For example, a parent can say to a child, "Oh, you are holding your favorite Teddy. Teddy loves you!" (The parent makes the teddy bear hug the child.) "Teddy is happy to be with you. Here, take this medicine." (The parent gives the child a measured dose of an antibiotic the child doesn't like.)

Meaningful, Interesting, and Predictable Routines and Activities Just as the above strategy of positive social comments can put a child in a good mood and thereby decrease challenging behavior, constructing a child's experiences so that they are filled with meaningful, interesting, and predictable routines and activities can also promote a good mood and appropriate behavior (Hemmeter & Ostrosky, 2003). For an infant, toddler, or young child, meaningful and interesting routines and activities might include play situations (home, early childhood programs, parks, infant/toddler exercise groups), accompanying parents on errands, and typical activities of daily living. Although daily living activities such as mealtimes, bathing, and dressing may not seem inherently interesting, these activities can be done in ways that are sociable and enjoyable. Furthermore, when they are done in preparation for play or an outing, they may come to be associated with meaningful and interesting activities, and thus they become motivating.

Predictable routines and activities are associated with appropriate behavior because they provide order to the infant/young child's world. If the world is predictable, there is a feeling of control; the world is not full of unanticipated events and surprises. For example, if a child's morning routine is always the same—Mom or Dad wakes her up and cuddles her, changes her diaper and plays a little, gives her a morning bottle, and dresses her—the child will learn from the daily repetition that her bottle will be coming shortly after playtime. The child may not be aware that she knows this, but if the routine were not in place, she would feel uncertain as to when and if she would be fed each morning. Predictable routines are also an important foundation for language comprehension: The child is more likely to learn the meaning of "Time for breakfast!" if the phrase is said in the same context each day and is immediately followed by her bottle and some cereal. Improving language comprehension contributes to creating predictable routines and activities. It has also been shown to be associated with decreases in challenging behavior (Carr et al., 1994).

As children reach age 1, they usually begin to learn simple rules, such as where they may and may not play, things they may and may not touch, and so on. Simple rules teach children the expectations for appropriate behavior. Most children are highly reinforced by positive attention from their family members and other adults and thus are motivated to "be good," that is, to comply with expectations for appropriate behavior. Consistent enforcement of simple rules results in predictable responses from adults and thus promotes appropriate behavior. Having rules for young children does not imply that punishment or harsh consequences must be imposed for infringements. It does imply, however, that the child's behavior should be corrected (e.g., a firm "No") and redirected to appropriate behavior when rules are not followed.

Supported Routines, Task Simplification, and Preteaching Whether at home or in an early childhood education setting, if young children are being asked to perform tasks that are new and difficult, appropriate behavior during the tasks can be encouraged by providing assistance. Assistance can include *supported routines, task simplification,* or *preteaching.* Each of these strategies eases the demands being placed on the child. In supported routines, children are assisted in doing the most difficult parts of tasks that they are learning (Cameron, Maguire, & Maguire, 1998). Teaching is focused on the easiest portions of the task to minimize frustration and encourage participation. In task simplification, teaching an alternative, easier way to do a difficult task minimizes frustration (Kern & Dunlap, 1998). Preteaching (also known as *priming*) is practicing or rehearsing a task before it is required in a more demanding or independent situation (Koegel, Carter, & Koegel, 1998).

Supports to Teach Effective Replacement Behaviors

Antecedent approaches—supports to prevent challenging behavior and supports to encourage appropriate behavior—for the PBS plan have been described. Although these approaches are essential elements of a comprehensive PBS plan, they do not address the purpose or function of challenging behavior. A PBS plan must include a section on teaching an appropriate behavior that serves the same function as the challenging behavior. If the child accomplishes the desired effect with the new replacement behavior, challenging behavior is not needed. Replacement behaviors that serve the same function/purpose as challenging behaviors recruit the same reinforcement that maintained the challenging behaviors. A very powerful PBS plan can be created by implementing antecedent strategies (supports to prevent challenging behavior and supports to encourage appropriate behavior) in conjunction with teaching functionally equivalent replacement behaviors.

Proactive Instruction As noted throughout this chapter, the three major functions (purposes) of challenging behavior are to gain attention, to obtain something, and to escape/terminate something. Replacement behaviors for these functions must communicate "I want attention," "I want something," or "I don't want (to do) something." Teaching one or more of these replacement behaviors is *functional communication training* (Carr & Durand, 1985). To be effective, the function of the replacement behavior must match the function of the challenging behavior. In addition, effective replacement behaviors have the following characteristics:

- They are relatively simple responses for the child to make.
- They result in immediate reinforcement.
- The resulting reinforcement is more powerful than that for the challenging behavior (Horner & Day, 1991).

Replacement behaviors must be simple because the child is already skilled at responding with challenging behavior. If the new acceptable response is more difficult than the challenging behavior, the child's perspective may be that it is not worth the effort to use the new response—the same reinforcement can be obtained by using the easier challenging behavior. Challenging behavior, because of its intensity and seriousness, usually produces an immediate and powerful result. Therefore, if a socially appropriate behavior is going to be an effective replacement for challenging behavior, it must also produce an immediate effect. Finally, the reinforcement for the replacement behavior must be more powerful than that for the challenging behavior; otherwise the child will opt for using challenging behavior. Imagine the immediacy and strength of a parent's response when Chelsea hits herself in the head and begins to cry: Chelsea's mom calls from the park bench, "No, Chelsea!" as she runs to her. If Chelsea is taught to say "Please" as a replacement for self-injury when she wants something, her mother must respond as quickly and strongly as she would had Chelsea hit herself in the head: "Yes, Chelsea! You may play with the shovel." In this way Chelsea will learn that the replacement behavior can be more effective than the challenging behavior.

Socially appropriate replacement behavior must be taught proactively. The most effective instructional times will be situations in which the challenging behavior is likely (Carr et al., 1994). In our example of Chelsea playing in the sandbox, the PBS plan could include teaching the replacement behavior of saying "Please" in close proximity to toddlers playing with toys on the playground. The plan might state that Chelsea's mother will bring a bag with a number of high-preference and playground-type toys (sand toys, balls, sidewalk chalk, and so forth) and situate Chelsea near a group of toddlers each time they visit the playground. When Chelsea shows interest in the toddlers' toys (stares at the toys or the toddlers, moves closer to the toys or the toddlers, or reaches in their direction), her mother whispers "Please" in her ear. If Chelsea imitates "Please" or approximates it, her mother observes the toddlers' response. If the toddlers don't immediately pass Chelsea a toy, Chelsea's mother quickly offers her an appropriate toy and says, "Yes, Chelsea, you may play too." At any time, if Chelsea reaches for a toy that the toddlers are playing with, her mother immediately guides Chelsea's hand away from the toddlers and their toys, whispers "Please," hands Chelsea an appropriate toy, and says, "Yes, Chelsea, you may play too."

Responding immediately and with equal power reinforcement to new replacement behavior will initially place significant demands on the adults involved in a child's PBS plan. This is a necessary first step in teaching the child that his or her new responses are very effective. For the obvious reasons of making PBS a practical approach, it is also necessary to teach children to wait a short time for reinforcement and to use socially acceptable behavior even when every response is not reinforced (Carr et al., 1994). These concerns are addressed by supports to maintain and generalize behavior changes (discussed below).

Redirection Although a PBS plan will include a number of strategies to prevent challenging behavior and render it ineffective and unnecessary, the behavior may still occur on occasion. As indicated in the discussion of crisis management procedures, there must be a plan for responding to it. Janney and Snell (2000) suggested that the response to challenging behavior should be neutral (i.e., the content of the behavior is not responded to) and the child should be redirected to appropriate behavior. Redirection is modeling or prompting the child to engage in appropriate behavior that serves the same function as the challenging behavior. Ignoring without redirection may be ineffective because the child is not being taught the appropriate response for the situation.

Supports to Maintain and Generalize Behavior Changes

The final components of a comprehensive PBS plan are strategies that support the absence of challenging behavior and the use of new replacement behaviors over time (maintenance) and in new situations (generalization). If the new functional communication skills (replacement behaviors) are more effective and result in stronger reinforcement, they will maintain and replace challenging behavior. Maintenance can be further enhanced by gradually introducing intermittent and delayed reinforcement as is more common to natural situations (Carr et al., 1994). Naturalistic schedules of intermittent and delayed reinforcement will be more practical than the immediate and continuous schedule of reinforcement that is necessary when first teaching a replacement behavior. Furthermore, intermittent and unpredictable schedules of reinforcement are more powerful schedules of reinforcement and result in responses that are more difficult to extinguish.

Maintenance There are two strategies that are useful in helping a child accept delayed and less frequent reinforcement. The first strategy is to acknowledge the child's request, ask her to wait a few moments, and suggest that she do a simple, known task or activity while waiting (Carr et al., 1994). For example, if Chelsea says, "Please" while playing with her cousins, her mother may say, "Yes, Chelsea. I'll be right there with some toys for you. While you wait, please look through the book next to you." Using an activity to mark the duration of the delay in reinforcement provides the child with a concrete measure of time as well as a clear indication that reinforcement is imminent. It is imperative, of course, that Chelsea's mom follows through and gives Chelsea the requested toys as soon as Chelsea completes the book activity.

A second strategy for reducing the immediacy and consistency of reinforcement is behavioral chaining. This strategy is relevant when challenging behavior serves the purpose of escaping or ending an activity that the parents and professionals have decided is important and cannot be eliminated. In behavioral chaining, the required number of activity steps is gradually increased before providing reinforcement (Lalli, Casey, & Kates, 1995). For example, if a child engages in challenging behavior to avoid toothbrushing (and dental health problems have been ruled out as the reason he dislikes this activity), he may initially be required to brush just his front teeth. Once he has been doing this successfully and requesting "No more brushing" by shaking his head side to side, a second step of brushing his teeth on one side may be added. Thus, he is now required to brush his front teeth and his teeth on one side before he may request, "No more brushing." In this fashion, additional steps may slowly be added so that the child learns to complete the entire toothbrushing task before requesting a break.

Generalization A true measure of learning is when a child demonstrates a skill in an appropriate situation other than where it was taught. This is *generalization*. Generalization of replacement behaviors is critical to eliminating challenging behavior. But generalization of new skills cannot be assumed. Instead, planning and implementing specific strategies are required to ensure that generalization occurs.

Generalization may be facilitated from the onset when teaching functional communication skills (some approaches to generalization assume that new skills must first be acquired before generalization can be addressed). A well-proven strategy is to teach the new skill across naturalistic conditions and a range of people, places, and activities, rather than first teaching under isolated conditions (Kazdin, 2001). Teaching situations should be chosen carefully to represent the range of naturalistic situations that the child is likely to encounter. This means that when teaching Chelsea to say "Please" when she wants a toy, the instruction should be conducted by her mother, father, grandparent, and early intervention professional. A range of play situations with young peers should also be selected: at the park, at home with her siblings, at her grandparents' home with her cousins, and during her weekly neighborhood playgroup. Similarly, a range of play activities and materials should be represented (e.g., sand toys, books, crayons, small figurines, blocks).

The likelihood of generalization will also be enhanced if instruction addresses all functions of the challenging behavior concurrently (Carr et al., 1994). If the complete assessment of Chelsea's challenging behavior indicated that her self-injury served the purposes of requesting adult attention and obtaining something, instruction should address both concurrently. In situations in which Chelsea seems to be requesting a toy, her use of "Please" should be responded to with a toy and very positive and enthusiastic attention. And in situations when she does not seem to be requesting a toy, her use of "Please" should be followed with positive and enthusiastic adult attention.

If challenging behavior is particularly difficult to prevent in one or more situations, it is helpful to start with the easiest, most "controlled" situations (Carr et al., 1994). Controlled situations are those that have relatively few triggers for challenging behavior. For example, Chelsea's home and small neighborhood playgroup may be initial teaching situations with fewer distractions and triggers for challenging behavior than Chelsea's grandparents' home or the park. Once Chelsea is regularly using her new replacement communication skills at home and the neighborhood playgroup, instruction can be extended to her grandparents' home and the park.

Data-Based Monitoring

The final element of a comprehensive PBS plan is monitoring the results of implementation. Data collection procedures (as described in Chapter 6) should be conducted to monitor the elimination or decrease in challenging behavior and the acquisition or increase in functionally equivalent replacement behaviors. If the family chooses, they may participate in data collection; otherwise, the professional can collect data as feasible. The data should be reviewed regularly (every 1 to 2 weeks) and intervention plans modified if progress is not judged to be sufficient.

SUMMARY

Because of efficacy and ethical concerns, the traditional behavioral approach to challenging behavior has been replaced by a positive behavior support model. The PBS model is superior to the traditional behavior model because it is more likely to have durable effects and it relies on positive and preventive methods rather than on methods that are reactive and punitive. At the heart of the PBS model is the use of functional assessment to identify the purpose (or function) of challenging behavior. Generally, challenging behavior serves a communication function: gaining attention; obtaining something tangible; or escaping, terminating, or avoiding something. Knowing the purpose of challenging behavior provides direction for developing a PBS plan. All PBS plans include strategies to prevent the occurrence of problem behavior, to increase the likelihood of appropriate behavior, to teach socially appropriate behaviors that replace the challenging behaviors, and to promote maintenance and generalization of newly acquired skills.

STUDY QUESTIONS

1. Identify and describe the levels of intervention for challenging behavior.
2. Compare and contrast the traditional behavioral approach and the PBS approach to assessment and intervention for challenging behavior.
3. Discuss the efficacy and ethical issues associated with traditional behavioral approaches.
4. Discuss how *social judgment* influences whether challenging behavior exists.
5. Define *function* as it applies to understanding challenging behavior.
6. Identify and provide an example of the four functions of challenging behavior.
7. Define and provide an example of a *trigger* for challenging behavior.
8. Discuss how contextual influences affect challenging behavior.
9. Define and describe the crisis plan component of PBS.
10. What is the purpose of conducting a *functional assessment*?
11. Discuss and compare what is learned through interviews and direct observation methods of functional assessment.
12. Identify and describe the components of the notecard format for recording direct observations of challenging behavior.
13. How and why are hypotheses of challenging behavior developed?
14. List the components of a PBS plan.
15. Discuss how culture can affect judgment concerning whether a behavior problem exists, interpretation of assessment information, and acceptability of intervention procedures.
16. Identify and describe at least three strategies for preventing challenging behavior.

17. Describe the characteristics of *effective replacement behaviors* for challenging behavior.
18. Discuss two approaches for promoting *generalization* of behavior changes.

REFERENCES

Benedict, E.A., Horner, R.H., & Squires, J.K. (2007). Assessment and implementation of positive behavior support in preschools. *Topics in Early Childhood Special Education, 27*(3), 174–192.

Bijou, S.W., Peterson, R.F., & Ault, M.H. (1968). A method to integrate descriptive and experimental field studies at the level of data and empirical concepts. *Journal of Applied Behavior Analysis, 1,* 175–191.

Brennan, L.M., Shaw, D.S., Dishion, T.J., & Wilson, M. (2012). Longitudinal predictors of school-age academic achievement: Unique contributions of toddler-age aggression, oppositionality, inattention, and hyperactivity. *Journal of Abnormal Child Psychology, 40,* 1–12.

Cameron, M.J., Maguire, R.W., & Maguire, M. (1998). Lifeway influences on challenging behaviors. In J.K. Luiselli & M.J. Cameron (Eds.), *Antecedent control: Innovative approaches to behavioral support* (pp. 273–288). Baltimore, MD: Paul H. Brookes Publishing Co.

Carr, E.G. (1977). The motivation of self-injurious behavior: A review of some hypotheses. *Psychological Bulletin, 84,* 800–816.

Carr, E.G., Carlson, J.I., Langdon, N.A., Magito-McLaughlin, D., & Yarbrough, S.C. (1998). Two perspectives on antecedent control: Molecular and molar. In J.K. Luiselli & M.J. Cameron (Eds.), *Antecedent control: Innovative approaches to behavioral support* (pp. 3–28). Baltimore, MD: Paul H. Brookes Publishing Co.

Carr, E.G., & Durand, V.M. (1985). Reducing behavior problems through functional communication training. *Journal of Applied Behavior Analysis, 18,* 111–126.

Carr, E.G., Levin, L., McConnachie, G., Carlson, J.L., Kemp, D.C., & Smith, C.E. (1994). *Communication-based intervention for problem behavior: A user's guide for producing positive change.* Baltimore, MD: Paul H. Brookes Publishing Co.

Carr, E.G., Reeve, C.E., & Magito-McLaughlin, D. (1996). Contextual influences on problem behavior in people with developmental disabilities. In L.K. Koegel, R.L. Koegel, & G. Dunlap (Eds.), *Positive behavioral support: Including people with difficult behavior in the community* (pp. 403–423). Baltimore, MD: Paul H. Brookes Publishing Co.

Davis, C.A., Brady, M.P., Williams, R.E., & Hamilton, R. (1992). Effects of high-probability requests on the acquisition and generalization of responses to requests in young children with behavior disorders. *Journal of Applied Behavior Analysis, 25,* 905–916.

Gilliam, W.S. (2005). *Prekindergarteners left behind: Expulsion rates in state prekindergarten systems.* Foundation for Child Development. Retrieved from http://www.plan4preschool.org/documents/pk-expulsion.pdf

Hemmeter, M.L., Fox, L., Jack, S., & Broyles, L. (2007). A program-wide model of positive behavior support in early childhood settings. *Journal of Early Intervention, 29*(4), 337–355.

Hemmeter, M.L., & Ostrosky, M. (2003). Classroom preventive practices. In G. Dunlap, M. Conroy, L. Kern, G. DuPaul, J. VanBrakle, P. Strain, et al. (Eds.), *Research synthesis on effective intervention procedures: Executive summary* (pp. 11–12). Tampa, FL: University of South Florida, Center for Evidence-Based Practice: Young Children with Challenging Behavior.

Horner, R.H., Albin, R.W., Todd, A.W., & Sprague, J.R. (2006). Positive behavior support for individuals with severe disabilities. In M.E. Snell & F. Brown (Eds.), *Instruction of students with severe disabilities* (6th ed., pp. 206–250). Upper Saddle River, NJ: Prentice-Hall.

Horner, R., Day, M., Sprague, J., O'Brien, M., & Heathfield, L. (1991). Interspersed requests: A nonaversive procedure for reducing aggression and self-injury during instruction. *Journal of Applied Behavior Analysis, 24,* 265–278.

Horner, R.H., & Day, H.M. (1991). The effects of response efficiency on functionally equivalent competing behavior. *Journal of Applied Behavior Analysis, 24,* 719–732.

Iwata, B.A., Dorsey, M.F., Slifer, K.J., Bauman, K.E., & Richman, G.S. (1982). Toward a functional analysis of self-injury. *Analysis and Intervention in Developmental Disabilities, 2,* 3–20.

Janney, R., & Snell, M.E. (2000). *Behavioral support: Teachers' guides to inclusive practices.* Baltimore, MD: Paul H. Brookes Publishing Co.

Kalyanpur, M., & Harry, B. (1999). *Culture in special education: Building reciprocal family-professional relationships.* Baltimore, MD: Paul H. Brookes Publishing Co.

Kazdin, A.E. (2001). *Behavior modification in applied settings* (6th ed.). Belmont, CA: Wadsworth/Thomson.

Kennedy, C.H., & Souza, G. (1995). Functional analysis and treatment of eye-poking. *Journal of Applied Behavior Analysis, 28,* 27–37.

Kennedy, C.H., Itkonen, T., & Lindquist, K. (1995). Comparing interspersed requests and social comments as antecedents for increasing student compliance. *Journal of Applied Behavior Analysis, 28,* 97–98.

Kern, L., & Dunlap, G. (1998). Curricular modifications to promote desirable classroom behavior. In J.K. Luiselli & M.J. Cameron (Eds.), *Antecedent control: Innovative approaches to behavioral support* (pp. 289–307). Baltimore, MD: Paul H. Brookes Publishing Co.

Koegel, R.L., Carter, C.M., & Koegel, L.K. (1998). Setting events to improve parent-teacher coordination and motivation for children with autism. In J.K. Luiselli & M.J. Cameron (Eds.), *Antecedent control: Innovative approaches to behavioral support* (pp. 167–186). Baltimore, MD: Paul H. Brookes Publishing Co.

Kupersmidt, J.B., Bryant, D., & Willoughby, M.T. (2000). Prevalence of aggressive behaviors among preschoolers in Head Start and community child care programs. *Behavioral Disorders, 26*(1), 42–52.

Lalli, J.S., Casey, S., & Kates, K. (1995). Reducing escape behavior and increasing task completion with functional communication training, extinction, and response chaining. *Journal of Applied Behavior Analysis, 28,* 261–268.

Lewis, T.J., Beckner, R., & Stormont, M. (2009). Program-wide positive behavior supports: Essential features and implications for Head Start. *NHSA Dialog, 12*(2), 75–87.

Luiselli, J.K., & Cameron, M.J. (1998). *Antecedent control: Innovative approaches to behavioral support.* Baltimore, MD: Paul H. Brookes Publishing Co.

Muscott, H.S., Pomerleau, T., & Szczesiul, S. (2009). Large-scale implementation of program-wide positive behavioral interventions and supports in early childhood education programs in New Hampshire. *NHSA Dialog, 12*(2), 148–169.

Neilsen, S.L., & McEvoy, M.A. (2004). Functional behavioral assessment in early education settings. *Journal of Early Intervention, 26,* 115–131.

O'Neill, R.E., Horner, R.H., Albin, R.W., Sprague, J.R., Storey, K., & Newton, J.S. (1997). *Functional assessment and program development for problem behavior: A practical handbook.* Pacific Grove, CA: Brooks/Cole.

Park, K.L., & Scott, T.M. (2009). Antecedent-based interventions for young children at risk for emotional and behavioral disorders. *Behavioral Disorders, 34*(4), 196–211.

Powell, D., Dunlap, G., & Fox, L. (2006). Prevention and intervention for the challenging behaviors of toddlers and preschoolers. *Infants & Young Children, 19*(1), 25–35.

Sugai, G., Horner, R.H., Dunlap, G., Hieneman, M., Lewis, T.J., Nelson, C.M., Turnbull, A.P., Turnbull III, H.R., Wickham, D., Wilcox, B., & Ruef, M. (2000). Applying positive behavior support and functional behavioral assessment in schools. *Journal of Positive Behavior Interventions, 2*(3), 131–143.

Appendix 10.1

Positive Behavior Support Plan for Chelsea

Positive Behavior Support Plan

Child: Chelsea C. **Start Date:** 5/22/13

PBS team: Toni (early intervention program), Mom, Dad, Grandpa, Kelli (babysitter)

Behavior of concern: Chelsea hits her forehead with her fist.

Hypotheses

Functions

1. Chelsea hits her forehead to obtain adult attention.
2. Chelsea hits her forehead to obtain a desired object.

Contexts and Triggers

3. Chelsea is most likely to hit her forehead when playing with younger children.
4. Chelsea is most likely to hit her forehead when she is in a crowded situation.
5. Taking something from Chelsea is a trigger for her to hit her forehead.

Crisis Management Plan

If Chelsea hits her forehead, follow the steps listed below:

1. Pretend you didn't see it or hear her. If it occurs a second time, proceed to step 2.
2. Approach Chelsea slowly, and calmly redirect her to move to a less crowded area and to play with a favorite toy. If she continues to hit herself, proceed to step 3.
3. Firmly hold Chelsea's hands down and away from her head. Talk quietly and calmly to her about the new toy you have placed in front of her. As she seems to relax her arms, ease your hold on her hands and guide her hands to the toy. As she shows interest in the toy, release your hold on her hands. If she shows interest in another toy or other kind of play during this time, ease your hold on her and follow her lead for play. If Chelsea doesn't calm easily, quietly sing some of her favorite songs ("Itsy Bitsy Spider," "You Are My Sunshine") and slowly rock her.

Teaching Young Children in Natural Environments, Second Edition by Mary Jo Noonan, Ph.D. and Linda McCormick, Ph.D. Copyright © 2014 by Paul H. Brookes Publishing Co., Inc. All rights reserved.

Positive Behavior Support

Behavior Support Strategies	Prevent problem behavior			Encourage appropriate behavior					Teach replacement behaviors			Maintain and generalize behavior changes			
	Modify/eliminate contextual variables	Modify/eliminate triggers	Interrupt escalating behavior chains	Provide choice and preferred situations	Embed cues	Present positive social comments	Create positive routines and activities	Use supported routines, task simplification, and preteaching	Teach functionally equivalent communication responses	Teach more effective behaviors	Teach proactively	Use delayed and intermittent reinforcement	Teach across people, places, and activities	Address functions of problem behavior concurrently	Move from controlled to less controlled situations
Avoid crowds, especially if a number of toddlers are present; seek out areas that are not crowded and/or areas with older children (ages 4+).	✓														
Bring toys that are the same or similar to those that other children are likely to have at play areas (playground and park: balls, sand toys, small bike; pool: beach ball, swim ring, goggles, and so forth).		✓					✓								
Stay close and observe if Chelsea asks to play with toys that her peers have. If she makes a request that is unsuccessful (peer ignores her or says "no"), approach Chelsea, acknowledge her request ("Oh, you want to play with a ball"), and give her the type of toy she requested.			✓						✓						
Stay close in crowded situations. Quietly sing her favorite songs and rub her back.					✓		✓								

Teaching Young Children in Natural Environments, Second Edition by Mary Jo Noonan, Ph.D. and Linda McCormick, Ph.D. Copyright © 2014 by Paul H. Brookes Publishing Co., Inc. All rights reserved.

✓	✓												
	✓												
		✓											
			✓	✓		✓							
					✓		✓	✓					
							✓	✓	✓	✓	✓	✓	✓

Invite older peers (age 4+) for play.

Gradually introduce young peers to Chelsea. First have her play close to one toddler and same-age peer. Provide requested toy if she is unsuccessful in requesting it and redirect if she hits her forehead. As she is successful in this situation, add another peer to the group. Repeat until she is able to play with three or four young peers in close proximity.

Let Chelsea choose where and with what she wants to play on arrival at a play area. Have her choose among peers and toys.

Teach Chelsea to say "please" audibly and point to a desired toy. Sit close when she plays near peers with toys. If Chelsea looks at a toy intently (more than 5 seconds), whisper "Please" in her ear. If she doesn't imitate, model it and guide her to point to the desired toy. If the peer does not share, redirect Chelsea to play with a similar toy.

Provide enthusiastic attention whenever Chelsea makes a request by saying "Please."

Teach chelsea to wait. Once Chelsea has been making requests by saying "Please" (for at least 2 weeks), begin asking her to do something else before her request is honored. (Yes, Chelsea, you may have a ball. Please drink this juice while I get the ball.)

Teaching Young Children in Natural Environments, Second Edition by Mary Jo Noonan, Ph.D. and Linda McCormick, Ph.D. Copyright © 2014 by Paul H. Brookes Publishing Co., Inc. All rights reserved.

11

Small-Group Instruction

Mary Jo Noonan

FOCUS OF THIS CHAPTER

- Rationale for small-group instruction
- The characteristics of small groups
- Group-participation skills and objectives
- Teaching group skills, organizing groups, and facilitating participation
- Using groups to support the instructional process
- Cooperative learning groups

Children are often among peers, particularly if they spend time in child care, preschool, or kindergarten settings. Peer groups may also be present at home (if there are two or more siblings who are close in age), at family gatherings, in neighborhoods, and in public recreational environments such as the beach or playground. These situations provide opportunities for children with disabilities to learn to play and socialize with their age-mates (Garfinkle & Schwartz, 2002). Skills associated with small-group play and socialization are important instructional objectives for children with disabilities, especially for children with autism and others who have significant social needs (Heflin & Alberto, 2001).

RATIONALE FOR SMALL-GROUP INSTRUCTION

Instruction with two or more children simultaneously is *group instruction.* Successful participation in educational and social groups requires a wide range of skills, such as following group directions, responding to group-directed teaching techniques, following rules and routines, working and playing independently in close proximity to others, working and playing cooperatively with peers, turn taking, sharing, and waiting. These skills can be taught only in group situations. Small-group instruction has been shown to be an effective instructional arrangement for children of all ability levels, including those with severe disabilities (Bambara, Warren, & Komisar, 1988; Brown & Holvoet, 1982) and autism (Garfinkle & Schwartz, 2002; Taubman et al., 2001). While small-group instruction is advocated for young children with disabilities as an alternative to the predominance of one-to-one instruction, it is also recommended for young children without disabilities who receive instruction primarily in large groups. As an alternative to large groups, small-group instruction allows for more individualized assessment and instruction for all children (Camilli, Vargas, Ryan, & Barnett, 2010; Morrow, 2010; Wasik, 2008) and affords children with more opportunities for active participation (Phillips & Twardosz, 2003).

One reason that small-group instruction is effective is that it provides opportunities for observational learning, particularly when children of differing ability levels are grouped together (Colozzi, Ward, & Crotty, 2008; Whalen, Schuster, & Hemmeter, 1996). In a toddler group, for example, Tommy, who does not say words, learns to vocalize for adult attention when he observes Kimi gaining attention by speaking. One study found that observational learning is enhanced when peer models verbalize each step of a task they are modeling (Werts, Caldwell, & Wolery, 1996). Another benefit of small-group instruction is that it can increase the total amount of time in which children are actively engaged in instruction (Carnahan, Musti-Rao, & Bailey, 2009). Rather than divide 30 minutes into three 10-minute individual instructional sessions for three children, all three children receive instruction for the entire 30 minutes. The increased engaged time associated with small-group instruction has been shown to be associated with cognitive and social skill gains (Camilli et al., 2010).

Group instruction also benefits families and interventionists. In infant and toddler programs, it creates opportunities for families to meet one another and form relationships and support networks. Families might otherwise meet only program staff. Small-group instruction is a more efficient use of professionals' time (Collins, Gast, Ault, & Wolery, 1991; Rothholz, 1987). A one-to-one staff–child instructional arrangement is costly and time intensive in terms of staff resources.

THE CHARACTERISTICS OF SMALL GROUPS

Participation in small-group instruction should be considered for all children with disabilities. The task is to match the child with the group. Groups can be characterized by their composition, interaction, and content.

Group Composition

The number and types of children included in a small group are group composition considerations. Instructional group size can be as small as two children; a maximum of five is recommended for small groups to allow for individualized attention (Wasik, 2008). Larger groups can occur in child care and preschool programs serving a majority of children who do not have disabilities: Group size in these settings may approach 25 to 30. For a particular child, the decision on the size of the group is based on the following questions:

- What size group is needed for the child to participate in the activities associated with the instructional objectives?
- What size group is typical of the targeted activities and age peers?
- For what size group does the child possess group skills?
- What size group can the professional effectively manage?

Expectations for group skills should consider each child's current abilities related to group participation, instructional objectives, and developmental norms. Current abilities provide information for individualizing expectations. For example, a 3-year-old child who becomes upset in noisy situations may initially participate in a group with only two other children. When the child becomes comfortable in the small-group situation, participation in slightly larger groups may be considered. If a 4-year-old child has instructional objectives for participating in a community preschool program, she may receive instruction in a variety of small- and large-group situations typical of the preschool classroom. If her current ability levels suggest that large groups may be challenging for her, extra supports (e.g., sitting with a special friend) may be provided, or a schedule for gradually increasing her time spent in the group may be implemented. Developmental norms must also be considered. Young children from 6 to 24 months of age typically engage in simple social interactions (e.g., smiling, turn taking in games such as peekaboo); from 24 to 30 months of age they tend to play alone with toys; from 30 to 42 months they continue to play alone but near other children; and from 42 months of age and on, children play with their peers cooperatively (Wolery, McWilliam, & Bailey, 2005).

Small-group composition may be homogeneous or heterogeneous (Collins et al., 1991). *Homogeneous groups* include children who have similar skill levels and concerns or are close in age (within 6 to 12 months of one another).

Heterogeneous groups include children with varied skill levels and concerns or children who are not close in age. Other child characteristics such as gender, temperament, and cultural and/or linguistic backgrounds also contribute to a group's homogeneity or heterogeneity.

Homogeneous groups are easier for instruction because the children are likely to have similar goals. Furthermore, an activity that is of interest to one child in a homogeneous group is likely to be of interest to the others. Homogeneous groups have a major disadvantage: They do not include children who could serve as more competent models for others in the group. In addition, if all children in the group have significant learning needs, severe physical disabilities, or limited expressive communication skills, active group participation may be difficult to accomplish. Planning and implementing instruction for heterogeneous groups may be more challenging for the professional, but the availability of competent peer models and varied group-participation abilities are important advantages that can be used to promote learning (Sharan, 1980). The assignment of children to groups should be deliberate and should contribute positively to the instructional activity (Wasik, 2008).

Group Interaction

A major rationale for small-group instruction is teaching social interaction skills. These skills are easily embedded and taught in the group. For example, Joseph can be taught to turn toward a named peer. And if the children already possess simple social interaction skills, the skills can be included within the group activity, as when children hand materials to one another or peers reinforce one another (Brown, Holvoet, Guess, & Mulligan, 1980; Zanolli, Daggett, & Adams, 1996). Some form of group interaction should be considered for all small-group instruction because it is a form of engagement that promotes attention to the activity and peers.

Instructional Content

Most small groups have a theme or purpose (also called a *unit approach*). Whatever the topic or purpose of the group, it should always be age appropriate. A theme is selected for a specified period of time (e.g., 1 week, 2 weeks, 1 month) and carried out in activities, materials, and songs. For example, weather may be the theme in March. Bulletin boards depicting a variety of weather conditions are designed; numbers for the calendar are written on sun and cloud cutouts; songs about sunshine, rain, and wind are sung during morning circle; stories about rainbows, summer fun, and snowy day adventures are placed in the book corner; and science and art activities addressing the weather theme are conducted. In addition to nature, common unit themes for early childhood settings include seasons, holidays, animals, birds, transportation, family, neighborhood, occupations, and so on. Many curriculum guides with ideas for implementing a unit approach are commercially available (cf. Charner, Murphy, & Clark, 2006; Dodge, 2010; Dodge, Rudick, & Berke, 2010; Herr, 2012; Jackman, 2011; Wortham, 2010).

Group instruction is conducted in the context of an activity, with individual objectives addressed for each group member. In a toddler group, for example, an activity with apples and oranges involves naming, identifying color, feeling texture, and tasting. One toddler practices his objectives of reaching and touching when the apple and orange are presented; another toddler is encouraged to imitate the names of the fruit, and point to her peer when her turn is finished.

In general, small groups are more effective than large groups for teaching content in early childhood settings (Wasik, 2008). In a kindergarten or first grade classroom, small-group instruction may focus on content in early literacy, mathematics, or science that is appropriate to the entire group. While providing instruction to the small group, the teacher has abundant opportunities to observe and listen to the children and judge their learning and understanding of the lesson's content.

It is possible to organize children into groups even though each child may be participating in a different activity. This occurs in child care and preschool when children are allowed to select activities for independent activity times. Although the children are working independently, they are physically in a group (either at a table or on the floor). Learning to work independently and behaving appropriately while in close proximity to peers is an expectation of preschool and kindergarten classrooms.

GROUP-PARTICIPATION SKILLS AND OBJECTIVES

Among the social and communication skills acquired during the early childhood years are a number that are relevant to participation in groups. Children learn skills for at least three types of group situations: 1) social play groups, 2) independent activities play groups, and 3) instructional-recreational groups. The following are examples of the types of skills required for each type of group situation:

- Social play groups
  - Sharing
  - Turn taking
  - Helping
  - Cooperating
- Independent activities play groups
  - Attending to task
  - Working or playing without assistance
  - Not bothering peers
- Instructional-recreational groups
  - Following group directions
  - Following rules and routines
  - Asking questions at appropriate times
  - Speaking at appropriate times

- Staying with the group
- Waiting and walking in lines

Many of the group skills listed here are learned in the toddler years; the others are learned later with increasing competence into the school years and through adulthood. Table 11.1 lists the group skills identified by teachers as important for success (*survival skills*) in preschool (Noonan et al., 1992) and kindergarten (Vincent et al., 1980). Note that the preschool group skills were validated via the repertoire of 3-year-olds who did not have disabilities. If a child does not demonstrate the group skills in Table 11.1, the skills may be appropriate instructional objectives. Also, group-participation objectives may be identified through the person-centered planning and ecological assessment process described in Chapters 3 and 4.

TEACHING GROUP SKILLS, ORGANIZING GROUPS, AND FACILITATING PARTICIPATION

There are many considerations to take into account when planning small-group instruction. Decisions about when and how objectives will be included must be made, and instructional techniques that facilitate group participation and take advantage of learning opportunities must be selected. Each of these important elements of groups—teaching group skills, organizing groups, facilitating group participation, and using group situations to support the instructional process—is discussed below.

Table 11.1. Group skills included on survival skills lists

Preschool group skills
Makes transitions from one activity to another
Complies with directions
Follows rules and routines
Focuses on task
Focuses attention on speaker
Socializes with others
Communicates with peers
Communicates with adults
Takes turns
Shares materials and toys with peers
Cooperates with and/or helps others
Does not disturb others
Uses voice appropriate to activity

Kindergarten group skills
Initiates interactions with adults and peers
Interacts with adults and peers when not the initiator
Listens and attends to speaker in large group
Demonstrates turn taking in a small group
Attends to task for minimum of 15 minutes
Adapts to transitions between activities throughout the day
Communicates with peers and adults
Asks questions of others
Lines up and stays in line
Raises hand and/or gets teacher's attention when necessary
Waits to take turns and shares
Controls voice in classroom
Stays in "own space" for activity

Sources: Noonan et al. (1992) and Vincent et al. (1980).

Teaching Group-Participation Skills

Children as young as age 2 can be taught group-participation skills, such as those listed above, using the direct instruction and naturalistic teaching strategies explained in Chapters 6 and 7. Caregivers should begin with an objective that explicitly defines a group-participation skill. For example, "Allana will approach two peers and play with them in a 15-minute small-group play session (e.g., take a turn adding blocks to a tower, play a role in a game of "house," join in working on a puzzle) at least 3 times per week for 4 consecutive weeks." Then define the strategies that will be used to assist and encourage the desired behavior. For example, an adult may prompt Allana during the first 5 minutes of each playgroup by whispering a brief direction for participating in the activity ("Choose a puzzle piece"). Each time Allana demonstrates a correct response, prompted or unprompted, the adult makes a positive comment to the group about how nice they are playing. As Allana makes progress, the prompt can be faded by initially whispering her name. The remainder of the prompt ("Choose a puzzle piece") is provided if Allana does not respond within 5 seconds. This example includes the instructional strategies of a verbal prompt, time delay, and verbal reinforcement. As in all instruction, the child's progress should be monitored by frequent data collection.

When children have difficulty staying with a group or participating in a group, begin by rewarding the child for interacting and participating with only one other child. As the child learns to participate in this smallest group arrangement, add other children, one at a time (Collins et al., 1991; Koegel & Rincover, 1974). If the child participates appropriately in a group situation but is not making progress with individual goals, it may be necessary to also conduct individual teaching sessions (Collins et al., 1991). This is an alternative to discontinuing the child's participation in the group when he or she is not progressing. It may provide enough extra help to allow the child to benefit from group instruction. The individual teaching sessions are discontinued when the child demonstrates adequate progress.

Organizing Group Instruction

Ideally, all children with disabilities receive instruction on at least one goal during a group activity. As noted above, children in the group may have the same instructional goals or they may have different goals. There are two approaches to incorporating instruction of specific objectives into groups: *skill embedding* (Harris & Delmolino, 2002)—also known as embedded learning opportunities (Dunst et al., 2001; Horn, Lieber, Li, Sandall, & Schwartz, 2000)—and *skill sequencing* (Brown & Holvoet, 1982).

Skill Embedding Skill embedding is much like the activity-based approach to instruction described in Chapter 7. The first step is to select a small-group activity. The activity may be a self-care or play activity (e.g., brushing teeth, playing house), an early childhood curricular activity (e.g., science activity), or a daily routine (e.g., circle time). The activity may also be a child's instructional goal. After selecting a group activity, review the child's objectives and select one or more objectives that fit logically into the activity. If there is more than one child with a disability in the group, select only two to four objectives per child. Imagine, for example, how Kimi's objectives of "grasping," "asking for more," and "manipulating objects" could be embedded in the activity of "playing with the kitchen bowls and utensils." All three skills can be taught during the activity: Kimi grasps the bowls and utensils when passing or receiving them from another child in the group, and she grasps the utensil while "stirring" in the bowl. Kimi asks for "more" when the bowl is out of reach and she manipulates objects by examining the utensils and bowls when they are given to her.

After selecting the activity and each child's objective(s), the next task is to write out the group activity as one would a script and indicate when each child's instructional trials will be presented. Figure 11.1 is an example of a group instruction plan that includes Kimi and the kitchen play activity. For each skill in italics, systematic instruction is implemented. Skill embedding may be used with traditional group instruction or with cooperative learning groups, described later in this chapter.

Skill Sequencing   Skill sequencing (Bambara et al., 1988; Guess et al., 1978) is similar to skill embedding. The difference is that objectives are chained and taught consecutively rather than distributed throughout the activity. Group skill sequences are constructed by first listing the objectives of the children who will be in the group. An age-appropriate activity or theme is then selected. Next, one to three objectives for each child are identified on the basis of their

Group lesson: Kitchen play
Group: Kimi (12 months), Darron (14 months), and Kawika (11 months)
Lesson time: Mondays, 9:00–9:30
Interventionist: Allen
Start date: 5/20/13   End date:_____
Give each child two metal mixing bowls and two wooden spoons. Call each child by name and talk about the bowls and utensils as they are distributed. 　Darron: *Visually tracks* the utensils and bowl when they are given to him. 　Kawika: *Looks at the person calling his name* (when bowls and utensils are distributed). Encourage the children to look at and pick up the bowls and utensils, assisting as necessary. Demonstrate different ways to play with the bowls and utensils, turning them over, banging them on the floor, banging a utensil outside and inside a bowl, "stirring" with a spoon, and so forth. 　Kimi: *Grasps* the spoon and *manipulates* it. 　Kimi: As she repeatedly bangs on the bowl, move the bowl out of reach and look at her expectantly. Kimi will *ask for more*. 　Darron: *Visually tracks* the bowl and spoon as the interventionist bangs them together and moves them slowly in an arc, from right to left and then left to right. 　Kawika: *Points to named objects* when the interventionist holds up the bowl and spoon. Continue to encourage the children to play with the bowls and spoons. Repeat the above sequence (Kimi grasping and manipulating, Kimi asking for more, Darron tracking, and Kawika pointing to named objects) at least two more times.

Figure 11.1.   Sample group instructional plan with embedded objectives.

logical relationship to one another. The final step is to write the sequence as a script, indicating the order in which instruction will be conducted for each objective. If the kitchen play group in Figure 11.1 was reconstructed as a skill sequence, the plan might be as follows:

1. Kawika: Looks at the adult calling his name
2. Kawika: Points to named objects
3. Darron: Visually follows the spoon and bowl (when given to Kawika)
4. Darron: Visually follows the spoon and bowl (when given to Darron)
5. Darron: Visually follows the spoon and bowl (when given to Kimi)
6. Kimi: Grasps the spoon
7. Kimi: Manipulates the spoon
8. Kimi: Asks for more (e.g., "More play" when the bowl is removed)

In this skill sequence, after Kawika looks at the adult calling his name, he is asked to point to something. There is a logical progression from the skill of looking to a skill that requires participation in the group (point to something). Darron visually follows the spoon and bowl as they are given to Kawika. It is meaningful for him to do this after Kawika has pointed to the objects and is receiving them. The relationship between the skills enhances motivation to perform the skills. In skill sequencing, children have opportunities to learn the logical relationships among skills they are learning—relationships that are likely to be present under natural conditions.

The group activity may not always occur exactly as scripted in the instructional plan. The behavior and needs of children may vary considerably from day to day. The script, therefore, is to be used as a guide.

Facilitating Group Participation

Effective instruction requires frequent and appropriate participation by all children in the group. Participation is evidence that the child is actively engaged. Techniques to enhance group participation include quick pacing, selective attention, partial or adapted participation, peer interaction, group responding, and group contingencies.

Quick Pacing *Pace* refers to the speed with which instruction is directed from one child to the next in the group. Quick pacing has three advantages: It results in frequent instruction for all children, it helps children attend to the activity, and it decreases the likelihood of boredom and problem behaviors. To implement quick pacing, focus attention on each child for several moments, one at a time, to instruct specific skills. With practice, a teacher can become skilled at quick pacing.

Periodic attention is a technique associated with pacing. Occasionally during instruction, a teacher should call children by name in no particular order, or use some other strategy such as eye contact, pointing, or smiling to maintain or regain their attention. In addition to assisting children to focus on the group activity, periodic attention rewards children for attending.

Selective Attention Selective attention is another way to promote group participation. Praise children specifically for attending and participating. Social reinforcement should be delivered quickly and individually. In addition to praise, eye contact, smiling, gentle touching, or other social reinforcers may be used. Ideally, children who are not attending or participating will notice that they have been bypassed for reinforcement and will attempt to imitate peers who were successful in obtaining reinforcement.

Partial Participation and Adaptations Some children are not able to independently participate in typical group activities. Requirements for participation may be modified through *partial participation* or *adaptations*. Partial participation and adaptation are slightly different from each other. When a response requirement is limited to a portion of the response, it is partial participation (Baumgart et al., 1982). An adaptation is when response requirements are changed and a modified or alternate response that serves the same purpose is substituted (Janney & Snell, 2005). For example, when children are expected to select their materials from a tray and one child is unable to grasp, partial participation may require that the child reach for the materials and open her hand. An adult or peer then assists her to grasp the materials and set them on a table. An adaptation is another option for this child. She could wear a strap on her hand fitted with Velcro, and the materials she reaches for could also have a Velcro strip. After reaching and aligning the Velcro on her hand with that on the materials, she completes the task independently. Partial participation and adaptations are discussed in greater detail in Chapter 13.

Peer Interaction To take full advantage of opportunities provided in group instruction, social interaction among the group members should be promoted. As noted in the rationale for instruction, group activities are the only context in which it is possible to teach social interaction with peers. The most direct way to promote interaction is to identify and target one or more social interaction skills for children in the group. These skills may or may not be objectives on the individualized family service plan (IFSP) or individualized education program (IEP). Socialization skills are taught by embedding them in the group activity or through skill sequencing.

Figure 11.2 shows a group activity in which preschoolers are passing materials one at a time (IFSP and IEP objectives are designated with an asterisk in the figure). In this example, passing materials is not an IFSP or IEP objective; it is included to encourage social interaction and to teach turn taking. Specific social interaction objectives are also included in the group sequence for three of the four preschoolers (indicated in bold print in the sequence). The fourth child, Daria, practices attending to the activity four times each time the sequence is conducted.

Group instruction can also be planned to include *interdependence* among group members. Interdependence occurs when each child's participation in the activity is dependent on another group member's participation (Brown et al., 1980). Each child has a clear and necessary role. Group members must attend to what their peers are doing to know when it is their turn. In the example in Figure 11.2, the requirement that children pass the materials so that their peers can take turns sets up an interdependent situation. Usually, however, interdependence involves a more complex activity. For example, if preschoolers are

Group skill sequence: Sand or water play			
Group: Tomiko (36 months), Sean (32 months), Matthew (40 months), and Daria (36 months)			
Lesson time: Tuesdays, 10:00–10:20 a.m.			
Interventionist: Anisa			
Start date: 7/07/13 End date:			
Tomiko	Sean	Matthew	Daria
Pours from one container into another (uses both hands in fine motor activity)* Passes containers to Sean	**Says "Thank you"*** Imitates Tomiko Passes containers to Matthew*	Pours from one container into another **Identifies named peer*** Passes containers to Daria	Attends to activity (watches peer)* Attends to activity (watches peer)* Attends to activity (watches peer)* Attends to activity (receives containers)* Pours from one container into another Passes containers to Tomiko

Figure 11.2. Sample group skill sequence with social interaction. Repeat sequence four times using different actions requiring Tomiko to use both hands with objects in the sand or water play. Social skill objectives are in bold; instructional objectives are indicated with an asterisk.

setting a table, one may have the task of wiping the table clean; another may be required to count out the appropriate number of dishes, cups, and napkins; and the third may be assigned to set the table. The group is interdependent because dishes, cups, and napkins cannot be placed on the table until the table has been cleaned by the first group member and the second group member has given the materials to the third.

Group Responding In the examples of group instructional plans presented thus far, most participation has been one child at a time. Group members may respond together. *Group responding,* also known as *unison* or *choral responding,* increases each child's opportunities for active participation (Beneke, Ostrosky, & Katz, 2008; Sainato, Strain, & Lyon, 1987). Group responding can be verbal, with children answering questions, singing songs, or rote reciting (e.g., counting), or nonverbal, with children performing motor responses. Making hand motions to a song, imitating the teacher (e.g., demonstrating folding a paper in four), or playing with the activity materials (e.g., musical instruments) are examples of nonverbal group responding.

During group responding, the teacher should shift eye contact and attention quickly among the children to let them know that their participation is appropriate. This requires that the group members be in close proximity to one another. Whether the response is verbal, nonverbal, or both, group responding has two important advantages: 1) it assists children to attend and participate in the activity and 2) it minimizes the time that children must wait for a turn.

Group responding is more difficult to plan when group membership is heterogeneous, but it may still be feasible. For example, all children may be asked to point at pictures as they are named in a story. Then there may be individualized response requirements: one child is required to vocalize and another to say a word during the group response. Individualized response requirements may include partial participation or adaptive participation. Chapter 13 discusses partial participation and adaptive participation in detail. Partial participation refers to performing one or more components of a skill or task but not the skill or task in its entirety. It is important that the child's participation in the task include meaningful and important components. For example, if a child needs adult assistance to drink from a cup, he may nod his head toward the cup to indicate that he wants a drink, and he may nod his head to indicate when he is finished drinking. Partial participation in this manner meets the criteria of being meaningful and important because it provides the child with control over when he takes a drink and how much he drinks. In contrast to partial participation, adaptive participation involves changing how the skill or task is performed and may involve the use of alternative or special equipment or devices. Instead of having an adult assist a child with drinking from a cup, the child may drink from a straw as a form of adaptive participation. Furthermore, the cup may be in a weighted cup holder to hold the cup steady (another adapted component).

Group Contingencies A group contingency is an instructional arrangement whereby reinforcement is provided when all group members demonstrate a required response (Alberto & Troutman, 2012). Most teachers are familiar with group contingencies from elementary school experiences in which they lost or gained privileges depending on the behavior of the entire class. If the entire class did their spelling homework, for example, the class could earn 10 minutes of free time. If one or more members of the class did not do the homework, however, the class did not earn the free time or was otherwise penalized. Because group contingencies rely on peer pressure (anticipated peer acceptance or rejection) for their effectiveness, they may not be effective for infants or toddlers who have not yet acquired that level of social understanding. Group contingencies, however, have been demonstrated to be as effective as individual contingencies when teaching social skills to preschoolers with disabilities (Kohler, Strain, Maretsky, & DeCesare, 1990; Ling, Hawkins, & Weber, 2011; Murphy, Theodore, Aloiso, Alric-Edwards, & Hughes, 2007).

USING GROUPS TO SUPPORT THE INSTRUCTIONAL PROCESS

Group instruction offers unique teaching opportunities. In addition to teaching social interaction skills, group situations are well suited for enhancing the instructional process in providing assistance, encouragement, and generalization.

Assistance Procedures

Possibly the most important advantage of group instruction is the opportunity for *observational learning*. Observational learning, however, should not be left to chance. Instead, praise children who watch or imitate their peers ("I see you are doing it just like Carmen—that's good!"). Observational learning can also be facilitated by encouraging children to reinforce one another. Teachers can have children clap for one another or have a child give stickers to peers for correct responses. Delivering reinforcement to peers enhances attention to them and facilitates observational learning (Brown & Holvoet, 1982).

Peer modeling can be used to prompt desired behavior. For example, Jason is asked to demonstrate how to spread paste with his finger. Brendyn observes Jason spreading the paste on his artwork. He also sees that Jason gets praised for doing that, so Brendyn spreads paste in the same way. Children imitate peers they identify with, more competent peers, and those they observe receiving reinforcement. Peer modeling is a good technique to teach social and communicative interactions—skills that cannot be modeled by an adult.

Group instruction also provides opportunities for *peer tutoring*. Peer tutoring uses other children in the group (usually more competent children) to provide assistance and encouragement. This is discussed at length in Chapter 12. Research has demonstrated that young children can deliver prompts effectively if they are directly taught to do so (Kohler & Strain, 1997). Prompting is maintained through group reinforcement: All children are reinforced if the children learning the new skills are successful. A kindergarten teacher might use peer tutoring and a group contingency to teach children to walk to the cafeteria quietly and in a line. Peer tutors are assigned and told to remind their partners periodically to "use a quiet voice" and to "walk slowly and stay in line." The entire class earns an extra story during storytime if they all walk quietly in a line to the cafeteria.

In homogeneous groups in which more than one child has the same objective, the effectiveness of instruction is enhanced by repetition of the same (or similar) instructional procedures. This is in conjunction with observational learning. A child may observe instruction implemented one or more times before being required to respond. Repetition has the effect of providing additional instruction. Similarly, repetition of the prompt highlights it and increases its saliency and effectiveness. And if a peer is working on the same objective but receiving a less intrusive prompt, a child may learn to respond to the less intrusive prompt (Brown & Holvoet, 1982). For example, Jimmy, a toddler who needs hand-over-hand assistance to put on his sweater, observes his peer putting on his sweater after a demonstration. Jimmy attempts to imitate, thus responding to a less intrusive prompt.

Encouragement Procedures

Children's attention is critical for effective instruction. A teacher can use selective reinforcement to reward attention to instruction: If a child attends, give her a turn. Group instruction also provides opportunities for children to observe the consequences for not attending (losing a turn).

As noted earlier in the discussion on facilitating group participation, peers may be taught to provide reinforcement. There are several advantages for teaching peers to praise and encourage one another. First, in many cases peer attention and reinforcement are more powerful than adult attention. Second, when peers provide reinforcement, friendships develop (people tend to like individuals who reinforce them). Third, children often generalize the use of peer reinforcement beyond the group instruction setting. Fourth, children may imitate reinforcing behaviors because such behaviors, in turn, earn reinforcement for them (reinforcement begets reinforcement). Teachers should not teach peers to correct or otherwise punish one another for incorrect responding. This may be counterproductive to promoting friendships among the children.

Generalization Procedures

Group instruction can be used to enhance skill generalization. If group members are working on the same (or similar) objectives, teachers may use different materials and instructional stimuli for different children. This allows children to observe a range of stimuli associated with the target response and thus facilitates stimulus generalization (Stokes & Baer, 1977). When different materials and stimuli are used to teach the same response, slightly different responses may be appropriate to accommodate the differences in the materials and/or stimuli. Observing different appropriate responses assists children to learn the response class.

Most important, through group participation children *learn how to learn* in a group. Much of the instruction provided to children without disabilities is large-group instruction, and much of the instruction provided to young children with disabilities is in one-to-one situations. Thus it is valuable to include all children in groups of various sizes. Variation across groups increases the likelihood that the children will generalize their group-participation skills.

Snell and Brown (2011) offered the following guidelines for maximizing the benefits of group instruction:

1. Involve all members by using individualized instruction, teaching the same concept at multiple levels of complexity, and allowing for different response modes and modified materials.

2. Keep the group instruction interesting by keeping turns short, giving everyone turns, making turns dependent on attending, giving demonstrations, and using a variety of materials that can be handled.

3. Encourage students to listen and watch other group members as they take their turns. Praise them when they do. Actively involve students in the process of praising and prompting others.

4. Provide task-specific and individualized attention and praise to group members for turn taking and being on task. Also, use group reinforcement procedures in response to the performance of the entire group.

5. Allow students to participate in demonstrations and handle materials related to the skill or concept being taught.

6. Keep waiting time to a minimum by controlling group size, teacher talk, and the number of student responses made in a single turn.

7. Prompt cooperation among group members and discourage competition among them (p. 139).

While this chapter has focused primarily on group instruction delivered by a teacher, it is also possible to arrange groups to function somewhat independently with an adult preparing the activity and then monitoring rather than instructing the lesson. Cooperative learning groups are one such model.

COOPERATIVE LEARNING GROUPS

Described first by Johnson and Johnson (1975), the cooperative learning model has been shown to improve children's social interaction behaviors and promote positive peer interactions (Putnam, Rynders, Johnson, & Johnson, 1989). The model structures activities to teach children to encourage one another, celebrate one another's successes, and work toward common goals. It is well suited for use with heterogeneous groups in inclusive settings (McMaster & Fuchs, 2002).

Cooperative Learning Elements

Cooperative learning groups are instructional situations in which children can reach their learning goals if and only if peers in their group also reach their goals. The teacher's role is to teach requisite cooperative skills so that groups function effectively. Cooperative learning groups have four essential elements: 1) positive interdependence, 2) face-to-face communication, 3) individual accountability, and 4) group process.

Positive interdependence requires group members to work together to accomplish one or more common goals. Methods for promoting positive interdependence are divisions of labor; dividing materials, resources, or information among group members; assigning students different roles; and giving joint rewards. The second element, face-to-face communication, requires group members to interact with one another to accomplish a task and goal. In individual accountability, students are each responsible for mastering the assigned material and for contributing to the group's efforts. Finally, in the fourth element, group process, students are expected to use appropriate interpersonal and small-group skills.

Cooperative Learning Strategies

Although cooperative learning groups are most commonly used with school-age children, they are applicable to children in preschool and kindergarten. The following is an adaptation of cooperative learning for preschool and kindergarten children (Johnson & Johnson, 1986):

1. *Select or develop a unit with clear cognitive or preacademic objectives and list the cooperative skills to be taught.* Interpersonal and small-group skills, such as taking turns or assisting one another, are examples of possible cooperative skills to teach.

2. *Plan a series of lessons or activities.* The objective is to teach cooperative skills in the context of cognitive and preacademic lessons and activities.

3. *Assign children to dyads or three-member groups.* Do not include more than one child with disabilities in each group. Maintain the same groups for all the lessons and activities in the unit.

4. *Encourage cooperative effort by the way materials are distributed.* There are many ways to do this to encourage group effort. For example, consider providing each group member with only part of the materials needed to complete the activity or providing the group with only one set of materials.

5. *Introduce the lessons and activities by providing a clear and specific description (and demonstration if necessary) of what it means to be cooperative.* Define *cooperation* operationally by specifying the behaviors that are appropriate and desirable within the groups. Beginning behavior might include "staying near one another," "using quiet voices," and "taking turns." Contrast "working with a friend" and "working alone" by showing pictures of each and asking the children to discuss the pictures. Consider making a bulletin board with a "friends help each other" theme. It may require more than one session for the children to understand what it means to work with a partner to produce a single product. Stress that everybody is to have fun and that they will be successful if they work together and help one another.

6. *Assist and monitor.* Monitor groups carefully to see where assistance is needed, either related to the activity or to cooperation. Publicly praise children when they share and help one another and prompt collaboration and cooperation as needed. Say, for example, "What does taking turns mean? It means doing something one at a time." Intervene as necessary to clarify instructions or answer questions.

7. *Evaluate and provide feedback.* Take time at the end of each cooperative learning activity to provide positive feedback on each group's product. It is particularly important to talk about cooperation efforts. Ask for examples of cooperation and comment on how well group members worked together.

The basic premise of the cooperative learning model is that accomplishing a goal together leads children to invest in one another's learning. In turn, this helps children build more realistic and multifaceted views of one another and encourages acceptance and positive feelings. The cooperative learning model uses group dynamics as a means of encouraging social interactions and friendships (Johnson & Johnson, 1981).

SUMMARY

Group instruction is an important component of early intervention and early childhood special education. It is particularly important for 2- through 6-year-olds who need group-participation skills in inclusive early childhood settings. This chapter described strategies for facilitating participation in small groups: quick pacing, selective attention, partial and adaptive participation, group interaction, and group responding. Techniques for using group arrangements to support the instructional process (assistance, encouragement, and generalization strategies) were also described.

STUDY QUESTIONS

1. Write a list of benefits associated with small-group instruction for children with and without disabilities.

2. Identify and describe a range of group activities that 1-, 3-, and 5-year-olds typically experience. What types of skills support their participation in each activity?

3. Discuss the pros and cons of *homogeneous* and *heterogeneous* instructional groups.

4. Identify three preschool children with special concerns. Make a list of the skills targeted on their IEPs. Discuss how you might *embed* two skills for each child in a group lesson about "our community."

5. Referring to the children and skills identified in Question 4, develop a skill sequence for a lesson about "our community" using at least two skills for each of the three children. Include children without disabilities in your plan and describe how they will participate in the group lesson.

6. Referring to a group lesson discussed in Question 4 or 5, describe how you might apply each of the following strategies to facilitate group participation: quick pacing, periodic attention, selective attention, partial participation, adaptations, group interaction, group responding, and group contingencies.

7. Develop a group lesson about insects that includes one of the children from Question 4. The group is heterogeneous in a mixed-age preschool class (3-, 4-, and 5-year olds), and the child from Question 4 is the only child with a disability in the group. Discuss how you might use the group situation to enhance instruction with each of the following procedures: assistance procedures, peer modeling, peer tutoring and prompting, encouragement, and generalization. Discuss how you might structure this lesson for cooperative learning groups.

REFERENCES

Alberto, P.A., & Troutman, A.C. (2012). *Applied behavior analysis for teachers* (9th ed.). Upper Saddle River, NJ: Pearson Education.

Bambara, L.M., Warren, S.F., & Komisar, S. (1988). The individualized curriculum sequencing model: Effects on skill acquisition and generalization. *Journal of the Association for Persons with Severe Handicaps, 13*, 8–19.

Baumgart, D., Brown, L., Pumpian, I., Nisbet, J., Ford, A., & Sweet, M., et al. (1982). The principal of partial participation and individualized adaptations in educational programs for severely handicapped students. *Journal of the Association for Persons with Severe Handicaps, 7*(2), 17–27.

Beneke, S., Ostrosky, M., & Katz, L. (2008). Calendar time for young children: Good intentions gone awry. *Young Children, 63*(3), 12–16.

Brown, F., & Holvoet, J. (1982). Effects of systematic peer interaction on the incidental learning of two severely handicapped students. *Journal of the Association for Persons with Severe Handicaps, 7*(4), 19–28.

Brown, F., Holvoet, J., Guess, D., & Mulligan, M. (1980). The individualized curriculum sequencing model: III. Small group instruction. *Journal of the Association for the Severely Handicapped, 5*(4), 352–367.

Camilli, G., Vargas, S., Ryan, S., & Barnett, W.S. (2010). Meta-analysis of the effects of early education interventions on cognitive and social development. *The Teachers College Record, 112*(3), 579–620.

Carnahan, C., Musti-Rao, S., & Bailey, J. (2009). Promoting active engagement in small group learning experiences for students with autism and significant learning needs. *Education and Treatment of Children, 32*(1), 37–61.

Charner, K., Murphy, M., & Clark, C. (2006). *The encyclopedia of infant and toddler activities: Written by teachers for teachers.* Beltsville, MD: Gryphon House.

Collins, B.C., Gast, D.L., Ault, M.J., & Wolery, M. (1991). Small group instruction: Guidelines for teachers of students with moderate to severe handicaps. *Education and Training in Mental Retardation, 26,* 18–32.

Colozzi, G.A., Ward, L.W., & Crotty, K.E. (2008). Comparison of simultaneous prompting procedure in 1:1 and small group instruction to teach play skills to preschool students with pervasive developmental disorder and developmental disabilities. *Education and Training in Developmental Disabilities, 43*(2), 226–248.

Dodge, D.T. (2010). *The creative curriculum for preschool.* Bethesda, MD: Teaching Strategies.

Dodge, D.T., Rudick, S., & Berke, K. (2010). *The creative curriculum for infants, toddlers and twos* (Revised). Bethesda, MD: Teaching Strategies.

Dunst, C.J., Bruder, M.B., Trivette, C.M., Hamby, D., Raab, M., & McLean, M. (2001). Characteristics and consequences of everyday natural learning opportunities. *Topics in Early Childhood Special Education, 21*(2), 68–92.

Garfinkle, A.N., & Schwartz, I.S. (2002). Peer imitation increasing social interactions in children with autism and other developmental disabilities in inclusive preschool classrooms. *Topics in Early Childhood Special Education, 22*(1), 26–38.

Guess, D., Horner, D., Utley, B., Holvoet, J., Maxon, D., Tucker, D., & Warren, S. (1978). A functional curriculum sequencing model for teaching the severely handicapped. *AAESPH Review, 3,* 202–215.

Harris, S.L., & Delmolino, L. (2002). Applied behavior analysis: Its application in the treatment of autism and related disorders in young children. *Infants and Young Children, 14*(3), 11–17.

Heflin, L.J., & Alberto, P.A. (2001). Establishing a behavioral context for learning for students with autism. *Focus on Autism and Other Developmental Disabilities, 16,* 93–101.

Herr, J. (2012). *Creative resources for the early childhood classroom.* Belmont, CA: Wadsworth Publishing.

Horn, E., Lieber, J., Li, S., Sandall, S., & Schwartz, I. (2000). Supporting young children's IEP goals in inclusive settings through embedded learning opportunities. *Topics in Early Childhood Special Education, 20*(4), 208–223.

Jackman, H. (2011). *Early education curriculum: A child's connection to the world.* Belmont, CA: Wadsworth Publishing.

Janney, R., & Snell, M.E. (2005). *Teachers' guides to inclusive practices: Modifying schoolwork* (2nd ed.). Baltimore, MD: Paul H. Brookes Publishing Co.

Johnson, D., & Johnson, R. (1975). *Learning together and alone: Cooperation, competition, and individualization.* Englewood Cliffs, NJ: Prentice Hall.

Johnson, D., & Johnson, R. (1986). Mainstreaming and cooperative learning strategies. *Exceptional Children, 52*(6), 553–561.

Johnson, R., & Johnson, D. (1981). Building friendships between handicapped and nonhandicapped students: Effects of cooperative individualistic instruction. *American Educational Research Journal, 18,* 415–423.

Koegel, R.L., & Rincover, A. (1974). Treatment of psychotic children in a classroom environment: I. Learning in a large group. *Journal of Applied Behavior Analysis, 7,* 45–49.

Kohler, F.W., & Strain, P.S. (1997). Merging naturalistic teaching and peer-based strategies to address the IEP objectives of preschoolers with autism: An examination of structural and child behavior outcomes. *Focus on Autism and Other Developmental Disabilities, 12*(4), 196–206.

Kohler, F.W., Strain, P.S., Maretsky, S., & DeCesare, L. (1990). Promoting positive and supportive interactions between preschoolers: An analysis of group-oriented contingencies. *Journal of Early Intervention, 14*(4), 327–341.

Ling, S., Hawkins, R., & Weber, D. (2011). Effects of a classwide interdependent group contingency designed to improve the behavior of an at-risk student. *Journal of Behavioral Education, 20*(2), 103–116.

McMaster, K.N., & Fuchs, D. (2002). Effects of cooperative learning on the academic achievement of students with learning disabilities: An update of Tateyama-Sniezek's review. *Learning Disabilities Research and Practice, 17,* 107–117.

Morrow, L.M. (2010). Preparing centers and a literacy-rich environment for small-group instruction in Early Reading First preschools. In M.C. McKenna, S. Walpole, & K. Conradi (Eds.), *Promoting early reading: Research, resources, and best practices* (pp. 124–141). New York, NY: Guilford.

Murphy, K.A., Theodore, L.A., Aloiso, D., Alric-Edwards, J.M., & Hughes, T.L. (2007). Interdependent group contingency and mystery motivators to reduce preschool disruptive behavior. *Psychology in the Schools, 44*(1), 53–63.

Noonan, M.J., Ratokalau, N.B., Lauth-Torres, L., McCormick, L., Esaki, C.A., & Claybaugh, K.W. (1992). Validating critical skills for preschool success. *Infant-Toddler Intervention, 2*(3), 187–202.

Phillips, L.B., & Twardosz, S. (2003). Group size and storybook reading: Two-year-old children's verbal and nonverbal participation with books. *Early Education and Development, 14*(4), 453–478.

Putnam, J.W., Rynders, J.E., Johnson, R., & Johnson, D. (1989). Collaborative skill instruction for promoting positive interactions between mentally handicapped and nonhandicapped children. *Exceptional Children, 55*(6), 550–557.

Rotholz, D.A. (1987). Current considerations on the use of one-to-one instruction with autistic students: Review and recommendations. *Education and treatment of children, 10,* 271–278.

Sainato, D.M., Strain, P.S., & Lyon, S.R. (1987). Increasing academic responding of handicapped preschool children during group instruction. *Journal of Early Intervention, 12*(1), 23–30.

Sharan, S. (1980). Cooperative learning in small groups: Recent methods and effects on achievement, attitudes, and ethnic relations. *Review of Educational Research, 50*(2), 241–271.

Snell, M.E., & Brown, F. (2011). *Instruction of students with severe disabilities* (7th ed.). Upper Saddle River, NJ: Pearson.

Stokes, T.F., & Baer, D.M. (1977). An implicit technology of generalization. *Journal of Applied Behavior Analysis, 10,* 349–367.

Taubman, M., Brierley, S., Wishner, J., Baker, D., McEachin, J., & Leaf, R. (2001). The effectiveness of a group discrete trial instructional approach for preschoolers with developmental disabilities. *Research in Developmental Disabilities, 22,* 205–219.

Vincent, L.J., Salisbury, C., Walter, G., Brown, P., Gruenewald, L.J., & Powers, M. (1980). Program evaluation and curriculum development in early childhood special education: Criteria of the next environment. In W. Sailor, B. Wilcox, & L. Brown (Eds.), *Methods of instruction for severely handicapped students* (pp. 308–328). Baltimore, MD: Paul H. Brookes Publishing Co.

Wasik, B. (2008). When fewer is more: Small groups in early childhood classrooms. *Early Childhood Education Journal, 35*(6), 515–521.

Werts, M.G., Caldwell, N.K., & Wolery, M. (1996). Peer modeling of response chains: Observational learning by students with disabilities. *Journal of Applied Behavior Analysis, 29,* 53–66.

Whalen, C., Schuster, J.W., & Hemmeter, M.L. (1996). The use of unrelated instructive feedback when teaching in a small group instructional arrangement. *Education and Training in Mental Retardation and Developmental Disabilities, 31,* 188–202.

Wolery, M., McWilliam, R.A., & Bailey, D.B. (2005). *Teaching infants and preschoolers with disabilities* (3rd ed.). Upper Saddle River, NJ: Pearson Prentice Hall.

Wortham, S.C. (2010). *Early childhood curriculum: Developmental bases for learning and teaching* (5th ed.). Upper Saddle River, NJ: Merrill/Prentice Hall.

Zanolli, K., Daggett, J., & Adams, T. (1996). Teaching preschool age autistic children to make spontaneous initiations to peers using priming. *Journal of Autism and Developmental Disorders, 26,* 407–422.

12

Interventions to Promote Peer Interactions

Linda McCormick

••••••••••••••• **FOCUS OF THIS CHAPTER** •••••••••••••••

- Types of social-skills interventions
- Classroom-wide interventions
- Naturalistic peer interaction interventions
- Explicit social-skills interventions

How well social skills are learned depends on the quality and quantity of a child's early opportunities to engage in social interactions with peers. By age 3, most children have participated in countless recurring routines where they have acquired the social skills (including the concomitant language and intellectual skills) for social competence. Socialization requires relatively little coaching when a child's development is progressing at a typical rate. This is not the case for children with disabilities. Many times they seem aloof, withdrawn and unaware of the initiations of peers, lacking the ability to share, take turns, get the attention of a peer, express their attention, ask for assistance, or communicate positive feelings.

The difficulties in peer-related social competence of young children with disabilities are compounded when they enter early childhood settings. The peer group may provide age-appropriate, competent, and positive models of social and communication competence, but if the children with disabilities are not socially accepted they cannot benefit from these models. The marginalization they experience in these settings can be potentially devastating to their future social development and educational achievements.

SOCIAL ACCEPTANCE AND REJECTION IN CLASSROOM SETTINGS

In examining the social environment in inclusive preschool settings, Odom, Zercher, Li, Marquart, and Sandall (2006) focused on two issues: 1) the social acceptance and rejection of young children with disabilities in inclusive settings and 2) characteristics of social behavior associated with social acceptance and rejection. They defined social acceptance as the generally positive appraisals of individual children by peers in reference to working or playing together. Social rejection was the active exclusion of children from peer-group activities. While a substantial percentage of the children in the study were well accepted in their inclusive settings, at least an equal proportion of the children with disabilities—those with disabilities such as developmental delay or autism that typically affect social problem solving and emotional regulation—were not well accepted by peers. The extent to which the social rejection by peers will affect their educational and social outcomes is a major concern.

Social Competence

Social competence is a composite of skills, each of which has many dimensions. Compared to competence in other skill areas, social competence seems to be an evaluative term and is based on subjective judgments by significant social agents rather than objective observations (Brown, Odom, McConnell, & Rathel, 2008). However, at the very least, most agree that it is the ability to be effective and appropriate in human interaction and relationships. More specifically, social competence includes the ability to use appropriate and effective social strategies to 1) gain entry to a peer group, 2) resolve conflicts, 3) maintain play interactions, and 4) initiate, develop, and maintain friendships (e.g., Guralnick, 2010; Odom, McConnell, & Brown, 2008). Additionally, it includes such communication skills as *joint attention, symbol use,* and *turn taking* (Prizant, Wetherby, Rubin, & Laurent, 2003).

Joint attention is the ability to consider the attentional focus of another person and to draw that attentional focus toward objects and events of mutual interest. This capacity is basic to the emergence of an understanding of the mind and, possibly, to the ability to have objective thought. It involves orienting and attending to a social partner, shifting gaze between people and objects, sharing affection or emotional states with another person, following the gaze or the pointing of another person, and drawing the attention of another person to objects or events for the purpose of sharing experiences. Evident in typically developing infants sometime around their first birthday, joint attention enables a child to coordinate and share attention and emotions, express intentions, and engage in reciprocal social interactions. Joint attention ability is often lacking in young children with autism and other severe disabilities (Greenspan & Wieder, 1997).

Symbol use refers to a child's understanding that meaning is expressed through gestures, words, and sentences. Young children with autism and other severe disabilities have difficulty learning and using conventional gestures. They also have difficulty learning the conventional meaning of words. The use of challenging behaviors for protesting or establishing social control may be a direct consequence of these limitations.

Turn taking is the ability to initiate, respond, and take turns in an exchange format. Successful turn taking requires children to continue their turns, which can be more challenging when interacting with peers than with adults. Turn-taking skills are frequently targeted in social skills interventions for children with disabilities.

This chapter describes intervention procedures used to promote the development of social and communication competence. In line with the tiered model suggested by Brown, Odom, and Conroy (2001), the types of social interventions are placed along a continuum from least intrusive to more structured and individualized. Some focus more specifically on language and communication targets, but they all involve communication as well as nonverbal social skills. There are three basic categories of social intervention:

- Classroom-wide interventions
- Naturalistic peer interaction interventions
- Explicit social skills interventions

Which procedure to use depends on the child and the circumstances, but the general rule is to begin with procedures that require minimal changes in classroom routines and few additional resources (the least intrusive and most normal type of peer interaction intervention), and then move to procedures that are more intense and individualized. While all of these interventions involve planning and preparation, the latter require more time and effort on the part of teachers.

CLASSROOMWIDE INTERVENTIONS

This category of interventions includes environmental structuring, affective interventions, and social competence curricula. These procedures are implemented with all the children in the class within the natural flow of classroom activities.

Structuring the Environment

Environmental-structuring strategies are adaptations to the classroom's physical environment, schedule, activities, and materials that promote engagement and prevent challenging behavior. An advantage of environmental strategies is that once planned and arranged they require little adult intervention.

There should be enough centers in the classroom to accommodate all of the children without crowding, which can lead to disruptive behavior. However, too many centers can be a problem in that there will be times where there is only one child in a center. This means limited opportunities for peer interactions. The only centers where the rule is "one child at a time" should be small, cozy, quiet areas with cushions on the floor.

Centers should be well defined so the boundaries are clear and materials are meaningful, responsive, and relevant to the children's needs and interests. Materials should be challenging enough to contribute to the children's feelings of competence but not so complex that they lead to frustration. Give priority to those toys and materials that promote peer interactions, particularly cooperation and sharing, both indoors and outdoors. In contrast to bikes and tricycles, playground items such as teeter-totters, rocking boats, and wagons are ideal in that they require two children to coordinate their actions. Even how children are positioned when in a center makes a difference. Arranging furniture and materials so that children face one another (e.g., across the water table, working with play dough, preparing something in the housekeeping center) encourages imitation and interaction as each child can see what the other is doing.

Affective Interventions

The goal of group-focused affective interventions is to gently challenge misconceptions and stereotypes about persons with disabilities. Photographs, books, and other printed materials, discussion groups, audiovisual materials, and puppetry are used to nurture children's positive attitudes about and perceptions of individuals with disabilities. Opportunities for the class to explore and experience adaptive equipment and to meet and talk with people with disabilities about their activities and aspirations are an important component of these activities.

Favazza and Odom (1997) suggest three specific components of affective interventions: 1) storytimes and discussions about children with disabilities, 2) structured free play with peer with disabilities, and 3) guided discussions at home. Books about disabilities are read and equipment related to the stories (e.g., a wheelchair, scooter board) is made available for the children to explore during storytimes. After reading the stories, there are questions on five topics: story content, disabilities, the similarities between children with and without disabilities, equipment related to story content, and playtime experiences. The questions on story content relate to factual information about the story (e.g., "Who was the girl in the story?"). The questions about disabilities focus on the cause of the disability and the reasons why the equipment is necessary (e.g., "If a person has to use a wheelchair because he has been in an accident, can he still do many things well?"). The next set of questions focuses on how the character in the story is similar to all children (e.g., "What are some things that Jason in the story likes to do that you also like to do?"). If the story introduced a special piece of equipment, the children are encouraged to explore it and then asked questions such as "What are the different parts of a wheelchair?" "How does someone make a wheelchair turn corners?" The last set of questions encourages the children to talk about their positive play experiences with their peers with disabilities and any issues or concerns such as communication difficulties or difficulties related to motor limitations (e.g., stacking blocks, moving from one learning/activity center or activity to another). All questions are answered in a factual manner.

The structured free-play sessions use environmental arrangement strategies as discussed above—limiting space, selecting materials and activities that promote social interaction, and rotating and limiting materials—to increase positive interactions. The emphasis is on ensuring that children with and without disabilities have fun playing with one another in small groups. No prompts or instructions are provided. The third component of affective interventions involves the parents. A copy of the story discussed in class is sent home for the parents to read again with their child. Parents are given the same questions used in class with the suggestion that they talk with their child about the story.

An additional advantage of this intervention strategy is the opportunity to integrate emergent literacy activities into the curriculum while at the same time promoting acceptance of children with diverse abilities. Another benefit is the increased self-esteem of all the children. Incorporating materials that celebrate and value all children is a positive and visible way to send the message that everyone belongs.

Social Competence Curriculum

There are many social competence curricula, some of which target specific skill domains while others are basically preventive interventions. Examples of curricula for preschool children include the Dinosaur School curriculum, which is part of the Incredible Years series (Webster-Stratton & Reid, 2004), the I Can Problem Solve curriculum (Shure, 2000), and the Emotions Course (Izard, Trentacosta, King, & Mostow, 2004).

Promoting Alternative Thinking Strategies, or PATHS (Domitrovich, Greenberg, Kusche, & Cortes, 2004), expands these curricula by including instruction in multiple skill domains delivered in a developmentally appropriate sequence. It is intended to prevent or reduce behavior and emotional problems in young children and enhance children's social-emotional competence. A unique aspect of this curriculum is its emotional component, which emphasizes affective awareness in oneself as well as in others. At the core of PATHS is the ecological concept that children's adaptation is a function of both their own skill level and the environmental context that surrounds them (Bronfenbrenner, 1979, 1992). Thus the curriculum emphasizes teaching new skills and creating meaningful real-life opportunities to ensure generalization of the newly acquired skills. The research findings are positive for these interventions and many others designed to help young children from birth to 5 years improve social-emotional functioning (Powell & Dunlap, 2009).

In addition to the above interventions, it is important to provide as many opportunities as possible for children to practice and consolidate their social and communication interactions skills within the natural flow of classroom activities. Teachers should begin with the assumption that the more interactions there are with peers who are good language, social, and play models, the more opportunities there will be for children with disabilities to acquire and practice language and communication skills. Use parallel talk to encourage and support children's understanding of the behavior of others in the social situation. Parallel talk is providing a running commentary about what the child is doing, usually beginning with "you" and essentially matching words to the child's actions. For example, Tyler is standing (almost hidden by a bookcase) watching a peer who is moving toy trucks and cars in and out of a small service station. Descriptive comments that include the children's names will draw their attention to one another. For example, one could say, "You are watching Jason move the cars up and down the garage ramp and you want to play too. You want Jason to let you put your car on the ramp beside his. To let Jason know that you want to play with him, you need to say, 'May I play too?'" This parallel talk highlights the action and the toy that are the focus of Tyler's attention, thus prompting and supporting joint attention. Tyler may not be able to imitate the verbal model, but the two boys look at each other and/or jointly attend to the play activity. The teacher moves quietly away once the boys begin playing.

NATURALISTIC PEER INTERACTION INTERVENTIONS

Naturalistic peer interaction interventions are implemented in a more systematic manner. Teaching opportunities are embedded within routine activities and use naturally occurring antecedents and consequences so they can easily be integrated into inclusive early childhood classrooms.

Friendship Activities

The goal of friendship activity interventions (also known as *group affection activities*) is to build affection and prosocial behaviors. They capitalize on the observation that preschool-age children typically respond positively to physical affection (e.g., high five, hugs, shaking hands) and prosocial responses such as friendly statements, compliments, smiles, and other forms of encouragement. Opportunities to experience affection and prosocial responses are embedded into common preschool games, songs, and other routine activities such as Simon Says, "The Farmer in the Dell," and "If You're Happy and You Know It." Children are taught a new song or game or they participate in one that is familiar. After they perform the song, game, or activity in the usual manner, they are told, "Now we are going to play this a little differently." Then some ways to exchange physical and other forms of affection (e.g., hug, pat on the back, high five, handshake, smile, taking turns with or sharing an object) are demonstrated. For example, the teacher would say, "After singing 'The Farmer in the Dell,' instead of singing 'the farmer takes a wife' or 'the wife takes a child,' we will sing 'the farmer hugs a wife' or 'the wife hugs a child' and then everyone will do it. We will all hug the friend standing next to us."

The children's game Musical Chairs also lends itself very well to adaptation as a friendship activity. There are multiple opportunities for children to interact socially with peers and to observe others socially interacting with peers. Each interruption of the music (the points at which children try to find a chair but chairs are inevitably one short) provides an opportunity for the children to interact by making friendly statements, complimenting one another, making high fives, or shaking hands. The prosocial behaviors of all the children are encouraged with special attention to maximizing positive exchanges of children with disabilities.

To be maximally effective, friendship activities should be conducted daily for about 10 to 15 minutes. These activities provide opportunities for children with disabilities to observe peer modeling of positive social behavior and then actually practice the behavior with positive feedback.

Enhanced Milieu Teaching of Social Behaviors

As noted in Chapter 7, enhanced milieu teaching (EMT) is a naturalistic instructional procedure wherein the environment is arranged to increase opportunities for social and communicative behavior. Rather than expecting the child to respond to prompts and directions, the adult follows the child's leads, matching instructional strategies to the child's ongoing actions and interests.

EMT is a hybrid approach in that it integrates aspects of both behavioral and social interactionist approaches for promoting social and communicative interactions. It incorporates 1) environmental arrangement to promote child engagement with activities and communication partners; 2) responsive interaction techniques to promote social and conversational interactions and to model desired behaviors; and 3) milieu teaching procedures to prompt, model, and appropriately acknowledge the use of new behaviors in functional contexts. The following steps are taken to implement EMT to facilitate social behavior:

- *Identify unstructured activities that engage the child with disabilities and include one or more peers without disabilities.* Routine activities that involve learning centers, outdoor play, meals and snacks, free play, and transitions are especially good contexts for teaching social behavior.

- *Plan the prompting procedures (modeling, mand model, time delay, or incidental teaching) to encourage social interactions during the identified activities or whenever the potential for peer interactions arises.* A teacher should also consider whether adults or peers will provide the prompts for appropriate social responses. For example, at snack they would give Taylor a double quantity of fruit or crackers and prompt him to share with a "friend." The way to find out if a situation is a good context in which to prompt social interactions is to observe the child and note whether he or she is interested in the materials and/or peers that are involved in the activity. If Taylor frequently watches Corey play with a particular set of cars and animals during manipulatives, he is probably interested in Corey, the toys, or both. If a child grabs a toy or other object from another child, it is safe to say that he is interested in that toy or object. Both situations provide good opportunities to prompt social interactions.

- *Implement the teaching procedures.* The objective is twofold: to teach new social responses and to provide opportunities for practice and elaboration of previously acquired social behaviors. For example, Jessie obviously enjoys the housekeeping center, but she never initiates interactions with peers. The teacher says to Jessie, "Remember how we ask our friends to play? I think Kaitlin would like to help you set the table. Say to Kaitlin, 'Want to help?'"

Jessie imitates the teacher's model. She says to Kaitlin, "Want to help?" and Kaitlin responds, "I'll put the cups out." Jessie and Kaitlin carefully set out the plastic dishes on the small table. Then they each sit in a chair and pretend to drink from the cups. Whenever her teacher sees Jessie playing alone, she prompts her to ask a peer to play. Over time Jesse begins to ask peers to play without the teacher's suggestion. Also, Jessie's peers are seeking her out and asking her to play with them during unstructured activities.

- *Acknowledge the peer or peers who reciprocally interact with the child with disabilities.* In the example above, Jessie's teacher commented to Kaitlin that it was nice of her to help Jessie set the table and to share the tea party (Brown, McEvoy, & Bishop, 1991).

Table 12.1 provides additional examples of contexts, teacher prompts, and anticipated social responses in EMT procedures. Friendship activities and/or EMT can be implemented concurrently with classroom-wide interventions. If these interventions are not accomplishing the desired peer interaction patterns, then the more individualized interventions described below should be implemented.

EXPLICIT SOCIAL-SKILLS INTERVENTIONS

Explicit social-skills interventions typically involve specialized instruction, prompts, and reinforcement for a particular child, but sometimes prompts and reinforcements are also extended to peers. Peer-mediated interventions focus on training peer confederates to support a specific skill in a peer with a disability.

Individual or Small-Group Lessons

Explicit social-skills interventions may involve individual or small group instruction of social skills for the children with disabilities, for the socially competent peers of children with disabilities, or both. Small-group lessons typically follow a standard format: the adult 1) describes the target skill (e.g., taking turns), 2) prompts two children to model the target skill, and then 3) separates the group into dyads and encourages them to practice the skill. After the small-group lesson, an activity is scheduled in which the children will have an opportunity to practice the new skill with others in the group. Initially, the adult stays very near the children to provide prompts and suggestions, moving away only when all the children are consistently demonstrating the skill.

Social Integration Activities

The goal of social integration activities is to bring children with social interaction difficulties in direct contact daily (for brief periods of time) with peers who are socially responsive and competent. Activities are carefully planned to provide opportunities for children with social interaction difficulties to 1) observe the socially competent play of their peers, 2) participate in social interactions with their socially competent peers, and 3) establish a positive history of peer interactions (Brown et al., 2001). Children soon learn that these activities are a regular part of their daily routine, similar to circle time, snacks, and so forth. The following are the steps in developing social integration activities:

Table 12.1. Examples: Enhanced milieu teaching procedures to promote social behaviors

Context	Teacher prompt	Child response	Peer response
Play			
Susie is standing and watching LiAn playing with the dolls.	"Susie, ask LiAn 'May I play too?'" "LiAn, could you let Susie dress the smaller doll?"	Susie sits down next to LiAn and says, "Me play too?"	LiAn gives Susie the smaller doll and says, "This is her dress."
Snack			
Jace needs help opening his milk carton.	"Jace, ask Angelica to help you. Say, 'Please help with my milk.'"	"Help please."	Angelica says, "I'll help you" as she twists the top of the milk carton.
Transition			
Christopher is having trouble moving his chair to the table for art activities. He watches Brandon push his chair to the table but does not speak.	"Brandon, ask Christopher if he would like you to help him with his chair."	Brandon says, "Do you want to sit here beside me?"	Christopher says, "Yes, sit beside Brandon."

Source: Brown, McEvoy, and Bishop (1991).

- *Identify children to make up the interaction groups.* Groups will typically include one or two children with social interaction difficulties and at least two or three socially responsive children.

- *Determine play areas.* Specific areas in the classroom in which the social integration activities will take place may change from one day to the next.

- *Select activities.* Select play activities that provide multiple opportunities for social interactions and positive play experiences.

- *Plan, arrange, introduce, and monitor the activities.* Assemble the identified children in the predetermined area, explain, and then lead the activity.

There are four play possibilities for the group: functional activities, constructive activities, sociodramatic play, and games with rules. Of these four possibilities, there is some evidence that sociodramatic play is the most supportive of peer interactions (DeKlyen & Odom, 1989). Activities should be selected, organized, and implemented with the goal of promoting sharing, talking, assisting, and playing. Each day, introduction of the selected activity includes suggestions to the children for how they might structure their play. In some activities, particularly sociodramatic play activities (e.g., making a birthday cake, playing storekeeper, preparing a tea party), children may be assigned roles. In others, ask the children to decide how they will play and which role each will take. After introducing and organizing the activity, teachers should withdraw partially but continue to monitor and support the activity. They may suggest a play idea, comment on the direction the play is taking, or, when indicated, directly prompt the children to interact with peers other than the ones with whom they have been interacting.

Peer-Mediated Interventions

Peer-mediated intervention is an evidence-based strategy in which peers assume an instructional role with classmates (e.g., Harris, Pretti-Frontczak, &

Brown, 2009). Socially competent peers are taught to initiate and respond to their peers with disabilities in an appropriate and respectful manner and draw them into play. They learn how to use social strategies such as establishing eye contact, asking a child to play or share a toy, suggesting play ideas, describing their own or other children's play, organizing play, and sharing, helping, and being responsive to the play of classmates with disabilities.

One well-researched peer-mediated intervention is the *buddy skills training package* developed by Goldstein and colleagues (Goldstein, Kaczmarek, Pennington, & Shaffer, 1992; English, Goldstein, Shafer, & Kaczmarek, 1997). The goal of this intervention is to teach social interaction skills to socially competent peers and to dyad partners with social interaction difficulties. There are two types of buddy skills training: peer training and dyadic training. Peer training includes sensitivity training and strategy-use training.

In sensitivity training, peers without disabilities are shown videotaped vignettes depicting the types of attention-getting and requesting behaviors that will help their peers with disabilities initiate interactions. The preschoolers in the vignettes use unconventional types of communicative behaviors such as gesturing and other nonverbal behaviors to request actions and attention. After viewing the vignette, the discussion focuses on what the child on the tape was trying to do or say and the importance of being sensitive to all of our friends' efforts to communicate. The strategy-use training teaches three "buddy" behaviors that can be condensed to the simple mnemonic "stay-play-talk."

- *Stay* near your assigned buddy—stand or sit beside your friend.

- *Play* with your friend—say your buddy's name, establish mutual attention, and talk or suggest playing together.

- *Talk* with your friend—continue to stay close and play and/or talk to him or her.

Once buddy pairs have been decided, individual training for the peers with competent social skills consists of five or six sessions (three direct-instruction lessons and two or three practice sessions). The standard procedures to follow in each training session are 1) discussion, 2) adult modeling, 3) guided practice, and 4) independent practice with feedback. Children have mastered the strategies when they are able to perform all three buddy steps without prompts in two consecutive turns.

After peer strategy training and practice sessions, dyadic training is conducted. These training sessions are conducted during classroom activities (e.g., free play, snack, large group). Depending on the needs of the child with disabilities in each dyad, there will be a need for two to four dyadic training sessions. During this training, the peers with disabilities in the dyads are taught a modified version of the stay-play-talk strategy. Most important, they learn to "stay and play" with their buddies. Dyadic sessions continue until the peers with disabilities are able to maintain proximity and interact with their buddies for 4 consecutive minutes in each of three activities in one day.

Harjusola-Webb, Hubbell, and Bedesem (2012) have combined peer-mediated intervention with social narratives to increase turn taking, which is one component of social competence. A social narrative is a simple story describing a particular social interaction activity. The goal is to teach the social responses the interaction requires. Social Story™ instruction is a teaching strategy with specific guidelines (Gray, 2000). Since roughly the start of the century, there has been considerable research investigating the use of the social narratives developed with these guidelines for improving social competence, specifically for such behaviors as responsiveness and initiation, joint attention, and turn taking (e.g., Delano & Snell, 2006; Scattone, 2008). The combination strategy described by Harjusola-Webb et al. has five steps:

1. *Select the target behavior.* The target behavior should be significant in the sense that mastery will contribute the child's access to and participation in a variety of social activities in his or her environment.

2. *Identify teaching opportunities.* Teaching opportunities should be embedded into activities in the daily schedule. An example would be free play: The socially competent peer asks the target child to help him assemble the tracks for the toy train. The target child nods or picks up a segment of track and the peer says, "Great, put that piece right here."

3. *Identify the peer helpers.* Select a peer who is compatible with the target child and competent in the target skill (in this case, turn taking).

4. *Create a social narrative.* There are many possibilities for the social narrative. They range from a simple booklet with stick figures or photographs to a digital story with video and narration. Most important is to match the narration to the level of communication skills of the target child. The story should describe the identified social situation, the desired behavior of the child in that situation, and peer responses. It should be short and simple enough for the child to memorize and recite it.

5. *Train the peer helpers.* Explain to the peer what his or her role is in helping the target child learn new behaviors. Read aloud the social narrative with emphasis on the expectations for the peer and the target child during the activity. Then role play the situation and consider possible responses. Stress the fact that learning new skills often takes a great deal of practice and that the interactions may need to be repeated many times before the target child learns the new response.

In addition to improving the social skills of young children with disabilities, this combined peer-mediated and social narrative intervention teaches peers how to interact with classmates who have not yet acquired the social skills. Not only does it promote friendships but it also contributes to awareness and acceptance of individual differences.

Young children with autism and other significant disabilities need the most intensive intervention. Often, initial social interaction training must focus on careful shaping of basic communication behaviors (e.g., requesting, commenting) using photographs, pictures, or gestures. Concurrently, peers without disabilities are taught to respond to the unconventional communication attempts of their classmates with disabilities.

A report by Stanton-Chapman and Snell (2011) describes a social communication intervention that fits in the category of explicit interventions. The purpose of this intervention is to teach turn taking. It incorporates a combination of methods: observational learning, reinforced learning (storybook scripting), and rehearsal, followed by live modeling during play. All of the participants (10 children in 5 dyads) in the study were receiving special education services under the diagnoses of specific language impairment, developmental delay, or behavior disorder. Intervention sessions were conducted 4 to 5 times a week. They were conducted in the context of one or another of five dramatic play themes: grocery store, doctor, construction worker, animal doctor, or hair designer/barber. Each intervention session had an advanced play organizer, the actual play session, and a review session. The advanced play organizer had four parts: 1) teaching target vocabulary words, 2) teaching the roles for each play theme, 3) reading the play theme storybook and teaching the communication strategies, and 4) planning the play. The storybooks—one for each play theme—were computer generated using a digital camera and a template for the format. They had pictures of the children and the exact materials and prompts used during the sessions. Four components of turn taking were taught:

1. Initiation: "Talk to your friend."
2. Responding: "Listen and then respond to your friend."
3. Naming: "Say your friend's name before talking to him."
4. Taking turns: "Take a turn and then give your friend a turn."

Evaluation of the turn-taking results in this study were stringent. The procedures effectively increased both initiations and responses in all five dyads. Initiations were followed by peer responses 75% of the time in the intervention condition. Where individual children were concerned, the intervention was highly effective for five children, moderately effective for three children, and mildly effective for two children. The generalization findings were especially encouraging. The generalization observations showed evidence of increased social play following the intervention, increased levels of engagement, and decreased levels of solitary play.

Stanton-Chapman and Snell (2011) speculated that one reason the intervention was not highly effective with all of the children was that they were not provided with enough experience with the scripted play. They were taught phrases to engage their peer in a social interaction but they did not have sufficient instruction as to how to maintain the interaction. They modified the program accordingly and are not using it in a Head Start setting. Rather than being instructed in dyads, the children are placed in small groups of five or six children. These are the elements of the intervention:

- *Advanced play organizers:* The children are taught the vocabulary words they need and the roles of the play themes. These sessions also include storybook reading and planning of play in the different themes.
- *Play themes:* There is a separate, stand-alone center in the classroom that is dedicated to the scripted play. The five themes are alternated every two weeks. Groups rotate through the center, where their play and social interactions in the play theme activities are facilitated by a teacher.
- *Review sessions:* During these sessions the teacher and the group review the thematic roles, the use of target vocabulary words, and the children's use of the social communication strategies.

This is an example of a structured intervention focused on the development of one particular social communication skill: turn taking.

In summary, the teacher's role in promoting peer interactions and friendships is to find a suitable social partner, create an environment conducive to positive peer relations, and provide frequent opportunities for children to play together and form mutually regulated friendships. A teacher may serve as an interactive partner, a social coach, or a provider of social opportunities. Being an interactive partner means playing with the child in a warm, responsive manner. This provides a model for the child on how to interact with a peer, and it provides opportunities for the child to learn social skills. Social coaching involves giving the child either a direction or the precise words to use to accomplish a social goal. Use social coaching to teach the child how to enter a peer playgroup and/or how to initiate social contacts with possible playmates. Being a provider of social opportunities requires careful attention to potential social dyads—noticing when children seem to show mutual interest in one another and whom they seem to like and then arranging play opportunities both within and outside the classroom.

Language and communication abilities and cognitive levels undoubtedly play a role in the development of friendships. Depending upon the child's skills, it is often a good idea to pair the child with a peer who is slightly younger and perhaps less developmentally advanced in some areas but who is socially competent. Create opportunities to highlight the special talents of the child (e.g., puzzles, computers, knowledge in a particular area), favorite activities, and favorite characters (e.g., Barney, clowns). Common interests and successful interaction in activities that build on these common interests can lay the groundwork for children to become friends.

SUMMARY

If inclusive environments are to afford the benefits of positive social interactions for children with disabilities, there must be planned and systematic opportunities throughout the day for the children to engage in and practice social and communicative interactions. Brown, Odom, and Conroy (2001) have provided a social relationship intervention hierarchy that can help teachers plan procedures to enhance the peer-related social competence of young children with disabilities. The least structured interventions, *classroom-wide approaches*, include environmental-structuring strategies, affective interventions, and social competence curricula. *Naturalistic peer interaction interventions* are more structured. This category of interventions includes friendship activities and enhanced milieu teaching EMT. Finally, the most structured interventions, *explicit social skills interventions*, include small-group lessons, peer-mediated interventions, and social integration activities.

Most important to remember is that missed opportunities for successful social experiences with peers are missed opportunities for learning language and communication skills. Peers in inclusive settings are more than natural partners—they are natural facilitators of language and communication.

•••••••••••••••••••• **STUDY QUESTIONS** ••••••••••••••••••••

1. What is *social competence* and why is definition of social competence so difficult?

2. Describe the three communication skills thought to be important for social competence.

3. Compare and contrast the three basic categories of social interventions.

4. Describe the components of and strategies involved in each of the three classroom interventions.

5. Describe the two types of *naturalistic peer interaction* interventions.

6. Describe the three types of explicit social skills interventions.

REFERENCES

Bronfenbrenner, U. (1979). *The ecology of human development: Experiments by nature and design.* Cambridge, MA: Harvard University Press.

Bronfenbrenner, U. (1992). Ecological systems theory. In R. Vasa (Ed.), *Six theories of child development: Revised formulations and current issues* (pp. 187–248). Philadelphia, PA: Kingsley.

Brown, W.H., McEvoy, M.A., & Bishop, J.N. (1991). Incidental teaching of social behavior: A naturalistic approach to promoting young children's peer interactions. *Teaching Exceptional Children, 24,* 35–58.

Brown, W.H., Odom, S.I., McConnell, S.R., & Rathel, J.M. (2008). Peer interaction interventions for children with developmental difficulties. In W.H. Brown, S.I. Odom, & S.R. McConnell (Eds.), *Social competence of young children: Risk, disability, and intervention* (2nd ed., pp. 141–163). Baltimore, MD: Paul H. Brookes Publishing Co.

Brown, W.H., Odom, S.L., & Conroy, M. (2001). An intervention hierarchy for promoting preschool children's peer interactions in naturalistic environments. *Topics in Early Childhood Special Education, 21,* 162–175.

DeKlyen, M., & Odom, S.L. (1989). Activity structure and social interactions with peers in developmentally integrated play groups. *Journal of Early Intervention, 13,* 342–352.

Delano, M., & Snell, M. (2006). The effects of social stories on the social engagement of children with autism. *Journal of Positive Behavior Interventions, 8,* 29–42.

Domitrovich, C., Greenberg, M., Kusche, C., & Cortes, R. (2004). *PATHS preschool program.* South Deerfield, MA: Channing Bete.

English, K., Goldstein, H., Shafer, K., & Kaczmarek, L. (1997). Teaching buddy skills in inclusive preschools. *Innovations* (monograph series of the American Association on Mental Retardation) *9,* 1–40.

Favazza, P.C., & Odom, S.L. (1997). Use of the Acceptance Scale with kindergarten-age children. *Journal of Early Intervention, 20,* 232–248.

Goldstein, H., Kaczmarek, L., Pennington, R., & Shafer, K. (1992). Peer-mediated intervention: Attending to, commenting on, and acknowledging the behavior of preschoolers with autism. *Journal of Applied Behavior Analysis, 25,* 289–305.

Gray, C. (2000). *The new social story book.* Arlington, TX: Future Horizons.

Greenspan, S.I., and Wieder, S. (1997). Developmental patterns and outcomes in infants and children with disorders in relating and communicating: A chart review of 200 cases of children with autistic spectrum diagnoses. *Journal of Developmental and Learning Disorders, 1,* 87–141.

Guralnick, M.J. (2010). Early intervention approaches to enhance the peer-related social competence of young children with developmental delays: A historical perspective. *Infants and Young Children, 23*, 73–83.

Harjusola-Webb, S., Parke Hubbell, S., & Bedesem, P. (2012). Increasing prosocial behaviors of young children with disabilities in inclusive classrooms using a combination of peer-mediated intervention and social narratives. *Beyond Behavior, 21*, 29–36.

Harris, K., Pretti-Frontczak, K., & Brown, T. (2009). Peer-mediated intervention: Implementing research-based practices within developmentally appropriate learning environments. *Young Children, 64*(2), 43–49.

Izard, C.E., Trentacosta, C.J., King, K.A., & Mostow, A.J. (2004). An emotion-based prevention program for Head Start children. *Early Education & Development, 15*(4), 407–422.

Odom, S.L., Zercher, C., Li, S., Marquart, J., & Sandall, S. (2006). Social acceptance and social rejection of young children with disabilities in inclusive classes. *Journal of Educational Psychology, 98*, 807–823.

Odom, S.L., McConnell, S.R., & Brown, W.H. (2008). Social competence for young children: Conceptualization, assessment, and influences. In W. Brown, S. Odom, & S. McConnell (Eds.), *Social competence of young children: Risk, disability, and intervention* (2nd ed., pp. 3–30). Baltimore, MD: Paul H. Brookes Publishing Co.

Powell, D., & Dunlap, G. (2009). Evidence-based social-emotional curricula and intervention packages for children 0–5 years and their families. *The Roadmap to Effective Intervention Practices Series.* Tampa, FL: Technical Assistance Center for Social Emotional Intervention for Young Children. University of South Florida.

Prizant, B.M., Wetherby, A.M., Rubin, E., & Laurent, A.C. (2003). The SCERTS model: A transactional, family-centered approach to enhancing communication and socio-emotional abilities of children with autism spectrum disorder. *Journal of Infants and Young Children, 16*, 4, 296–316.

Scattone, D. (2008). Enhancing the conversation skills of a boy with Asperger's disorder through Social Stories™ and video modeling. *Journal of Autism and Developmental Disorders, 38*, 395–400.

Shure, M. (2000). *I can problem solve: An interpersonal cognitive problem-solving program (preschool).* Champaign, L: Research Press.

Stanton-Chapman, T.L., & Snell, M.E. (2011). Promoting turn-taking skills in preschool children with disabilities: The effects of a peer-based social communication intervention. *Early Childhood Research Quarterly, 26*, 303–319.

Webster-Stratton, C., & Reid, J.M. (2004). Classroom social skills dinosaur program—strengthening social and emotional competence in young children—the foundation for early school readiness and success: Incredible years classroom social skills and problem solving curriculum. *Infants and Young Children, 17*(2), 96–113.

13

Environmental Arrangements, Adaptations, and Assistive Technologies

Mary Jo Noonan

·················· **FOCUS OF THIS CHAPTER** ··················

- Teaching independent behaviors
- Adaptations for functional independence, including assistive technology
- Functional independence in basic physical skills
- Physical development intervention procedures
- Independence in fine motor skills
- Establishing communication and environmental skills
- Independence in self-help skills
- Designing instructional programs to promote independence

Independent behavior is behavior performed in the presence of naturally occurring stimuli. This usually means that the behavior is achieved without the assistance of other people. There are many reasons why children with disabilities may not develop age-appropriate independent behaviors. First, failing to fade instructional prompts may inadvertently teach the children to "always wait for assistance." Second, adults may hold low expectations for children with disabilities and thus may not afford them opportunities to be independent (Stoneman & Rugg, 2004). Finally, significant physical, sensory, or communication needs may pose obstacles and interfere with achieving independence. It is important to systematically plan, teach, and provide adaptations and assistive technologies that promote independence.

TEACHING INDEPENDENT BEHAVIORS

Independent behavior goals for children with disabilities must be age appropriate. For example, 5 minutes of independent play could be a goal for a 1-year-old when placed on a blanket with some toys. Independent requesting might be an appropriate goal for a toddler. The toddler could be taught to point as a way of requesting desired objects, activities, and interaction. To construct a goal that fosters independence, caregivers should avoid stating performance conditions in which the behavior is initiated or prompted by an adult. Instead, the objective should specify natural conditions under which the skill is needed. Some examples include "When getting dressed in the morning, Sara will choose a T-shirt from the drawer," or "When playing with a friend in the free-play area, Tommy will choose a toy from the shelves." These are more natural conditions than "When given two T-shirts" or "When presented with three toys."

In addition to specifying independence as a performance condition, independence can be incorporated into the criterion of an objective. For example, when teaching a child to hold a spoon, the criterion might state that the child independently retrieves the spoon if it drops on the table. Criterion levels for independent behaviors should correspond to the standards or requirements of independence in natural environments. Once objectives have been formulated, the next step is to plan instruction.

Systematic Instruction

The concepts of systematic instruction were introduced in Chapter 6. Instructional prompts are used to help a child learn a correct response. The basic task of teaching is to fade the instructional prompt so that the child responds correctly to the natural prompt, that is, the child performs *independently* when the natural stimulus is present. To help a child achieve independence, systematic instructional plans should be 1) least intrusive, 2) naturalistic, 3) associated with routines and environmental modifications, and/or 4) designed to promote generalization. *Least intrusive* procedures are those that differ as little as possible from naturalistic learning experiences or do not interfere with ordinary routines. Least intrusive procedures have two advantages when teaching independent behavior. First, they are easily eliminated through fading because they are not very noticeable. Second, they are easy for others to implement because they are similar to what people would typically do to help a child.

Naturalistic instruction, particularly enhanced milieu teaching (EMT) (Kaiser, 1993; Kaiser, Hendrickson, & Alpert, 1991), was described at length in Chapter 7. Basic to systematic naturalistic procedures is the goal of independence—ensuring self-initiated rather than adult-prompted behavior. When planning EMT, a specific child behavior can be identified as an *occasion for instruction*. An occasion for instruction may be child behaviors as subtle as a child looking at an object or as obvious as reaching for a desired object or vocalizing for attention ("Watch me!").

Daily routines provide children with repeated and predictable sequences of events that help them anticipate what comes next. Repetition and anticipation promote learning. For example, a child's morning routine with a babysitter always begins with the child selecting some toys or books, playing with the sitter for a while, putting the toys or books away, and having a snack. After days or weeks of the routine, the sitter might arrive and be greeted by the child with a book for playtime. When the sitter stops playing and goes to the kitchen to prepare a snack, the child might put the book away, anticipating the snack.

Environmental modifications can be used to provide reminders to help children respond independently. Achieved by physically altering the environment, modifications can range from very intrusive to minimally intrusive. Consider this example: A preschooler is learning to distribute napkins and cups at snack time. Once she is reminded to do the task, she usually does it independently. Providing the napkins and cups at her place setting (rather than reminding her) is a natural, nonintrusive prompt for the child to begin distributing the napkins and cups.

Generalization Strategies

Although not always necessary when using naturalistic teaching procedures, including *generalization strategies* in instructional plans will promote independence (these were discussed in detail in Chapter 6). Several generalization procedures (Stokes & Baer, 1977) are well suited to promoting independence. Natural contingencies may be paired with instructional ones to facilitate generalization. Over time, instructional contingencies are faded. Sufficient *exemplar training* promotes independence because it teaches a stimulus class (the group of stimuli that are typically associated with the response). If a preschooler who uses a wheelchair is taught to ask a peer for assistance in maneuvering through a doorway, getting materials that are out of reach, or carrying his lunch tray (*exemplar training*), he is likely to generalize and ask a peer for assistance to retrieve a dropped toy (a response that was not taught). Encountering material from the instructional setting in natural environments (*program common stimuli*) may prompt a new behavior. Finally, self-prompting, a common strategy to mediate generalization, facilitates independence across settings and situations because it essentially "goes with" the child wherever he goes.

ADAPTATIONS FOR FUNCTIONAL INDEPENDENCE, INCLUDING ASSISTIVE TECHNOLOGY

White (1980) used the term *critical function* to distinguish the purpose of a behavior from the physical action used to accomplish it. Crawling, for example, serves the purpose of getting from one place to another—the critical function of mobility. Reaching and vocalizing may serve the purpose of obtaining more food—a critical function of communicating a request. A *functionally equivalent* response is a response that accomplishes the same critical function (purpose) as the target behavior, but by another means (Carr & Durand, 1985). For example, pointing may serve as a functionally equivalent response for grasping if pointing has the effect of the child obtaining the toy he pointed to (the same effect that would have been achieved if the child could grasp the toy). In general, instructional objectives should focus more on function than form; accomplishing an intended outcome is often more important than a specific behavior or form of behavior.

When a child uses functionally equivalent responses to do a task without assistance, she accomplishes *functional independence*. The following strategies teach an infant or young child to be functionally independent: 1) individualized participation, 2) environmental prompts, 3) learning centers, 4) peer assistance, and 5) assistive technology.

Individualized Participation

Group instruction was discussed in Chapter 11. Many activities in child care, preschool settings, and early intervention programs are conducted in small- or large-group situations. Group instruction, however, does not require that all children in the group participate at the same level or in the same way; participation can be individualized. Consider using a puppet activity to teach turn taking. Jason, a preschooler with a language delay and hearing impairment, can participate independently by manipulating the puppets while another group member speaks for the puppet.

Environmental Prompts

Another way to help an infant or young child achieve independence is to modify the environment or materials to provide extra clues or reminders. To assist a child to be independent in washing her hands, for example, a series of pictures illustrating task steps can be posted as reminders (Phillips & Vollmer, 2012). Color coding (e.g., cubbies, chairs, coats, rug squares, crayon boxes, toothbrushes) is another example of an environmental prompt that allows children to perform independently. An environmental prompt may be permanent (it remains in place) or temporary (it will be faded).

Learning Centers

One purpose of learning centers is to teach children to play without adult assistance. For example, a child care program may have a learning center that includes blocks and other building materials, or a preschool may have a learning center with science materials that change weekly (e.g., "dinosaur week" might include dinosaur coloring books, plastic dinosaur figures and habitats, a dinosaur egg game, a dictionary of dinosaurs, storybooks about dinosaurs). Learning centers provide opportunities for functional independence because children decide how they want to participate (within clearly established limits), interacting with materials in a manner that suits their interests and skills (McWilliam & Casey, 2008).

Peer Assistance

In many situations, peer assistance can help a child be independent of adult assistance. Peers can assist in a wide range of tasks, such as helping a child balance while walking, picking up items that a child drops, reminding a child what should be done next, and so on. Although one should be careful not to burden a sibling or young child with too much responsibility for another child, providing assistance in certain situations teaches children to be helpful and considerate. It also encourages empathy and nurturing, important attitudes for children to develop. At the same time, it helps children with disabilities to be independent of adults.

Assistive Technology

The Technology-Related Assistance for Individuals with Disabilities Act of 1988 (PL 100-407)—referred to as the Tech Act—and the Individuals with Disabilities Education Improvement Act (IDEA) of 2004 define and support the use of assistive technology (AT) for young children with disabilities. According to IDEA, AT is "any item, piece of equipment, or product system, whether acquired commercially off the shelf, modified, or customized, that is used to increase, maintain, or improve the functional capabilities of a child with a disability."

IDEA also requires that services necessary for selecting, obtaining, and using AT be provided. As with other IDEA requirements, AT devices and services must be included in a child's individualized education program and/or individualized family service plan if they are necessary in order for the child to benefit from his or her special education. To increase the likelihood that children with disabilities receive AT devices and services that they need, IDEA mandates that AT be discussed and considered for every child receiving special education and early intervention.

The purpose of AT is to improve a child's functional capabilities (Sadao & Robinson, 2010). For young children with disabilities, early childhood recommended practices note that AT should focus on "(1) enhancing development across all domains; (2) increasing independence and access; (3) enhancing individualized child and family interaction/instruction; (4) supporting professionals and families to ensure successful use of technology; and (5) increasing family and professional access to information and networking" (Sandall, Hemmeter, Smith, & McLean, 2005, p. 148).

When selected appropriately and used effectively, AT has the potential to increase a child's functional capabilities in communication and language, environmental access, social-adaptive skills, mobility and orientation skills, daily life skills, social interaction skills, health, and/or position/handling. It should also increase the availability of natural learning opportunities, participation in the general education curriculum, and access to diverse and less restrictive environments (Sandall et al., 2005).

Assistive Technology Devices Children with physical disabilities may benefit from special compensatory AT equipment such as a prosthetic device—a replacement or adaptation for a missing or nonfunctional limb (Hill, 1999). An artificial leg is a prosthesis for a child who is missing a leg. A splint with a Velcro band that secures a crayon in a child's hand is a prosthesis for a child who is otherwise unable to hold a crayon. If a child is not able to achieve functional independence immediately with the use of a prosthesis, guided practice may be used to teach the child to use the device.

Adaptive equipment is AT that refers to specialized furniture and other materials designed to assist individuals with disabilities, usually physical or sensory disabilities. Wheelchairs, walkers, positioning chairs, standers, adjustable tables, modified bicycles, and feeding equipment are examples of adaptive equipment for children with physical disabilities. For many children with special needs, physical support and therapeutically beneficial physical responses obtained with the use of appropriately selected and fitted adaptive equipment result in functional independence (Erwin et al., 2009). For children with vision impairments, a lighted magnifier is an example of adaptive equipment that may promote independence. And for children with hearing impairments or deafness, adaptive equipment to promote independence might include visual and tactile aids, such as an electric fan or flashing lights to signal the end of activity. Hearing aids and other amplification devices would also be considered AT.

Augmentative and alternative communication (AAC) devices include a range of adaptive equipment and approaches that aid a child who is unable to communicate effectively with speech. For example, a child with a neuromotor disability who lacks the oral-motor coordination required for speech may communicate by pointing to photographs on a cardboard communication board. A cardboard communication board, book, or set of cards is an example of low-tech AT. Many high-tech AAC devices are also available. High-tech devices are costlier, often electronic, and allow for more extensive and sophisticated communication exchanges. Among high-tech communication devices are ones that produce a synthetic or naturalistic voice that speaks for the child. These are called voice-output communication aids or speech-generating devices. A more in-depth discussion and examples of AT devices to support functional independence in motor, sensory, and communication skills are described later in this chapter. Intervention strategies to promote the use of communication skills—including skills in using AAC devices—are discussed in Chapter 7.

Assistive Technology Services In addition to devices, AT includes services related to selecting, acquiring, and using AT. Possible AT services are evaluation of AT needs by an AT professional, purchasing AT, customizing or repairing AT, coordinating AT with other interventions or services (such as physical therapy or early intervention), and training the child, family, or professionals in the use of the AT. While IDEA indicates that necessary AT must be provided as a part of special education for preschool- and school-age children at no expense to families, families of infants receiving services through early intervention need to first use their medical insurance or Medicaid to fund the cost of AT. Part C of IDEA will cover only costs that are otherwise not covered by other sources of funding available to families.

FUNCTIONAL INDEPENDENCE IN BASIC PHYSICAL SKILLS

Disabilities or delays associated with basic skills (gross motor, fine motor, communication, and self-help) may interfere with a child's development of independence in the home, community, play, and child care or school activities. Objectives may need to be formulated as functionally equivalent responses to provide opportunities for independence.

Independence in Gross Motor Skills

Gross motor skills involve large muscle movements. The developmental sequence of gross motor includes important developmental skills called *milestones* (e.g., head control, rolling, crawling, sitting, creeping, standing, walking). Movements in and out of these milestones (*transitional movements*) are also important gross motor skills.

Physical Development Difficulties

Motor development is linked to the development of the central nervous system, a process that begins before birth and continues until about age 5. An immature or injured central nervous system is often characterized by delayed motor development, atypical muscle tone, atypical reflexes, postural reaction deficits, and/or compensatory patterns (Pellegrino, 2002). The extent to which these characteristics are present and interfere with typical motor development varies from slight to severe.

Atypical Muscle Tone   Muscle tone, the "resistance to passive movement of a muscle" (Ratliffe, 1998, p. 433), may be too high (*hypertonia* or *spasticity*), too low (*hypotonia* or *flaccidity*), or fluctuating (*athetosis*). Atypical tone may result in too little or too much movement or movement that is too fast, too slow, or jerky. It also interferes with the development of typical postures and movement patterns and the ability to transition from one position to another (e.g., from creeping to sitting).

Atypical Reflexes   When the central nervous system is injured or immature, some reflexes tend to be atypical in three ways:

1. They *persist* beyond the usual developmental time frame; in typical development these reflexes fade or become integrated with voluntary movement.

2. They are *exaggerated*, easily elicited, and often fully demonstrated; they are *not fleeting* or *partial* as in typical development.

3. They are *obligatory*; once elicited, posture and movement are restricted and bound by the pattern. They are never obligatory in typical development (Pellegrino, 2002).

Postural Reaction Deficits   In young children with motor delays or an injured central nervous system, postural reactions (equilibrium and righting) do not develop or they develop incompletely (Pellegrino, 2002). Without righting reactions, there is not a strong physiological urge to establish aligned and upright postures and movements. And without equilibrium reactions that provide balance, typical postural and movement patterns are difficult to attain and maintain.

Compensatory Patterns Many children with motor disabilities do accomplish motor skills, but they may do so through atypical postures called *compensations*. Compensations allow a child to accomplish a useful position, such as holding his or her head up or sitting, but they restrict movement and block subsequent motor development (Bly, 1983). Examples of compensations include a neck block (holding the head upright by hyperextending the neck and resting the head between elevated shoulders) and a pelvic hip block (sitting by hyperextending the lower spine and using a "frog-legged" position).

PHYSICAL DEVELOPMENT INTERVENTION PROCEDURES

Motor interventions should be conducted within the context of functional activities. This is called *integrated therapy*; it teaches the purpose of new motor skills and enhances generalization (McWilliam, 1996). Intervention for children with mild physical delays or disabilities will usually target the typical sequences of gross and fine motor skills. For children with severe physical delays or disabilities, the functional use of selected motor skills and adaptive skills will usually be emphasized.

Mild Physical Disabilities

Intervention for gross motor skills when mild disabilities are present focuses on teaching the next skill in the developmental sequence and improving postural reactions, particularly the equilibrium (balance) reactions. Physical guidance and activities that encourage the child to practice a skill are common intervention procedures. For example, when a child is beginning to creep (move forward on hands and knees), encouragement is provided by enticing the child to creep toward desired objects held a short distance away. Guided practice assists the child to move her hips and legs back and forth in a creeping pattern. Balance reactions for creeping are encouraged by holding desired toys and objects off to the child's side, enticing her to lift one arm and reach to the side. Reaching requires the child to shift her weight to maintain the creeping position and avoid falling. If the child is unable to reach to the side, physical guidance to shift her weight is provided.

Severe Physical Disabilities

Usually, severe physical disabilities are due to a developmental disorder, such as central nervous system injury or a neuromuscular condition, rather than a delay. When a severe physical disability is present, the problems of atypical muscle tone, persistent primitive reflexes, delayed or absent postural reactions, and compensatory patterns are likely to characterize motor development. These problems affect the development of functional gross and fine motor skills.

Positioning and carrying procedures are therapeutic techniques that provide stable and aligned posture encourage, typical muscle tone, and inhibit atypical reflexes (Heller, Forney, Alberto, Schwartzman, & Goeckel, 2000).

Positions that appear to be opposite or counter to the atypical patterns are usually effective. For example, when a child is placed in his high chair and demonstrates an asymmetrical tonic neck reflex, his posture is characterized by too much muscle tone, asymmetry, and excessive extension (his trunk, neck, and head rotate to one side, extremities are extended on his face side, and the opposite extremities flex). This atypical pattern can be prevented or minimized by using pillows, positioning inserts, or a special chair that aligns his body, limbs, and head; flexes his hips, knees, and ankles; and brings his head and shoulders slightly forward. Figure 13.1 illustrates this positioning technique. Appropriate positioning and carrying procedures often facilitate typical movement patterns. This implies that positioning must not be too confining; if a child is over-positioned, movement will be restricted and opportunities to attempt and practice new motor skills will not be available.

Using furniture, pillows, or specialized adaptive equipment for positioning or carrying is called *static positioning*. The devices are fixed in place and cannot be readily adjusted in response to changes in muscle tone, movement, or situational demands. Static positioning and carrying procedures, however, provide the child with independence from an adult and free the adult for activities beyond the reach and confines of holding the child. The alternative to static positioning and carrying is *dynamic positioning*, in which an adult's body (instead of equipment) is used to support a child in a desired position. The advantage of dynamic positioning and carrying is that an adult can respond immediately to child and situational needs.

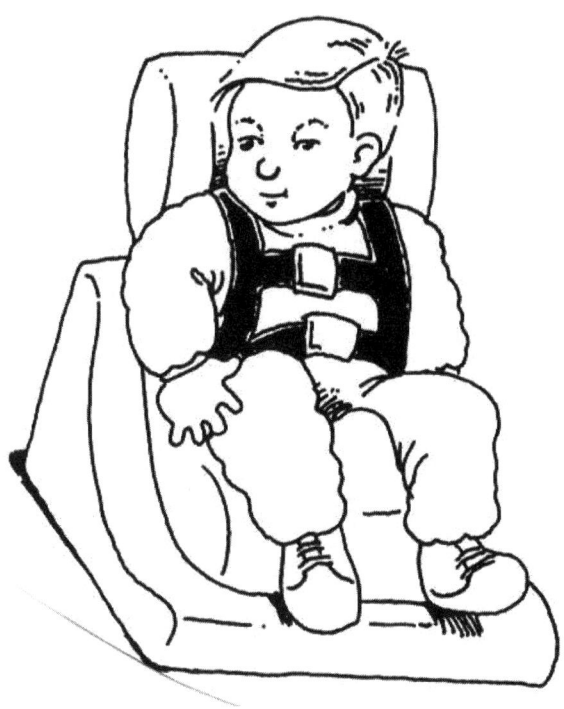

Figure 13.1. Example of positioning technique to inhibit asymmetrical extensor pattern.

Physical guidance and encouragement techniques that assist the child to accomplish typical postures and movements are called *facilitation techniques.* For example, while assisting with dressing, a father holds his 2-year-old daughter on his lap, helping her to prop herself with her hands on her knees. This position encourages and facilitates head and trunk control (holding her head and trunk upright) and discourages increased muscle tone. As her father helps her put on a T-shirt, he shifts her weight to one side, allowing her to lift her opposite arm into the T-shirt sleeve. As her weight is shifted to one side, she feels the weight bearing through her supporting arm. This facilitates an equilibrium reaction in sitting. It also facilitates a righting reaction associated with head and trunk control, encouraging her to realign and maintain her head and trunk upright. Appropriate positioning and carrying procedures (including the use of adaptive equipment) ideally function as facilitation techniques, allowing and encouraging increasingly more independent postures and movement.

Physical and occupational therapists typically have the responsibility of conducting motor evaluations, developing intervention plans, and teaching other team members to implement the plan. Although therapists have expertise in physical development, the team approach is critical to planning motor interventions that address children's movement needs associated with meaningful, functional activities.

Children with physical delays or impairments or neuromotor disabilities may not progress through the typical sequence of physical gross motor development. Motor skill development may be splintered (skills may be skipped), skills may be acquired partially, or they may develop in an atypical fashion (Illingworth, 1983). For example, a child with cerebral palsy may not crawl, but she may learn to scoot backward. When motor delays and disabilities preclude or interfere with independence, functionally equivalent gross motor objectives may be targeted. Several gross motor functions are critical for social and physical independence in home, community, child care, and school environments. These include postural and mobility functions. Table 13.1 presents examples of a few gross motor responses needed by children and some of the critical functions achieved by the motor responses. Note that AT considerations, therapeutic positioning and handling techniques, and adaptive equipment are included in the table.

INDEPENDENCE IN FINE MOTOR SKILLS

In the sequence of typical physical development, fine motor skills are refined following the accomplishment of gross motor skills. As previously mentioned, delays in gross motor skills are associated with delays in postural reactions. In turn, delays in postural reactions result in postural instability, that is, difficulty in maintaining proper joint, bone, and overall body alignment and balance (Bly, 1983). The problem of postural instability accentuates the problem of fine motor delays. For example, a preschooler with postural instability in sitting will have difficulty feeding herself because her trunk and shoulders are unsteady and she is continually at risk of falling.

Interventions that improve postural stability result in improved fine motor skills. These interventions can be provided through physical assistance or adaptations. For example, if a child is having difficulty controlling the movement of

Table 13.1. Examples: Gross motor responses, critical functions, and functionally equivalent responses

Gross motor responses	Critical functions	Functional equivalents
Head erect in midline	• Visual attending • Visual scanning • Oral-motor control	• Head rests on chair (with or without strap) • Head momentarily erect • Foam neck brace
Floor and chair sitting	• Arms free for fine motor tasks, materials, and toys • Upright position for eating and drinking • Upright position for adaptive, daily living, and other functional skills	• Propped sitting against wall or other surface for floor sitting • Kneeling (with/without support or adaptive equipment) • Communication of need for access or participation
Walking	• Access to locations, materials, and toys • Arms free for handling materials • Upright position for adaptive, daily living, and other functional skills • Participation with peers in movement activities	• Wheelchair (manual or electric) • Walker or cane(s) • Knee walking • Scooting in sitting position • Shoulder bag for carrying materials

his toothbrush, he may be guided to spread his feet apart for a more solid base of support. He may also be assisted to hold the edge of the sink for balance. With a steadier base of support and assistance in balance, controlling the movement of his toothbrush is an easier task. Functional independence can be further supported by providing the child with an electric toothbrush, a low-cost and commercially available AT device.

Many fine motor tasks are performed while seated. Postural stability is enhanced when the child is seated in a chair of the proper size (its seat length is the distance from her buttocks to her knees) and she can place her feet flat on the floor or on a footrest. If the child has difficulty sitting upright with her hips at the back of the seat, a wide strap holding her hips in the back of the seat will improve stability. In addition, the table height may be modified to improve postural stability. The table height should be at least a few inches above the height of the child's elbows. For additional support, the table may be raised to a level slightly below the child's armpits.

Fine motor skills are critical for independence in most daily living, adaptive, play, and school skills. If fine motor performance is delayed or impaired, functionally equivalent responses may provide alternatives for accomplishing independence. Examples of important fine motor responses, the critical functions they accomplish, and ideas for functionally equivalent responses are presented in Table 13.2.

ESTABLISHING COMMUNICATION AND ENVIRONMENTAL SKILLS

Infants communicate effectively long before they are able to speak. For example, they spit, purse their lips, gurgle, and smile to indicate their distaste or preference

Table 13.2. Examples: Fine motor responses, critical functions, and functionally equivalent responses

Fine motor responses	Critical functions	Functional equivalents
Reach	• Touch and exploration of toys and materials • Access to materials and locations	• Toys/materials within close proximity
Grasp	• Access to materials • Hold and carry materials • Play with toys • Engage in adaptive, daily living, and other functional skills • Indicate choice of objects or materials	• Shoulder and trunk stabilization through positioning, handling, or adaptive equipment • Attachments (e.g., strings) to eliminate need to reach • Prosthetic reaching stick • Communicating choice, verbally or through augmentative means
Point	• Indicate focus of interest • Clarify object of communication • Indicate desired object or event	• Shoulder and trunk stabilization through positioning, handling, or adaptive equipment • Adaptive feeding or marking utensils • Shoulder bag or adaptive tray to hold and carry materials • Materials strapped to hands (e.g., Velcro strap on pen) • Materials secured to surface to prevent them from slipping or falling • Holding materials with arms, mouth, or feet • Shoulder and trunk stabilization through positioning, handling, or adaptive equipment • Whole hand/fist use to indicate/clarify • Eye pointing • Augmentative communication to indicate/clarify (hand/fist, eye pointing, hand or head switch, and so forth)

for foods, or they smile and coo to urge a sibling to continue playing. From the earliest communicative responses, communication is a critical tool for meeting needs and desires, establishing social relationships, participating in family activities, and learning new skills and concepts. For example, an infant who reaches toward his father controls his environment if his father consistently responds by picking him up. Once an initial communication repertoire of environmental control skills is established, the young child's repertoire expands: communication becomes more refined and efficient. When children begin approximating words, their communication increases in effectiveness and efficiency.

The infant's earliest efforts to control the environment are simple, nonsymbolic communication behaviors such as eye contact, pointing, vocalizing, reaching, and touching. There are five phases in the development of environmental control skills:

1. *Attentional interactions:* indicating awareness, recognizing and/or anticipating persons, objects, or events (e.g., smiling in recognition of familiar person)

2. *Contingency interactions:* using simple behaviors to control reinforcing consequences (e.g., playing baby games such as "so big" to maintain interaction with an adult)

3. *Differentiated interactions:* controlling the behavior of others with responses that have socially recognized meanings (e.g., pointing, giving, other nonverbal gestures)
4. *Encoded interactions:* using behaviors that have precise meanings and are understood given the situation—using one- or two-word phrases or sign language in response to environmental stimuli or events (e.g., saying, "ball, Mommy" when a sibling comes into the room holding the ball)
5. *Symbolic interactions:* using behaviors that have precise meanings (e.g., language, pretend play) to communicate, without reliance on the situation to be understood (e.g., saying "Want drink") (Dunst et al., 1987)

Instructional goals are based on the child's communication needs in daily functional activities (derived from assessment strategies described in Chapter 5). The goals build on what a young child is doing and promote the child's development of skills at the next level of environmental control. For example, Timmy's parents indicated that they would like him to express his preferences at mealtimes and when playing with his sister. Presently, Timmy, who is unable to speak due to cerebral palsy, smiles and moves his arms excitedly when he sees his favorite foods and toys. One goal is for Timmy to look at a favorite food or toy for 5 seconds when given two choices. In requiring Timmy to look at a preferred food or toy, Timmy learns that looking controls getting what he wants. This goal moves Timmy from his present phase of awareness to the phase of contingent interactions.

There are five instructional approaches to assist infants and young children in progressing through the phases of environmental control skills: 1) enhance sensitivity, 2) increase opportunities, 3) structure predictable routines, 4) augment input, and 5) modify the environment (Noonan & Siegel, 2003). All five approaches can be used concurrently.

Enhance Sensitivity

Learn the ways in which a young child tries to communicate nonsymbolically and respond immediately when such behaviors are demonstrated. Also respond to the behaviors that *might* be attempts to communicate nonverbally (those that *infer intent*). For example, Sally's mom notices that Sally stares intently at her when she is enjoying an interaction and wiggles and looks away when she's tired. Mom responds immediately, continuing to talk and play with her when she stares, and ending the interaction and comforting Sally when she wiggles and looks away. As a result of Mom's immediate responsiveness, Sally is given control of the length of interactions. In turn, interactions become more satisfying to Sally and her mom. This strategy is particularly useful for enhancing adult–child interactions when the child's responses are difficult to detect, inconsistent, or infrequent.

Increase Opportunities

Be careful not to eliminate a young child's need to communicate by doing everything for him. Increase communication opportunities by altering the environment in such ways as placing things out of reach or delaying expected events. For example, place only two pieces of finger food (slices of an apple) on a toddler's high-chair tray. This will create the need to communicate a request for more food.

Structure Predictable Routines

Help a young child develop expectations by establishing predictable routines such as playing peekaboo during diapering. When the routine is well learned, change it or insert a pause to motivate a communication response. For example, hold the diaper above the infant but don't begin peekaboo until the infant demonstrates some expectation of the game such as giggling or reaching for the diaper.

Augment Input

Increase the communicative input a child receives by supplementing speech with additional modes. For example, point to photographs while talking to a child or use exaggerated facial expressions to support communications about feelings. The augmentative mode should correspond to the child's level of understanding. Such input may help increase a child's comprehension.

Modify the Environment

Environmental modifications can be used to assist a child to interact with others and to display more alert and responsive behavior. For example, a child may be taken out of his wheelchair and placed on the floor to play at the same level as his peers in the block area of a preschool classroom. Being at eye level with others and having easy access to materials can increase interaction. A child can be assisted to be more alert and responsive by enhancing the sensory qualities of an activity. For example, the visual appeal of a material can be enhanced by giving it a bright background.

Expanding Initial Environmental Control Skills

Once a child is demonstrating environmental control skills with simple, nonsymbolic behaviors (e.g., vocalizing for attention, pointing to a desired toy), the next goal is to expand the child's skills to include communication responses serving more uses or functions. Examples of communicative functions (*pragmatics*) include requesting, gaining attention, greeting, and protesting. These functions are typically demonstrated first through signals (e.g., specific gestures such as waving "bye-bye," or a vocalization that communicates, "I'm trying but I need help"). Later, these functions are demonstrated through symbols such as words or sign language.

When the child is using several communicative functions frequently and effectively, communication skills are expanded by increasing complexity. Complexity is increased in two ways. First, the content of what the child talks about can be expanded. Content or meaning is referred to as *semantics*. Children communicate about content such as people, places, events, and objects and about characteristics of people, places, events, and objects. Second, complexity is increased by expanding the structure of communication. The structure or grammar of language is *syntax* and includes such forms as nouns, verbs, and adjectives. Expanding what the child talks about and the structures used to communicate enables the child to communicate more precisely and thus more effectively.

Given the complexity of establishing goals that consider the pragmatic, semantic, and syntactic dimensions of communication, as well as needs related to home and community participation, a team approach is vital. As always, the family's role in decision making is central to the team process. A speech-language pathologist (a professional with expertise in assessing communication needs and planning interventions) is also an important team member.

The formulation of communication goals comes through a combined approach of ecological and developmental assessments. For example, a goal to "initiate requests for desired activities with siblings" may be identified in analyzing family routines. The ecological assessment is also the source for identifying needed vocabulary. In the play activity, for example, the names of games may be a vocabulary need.

The level or complexity of the goal is based on the child's present level of performance: syntax and semantics are expanded following developmental sequences. Returning to the example of requesting an activity, the child is using one-word utterances: he's using a grammar that consists of nouns or verbs, and he's talking about actions and people performing actions. A syntactic goal is to use a noun + verb form; a semantic goal is use of an agent + action expression (e.g., Tommy + catch).

Alternative Communication Modes Another consideration in formulating communication goals is deciding which communication mode would work best. Augmentative communication includes gestural, pictorial, or symbolic communication systems. Augmentative communication systems are alternative communication systems for some children who are unlikely ever to use speech; for others, the systems supplement and enhance oral communication and are not intended to replace it. Examples of alternative and augmentative systems include American Sign Language; common gestures (e.g., waving at someone to "Come here"); pictures, symbols, or words displayed in a book or on a large surface (communication board); pictures, symbols, or words displayed on an elevated Plexiglas surface for eye pointing (eye-gaze system); and electronic communication boards, some of which "talk" using voice-synthesizer microcomputer technology. Very often the best solution is to combine systems (McCormick & Wegner, 2003). For example, a child taps a bell attached to her wheelchair to call for attention. When someone responds, she points to the picture for "drink" on her communication board and nods yes when asked if she wants a drink of water. Figure 13.2 illustrates a communication board using line drawings arranged on the tray of a child's wheelchair.

The decision to use an augmentative system and the selection of a system are made by the early intervention team, including the family, speech-language pathologist, teacher or infant specialist, occupational therapist, and physical therapist. As noted throughout this text, parental preference should carry the most weight in decisions about their children. Decisions concerning the selection and use of an augmentative communication system are not one-time decisions. As the child develops and circumstances change, needs and the appropriateness of the system are continually evaluated.

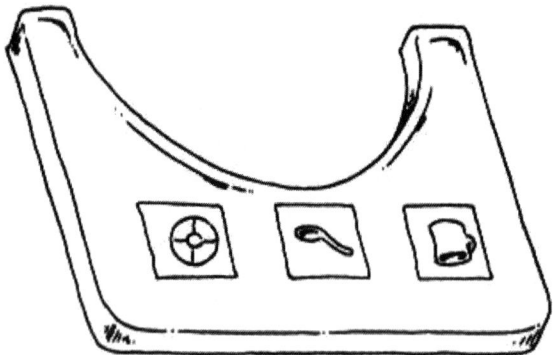

Figure 13.2. A communication board with line drawings (on a wheelchair tray).

Instructional Procedures EMT has been demonstrated to be particularly successful in assisting young children with disabilities to learn and use generalized communication skills (Kaiser, 1993; Kaiser et al., 1991). As reviewed in Chapter 7, EMT is a hybrid naturalistic approach to communication intervention that includes environmental arrangement, responsive interaction, and milieu teaching (McCormick, 2003). The procedures are well suited to inclusive settings because they follow the child's lead and instruction is embedded within ongoing routines and activities. Figure 13.3 is an instructional plan that illustrates assisting a child in learning to make requests using EMT procedures.

As with gross and fine motor skills, functionally equivalent responses can provide alternatives for accomplishing communication functions when

---

Child: Joseph K.
Objective: Make request ("Please")
Conditions: When Joseph wants something that is out of reach
Response: He will say "Please."
Criterion: So that it is clearly audible, 5 times within 3 days

Date begun: 6/3/13
Date completed:
Interventionist(s): Janet Yim

Intervention context	Prompting/ facilitation techniques	Consequences
Setting(s) At home, at preschool, and in stores or restaurants	*Positioning and handling; special equipment/ materials* n/a	*Reinforcement* Tell Joseph he can have what he asks for when he says "Please." Give him the item immediately; assist him in using, exploring, or playing with the item if he does not interact with it.
Routine(s)/activity(ies) During play times at home or preschool, during mealtimes, and while shopping	*Environmental modifications* Place several desired items or toys out of reach but within sight (leave a cup at the edge of the counter, toys on a top shelf of toy shelves, and books on top of an end table)	
Skill sequence(s) n/a		*Corrections* Say "Please," wait 5 seconds, reinforce if correct.
Occasions for incidental intervention Whenever Joseph focuses on an item for 10 seconds or whenever Joseph reaches for an item that is beyond his reach	*Prompts/facilitation* Approach Joseph, make eye contact, and ask, "What do you say, Joseph?" (wait 5 seconds)	If still incorrect or no response, say "Please" and give Joseph the item; do not praise him or interact further.

Figure 13.3. Instructional plan for "making request."

communication delays or impairments are present (McCormick & Wegner, 2003). Table 13.3 lists examples of communication responses, some of the functions accomplished by the responses, and suggestions for functionally equivalent responses. Most of the functionally equivalent responses are skill approximations or communication responses accomplished through alternative and augmentative communication systems.

INDEPENDENCE IN SELF-HELP SKILLS

Self-help skills are personal care skills such as dressing, bathing, tooth brushing, toileting, and eating. Sequences of development and the ages at which these skills are acquired by children without disabilities are contained in most developmental assessment scales such as the Assessment, Evaluation, and Programming System for Infants and Children (Bricker, 2002) and The Carolina Curriculum for Infants and Toddlers with Special Needs (3rd ed.) (Johnson-Martin, Attermeier, & Hacker, 2004). This information is useful in determining where to begin instruction and provides information on the age appropriateness of skills.

Many self-help skills are taught using task analysis and the assistance and encouragement procedures described in Chapter 6. For example, in teaching a

Table 13.3. Examples: Communication responses, critical functions, and functionally equivalent responses

Communication response	Critical functions	Functional equivalents
Cry or smile	• Request/maintain attention of others • Greet others • Express feelings and emotions • Terminate situations	• Visual or gestural signal for attention or greeting or to indicate feelings • Eye contact to maintain attention of others • Touch or hug to express emotion • Use of a switch attached to light or call device
Babble	• Experiment with or practice elements of speech, language, and oral-motor skills • Request/maintain attention of others	• Eye contact to maintain attention of others • Gestural/physical turn taking during social play • Use of switch attached to light or call device
Talk with single words, phrases, or sentences	• Practice elements of speech, language, and oral-motor skills • Request/maintain attention of others • Send specific messages • Fulfill needs and desires • Express feelings and emotions • Engage in social and conversational interactions	• Approximations of words, phrases, or sentences • Use of gestures, symbols, and/or signs • Visual or gestural signal to gain attention or indicate feelings • Eye contact to maintain the attention of others • "Yes" signaled with head nod when focus of interest/desired object or event is named • Activation of switch to indicate words, drawings, pictures, or symbols on a communication board

toddler to wash her hands, a task analysis assessment is first conducted. The steps of the task are as follows:

1. Turn on cold water faucet
2. Wet hands
3. Pick up soap
4. Lather palms
5. Replace soap
6. Lather back of hands
7. Rinse hands
8. Turn water off
9. Pick up towel
10. Dry hands
11. Replace towel

The toddler is helped to wash her hands, and her performance on each step is assessed. If she is unable to perform a step, prompting and motivation procedures are provided to identify teaching strategies that might be included in the instructional plan. The task analysis assessment also helps the teacher or infant specialist determine if the task has unnecessary steps that can be eliminated or combined or if steps are too broad and additional, smaller steps are needed. Following the task analysis assessment, the instructional plan is formulated with the task analysis included (revised according to the assessment results). Prompting and motivation procedures are specified for each step.

If a self-help goal is too difficult, or if it requires participation beyond the child's current abilities, a *partial participation task analysis* may be developed. In a partial participation task analysis, steps within the child's capabilities that enable him to participate meaningfully are delineated. For example, Snell (1987) described a partial participation task analysis for toothbrushing. The child's participation included opening his mouth for the teacher to brush one quadrant of his teeth and swallowing a drink of water after each quadrant had been brushed. A child holding his mouth open and swallowing are important steps in assisted toothbrushing that make the task of the adult much easier. Figure 13.4 illustrates an instructional plan for hand washing that includes a partial participation task analysis.

Toileting and feeding are each a complex set of self-help skills that are critical to independence. Therapeutic and specialized instructional procedures for facilitating these skills are drawn from the fields of nursing, psychology, occupational therapy, speech therapy, and physical therapy and are presented here.

Toileting

Toileting comprises several skills: recognizing the need, getting to the bathroom, lowering and raising clothing, getting on and off the toilet, sitting and voiding, wiping, flushing, washing hands, and drying hands. Among children

Child: Todd
Objective: Assisted hand washing
Conditions: Given a request to wash his hands
Response: Todd will assist in washing and drying his hands.
Criterion: 5 consecutive times

Date begun: 6/6/13
Date completed:
Interventionist(s): Selina and Mike

Intervention context	Prompting/ facilitation techniques	Consequences
Setting(s) At preschool, before lunch At home, before dinner *Routine(s)/activity(ies)* 1. Holds one hand up and keeps hand open with fingers apart (adult washes hand with washcloth) 2. Holds other hand up and keeps fingers apart (adult washes hand with washcloth) 3. Holds both hands out with fingers apart (adult dries both hands with towel)	*Positioning and handling; special equipment/ materials* n/a *Environmental modifications* Position Todd in his feeder seat *Prompting/facilitation* Tap hand(s) and say, "Let's wash (or dry) your hand(s)"	*Reinforcement* Smile and talk to Todd the entire time he is holding his hand(s) open *Corrections* Shake arm(s) to relax tone. Rub back of hand(s) and gently assist Todd to open his fingers

Figure 13.4. Participation intervention plan for self-help skill.

without disabilities, toileting is typically achieved between 24 and 30 months of age. Toileting is not usually learned earlier than this because the following entry requirements seem to be essential: 1) The child's schedule of urination and bowel movements occur on a predictable schedule, and 2) the child remains dry for 1 to 2 hours on a fairly consistent schedule from day to day (Farlow & Snell, 2006). Also note that daytime toileting is typically learned before nighttime toileting.

While the child is learning the prerequisites, toileting needs are most easily managed through *timed toileting* (also known as *toilet regulation*). Timed toileting is placing the child on the toilet for a few minutes (not more than 10 minutes) at the times she usually eliminates. If the child uses the toilet, reinforcement is provided. If the child does not eliminate, she is removed from the toilet without any consequences. Timed toileting helps the child learn why and when the toilet is used, and it eases the caregiving task, although accidents may still occur. Timed toileting may also be an appropriate goal for a young child with physical disabilities affecting mobility or fine motor skills that interfere with independence.

Teach children with mild disabilities who are delayed in toileting to recognize the need to use the toilet and to void in it by following a procedure similar to timed toileting. Keep a record of the times the child is dry and wet by checking her diapers frequently (every half hour). Ask her if she needs to use the toilet 5 to 10 minutes before she usually voids. If the child says yes, place her on the toilet for about 5 minutes. Praise her if she eliminates in the toilet; comment that she should try later if she did not use the toilet. Most children with mild delays will learn toileting with this simple procedure.

For children with more severe disabilities, toileting is usually taught by increasing the intake of liquids so that they need to use the toilet more often. This increases the number of teaching opportunities. The toilet-training approach that popularized this procedure is called the *rapid method* and is described in the paperback *Toilet Training in Less than a Day* (Azrin, 1989).

Medical clearance should be obtained prior to implementing toilet-training procedures that involve increased fluid intake. Care should be taken not to exceed typical daily water allowances: approximately one to four cups per day for children weighing between 4 and 22 pounds and approximately four to seven cups per day for children between 22 and 88 pounds (Thompson & Hanson, 1983). A substantial increase in fluids can cause overhydration. Symptoms include nausea, vomiting, muscle twitching, seizures, and coma. Some children have medical conditions for which increased fluid intake is contraindicated (e.g., hypertension, problems of the heart, liver, kidneys). Fluid intake procedures should *never* be used with children who have epilepsy, hydrocephaly, or a prior spinal injury.

Bedwetting (*nocturnal enuresis*) is common among young children. Children are ready to begin nighttime toilet training when they are successful through most of the day with daytime toileting. There are three major types of intervention strategies for nighttime toilet training. The simplest procedure requires that no fluids are provided 1.5 to 2.0 hours before bedtime. Awaken the child a few minutes before the times that he typically voids (most children will need to use the toilet only once during the night) and have him sit on the toilet for 5 minutes. Praise him for a dry bed and for eliminating in the toilet. If his bed is wet, change it without comment. Provide enthusiastic reinforcement in the morning if the child kept his bed dry. Gradually delay the wake-up (10 minute periods) to require that the child stay dry for increasingly longer periods of time.

The second procedure to eliminate nighttime bedwetting uses a *signaling device* placed under the bed sheet that sounds an alarm when the bed is wet. This procedure is most appropriate for children who are at least 5 years of age. When the alarm sounds, awaken the child and help him practice toileting skills (going to the bathroom and using the toilet, changing pajamas and bedding). Provide praise when the child sleeps through the night without wetting the bed.

The third procedure is a rapid bedtime method (Azrin, Sneed, & Foxx, 1973, 1974) and is much like the daytime rapid training method. The procedure includes increased fluids, use of a signaling device on the bed, hourly checks, toileting practice, and praise for dry bed and eliminating in the toilet. It is not necessary to implement the procedure throughout the entire night; it has been proven effective when used from bedtime until 1 a.m. (Azrin & Besalel, 1979).

Mealtime Skills

Eating and drinking involve a complex set of motor and oral-motor skills. The typical sequence of these skills is described in Table 13.4, which can be used as a guide for determining developmentally appropriate mealtime goals. For infants and young children with mild disabilities, mealtime skills are taught

Table 13.4. Typical development of eating and drinking skills

Birth
Sucking and swallowing
Incomplete lip closure

4 weeks
Opens mouth, waiting for food
Better lip closure
Active lip movement when sucking
Takes cereal from spoon

6 weeks
Pureed fruit from spoon

3 months
Anticipates feeding

4 months
Recognizes bottle, mouth ready for nipple
Cup feeding may be introduced—very messy but enjoys process
More control and movement of tongue is handled by child—not by reflexes
Appetite is more erratic
Will not consume three full feedings
Tongue thrust seen more with cup feeding than spoon feeding

5 months
Mouth opens ready for spoon
Uses hands to draw bottle to mouth but releases when nipple is inserted
Tongue reversal after spoon removed, ejecting food involuntarily

5.5 months
Good lip closure
Overhand grasp with both hands to feed self with cup

6 months
Good control with lips and tongue
Beginning definite chewing motion by gumming food

7 months
Spoon fed chunky foods
Feeds self soft foods (banana, vegetables, and so forth)
Drooling noticed with mouth activity
Reaches for food with head

8 months
Uses two hands on cup—messy
Holds own bottle
Picks up food with thumb and forefinger
Finger feeds most of food
Chokes easily when drinking from cup

9 months
Grows impatient when watching meal preparation
Enjoys chewing
Likes to finger feed self—messy
Appetite finicky

10 months
Lateral movement of jaw
Grasps and brings bottle to mouth
Food is to be felt, tasted, smeared, and dropped on floor
Cup feeding still messy—may want to play with it

11 months
Objects if mother tries to help complete feeding
Can use cup by self

12 months
More choosy about food
Independent about finishing meal—may dump remaining food on floor
Lunch is least motivating meal

(continued)

Table 13.4. *(continued)*

15 months
Holds cup with fingers—many spills
Grasps spoon—poor manipulation
Spoon inverted before insertion
Shows definite preference for certain foods

18 months
Drinks well from cup
Hands empty cup or dish to mother; if she doesn't see—child will drop item
Chews meat well
Better control with spoon

21 months
Handles cup well
Very regimented in eating—wants everything on a routine schedule and presented same way each time

2 years
Can handle small glass with one hand, partially filled
Moderate spillage from spoon
Refuses previous favorite food
Inserts food into mouth without turning over spoon
Food preference may stem from taste, consistency, or just color

3 years
Minimum spilling from spoon
Dawdles at mealtime
Likes to spear food with fork

4 years
Sets table well
Likes to serve self
Washes and dries own face and hands

5 years
Appetite may increase, prefers simple food
Beginning to use knife to spread
Talkative during meals
Doesn't always finish meals by self—may need assistance; often asks for help

6 years
Very active; cannot sit still
Asks for more food than can consume
Enjoys snacks more than mealtime
Spills with milk—common at this age
Breakfast may be most difficult meal
Not interested in dessert
May return to finger feeding

7 years
Appetite is less for girls; boys may have tremendous appetite
May eat formerly disliked dishes
Interested in desserts
Use of napkin is spotty

8 years
Girls hold fork in adult fashion; boys hold fork pronated
Starting to cut with knife
Shovels food into mouth
Asks for seconds, even thirds

9 years
Appetite under better control
Likes to help prepare meals
Still has difficulty controlling and knowing what to do with napkin
Difficulty in cutting food to appropriate size, tends to be too big

11 years
Has satisfied feeling after meals

12 years
Bottomless pit—eating constantly
13 years
Appetite more stable
14 years
More like adult balance

From Copeland, M., Ford, L., and Solon, N. (1976). *Occupational therapy for mentally retarded children* (pp. 146-147). Baltimore, MD: University Park Press. Data from Gesell and Amatruda (1947), Gesell and Ilg (1946), Ilg and Ames (1955), Rutherford (1971), Smart and Smart (1967), and Spock (1972).

using task analysis and direct instruction described in Chapter 6. For example, drinking from a cup may be task analyzed as follows:

1. Grasp cup

2. Lift cup to mouth

3. Drink a few swallows

4. Return cup to table

5. Release cup

Backward chaining may be used to teach the task analysis. For instance, assist the child to perform the first four steps and verbally prompt him to release the cup when it touches the table (the fifth step). When the child is successful with the fifth step, teach the fourth and fifth steps together. As each new combination of steps is learned, add the prior step until the entire set of steps is acquired. Figure 13.5 is an example of a systematic instructional plan using backward chaining. It also includes the use of adaptive feeding equipment to assist the child in acquiring independence. Another direct instruction procedure frequently used with self-feeding skills is hand-over-hand assistance. The adult lightly holds the child's hand and assists as necessary (e.g., to hold a spoon, to pick up a cracker).

For young children with severe disabilities, special feeding techniques may be necessary. Occupational, physical, and sometimes speech therapists are the professionals who collaborate as a team with families to address mealtime concerns. Mealtime intervention plans for young children with severe disabilities may include therapeutic positioning, adaptive equipment, prefeeding techniques, therapeutic feeding techniques, and systematic instruction. The purpose of therapeutic positioning for feeding, eating, and drinking is to foster typical muscle tone, inhibit atypical reflexes, and facilitate typical patterns of movement (including oral-motor patterns).

Several goals are particularly critical when positioning a young child for mealtimes. First, the child should be seated and as upright as possible (unless the child is still fed from a bottle or breast). The child's body should be symmetrical and aligned. Usually symmetry and alignment will inhibit atypical postural and tonal patterns. An exception to this may be positioning the child with trunk rotation to facilitate relaxation and decrease hypertonicity. The head should be a little forward with a slight downward tilt for swallowing. Alignment, symmetry, and an upright posture are critical to swallowing, the coordination of breathing and swallowing, and preventing food or liquids from passing into the trachea or lungs (*aspiration*) or choking. Next, the child's

Child: Francie	Date begun: 6/6/13
Objective: Scooping	Date completed:
Conditions: At lunch, when given a plate of ground and sticky food	Interventionist(s): Mom

Response: Francie will scoop and eat her lunch.
Criterion: Without assistance for 10 minutes, 2 consecutive lunches

Intervention context	Prompting/facilitation techniques	Consequences
Setting(s) Lunchtime *Routine(s)/activity(ies)* 1. Grasp spoon handle 2. Scoop food onto spoon 3. Raise spoon to mouth 4. Place spoon in mouth and remove food 5. Return spoon to bowl or table	*Positioning and handling; special equipment/materials, environmental modifications* Use plate with high rim and small plastic-coated spoon *Prompting/facilitation* 1. Point to spoon handle 2. (Wait 6 seconds) 3. Model opening your mouth 4. (Wait 6 seconds) Backward chain: Assist through steps not being taught; prompt and correct current step as noted in this plan (Criterion is 2 consecutive corrects for adding previous step to intervention chain)	*Reinforcement* Provide a sip of juice *Corrections* 1. Physically assist Francie to grasp and lift spoon 2. Assist Francie to start scooping 3. Physically assist Francie to make correct response

Figure 13.5. Intervention plan: Feeding skills with backward chaining and adaptive equipment.

feet should be flat on the floor or on a support to provide stability through the child's trunk. Shoulders and arms should be relaxed and free to move, so that the young child can accomplish hand-to-mouth movements and participate in self-feeding. Occupational and physical therapists on the early intervention or special education team are involved in identifying optimal mealtime positions for an infant or young child with neuromotor disabilities.

Therapeutic feeding techniques are strategies to inhibit atypical oral-motor patterns and to facilitate typical oral-motor patterns. The positioning techniques described above are important components of therapeutic feeding techniques. Prefeeding techniques include rubbing and stroking around and inside the mouth to decrease hypersensitivity and stretching techniques to facilitate typical tone and movement of the facial muscles. There are also techniques to assist a child with eating and drinking skills such as jaw control, lip closure, tongue control, chewing, and swallowing. An occupational, physical, or speech therapist can recommend and demonstrate appropriate therapeutic prefeeding and feeding techniques.

Infants and young children who need extensive supports for eating and drinking are often at risk for choking. Choking occurs when food or some other object or material obstructs the child's airway. Signs of choking include sudden coughing, gagging, or high-pitched noisy breathing; holding the neck (making the *choking sign*); or bluish lips or skin (American Heart Association, 2004). If the child can cough loudly or speak, the airway is not completely blocked. If the child's breathing is a concern, dial 9-1-1 for emergency assistance. If the child's airway seems to be completely blocked, in addition to calling 9-1-1, administer the Heimlich maneuver (abdominal thrusts). If the Heimlich maneuver is ineffective and the child becomes unresponsive, cardiopulmonary resuscitation must be provided (American Heart Association, 2004). Early interventionists and early childhood special educators should receive first aid and emergency care training (infant and/or child courses) annually so they can respond competently and quickly to choking and other emergencies that may arise.

For children who are unable to obtain adequate nutrition and hydration orally, feeding tubes (*gavage* feedings) may be used (Heller et al., 2000). A feeding tube is inserted through the abdominal wall (*gastrostomy*), nose (*nasogastric tube*), or mouth (*orogastric tube*). Food is administered through a gravity method or pump method (kangaroo bag). In the gravity method, food is placed in a large syringe attached to the feeding tube. The syringe is elevated 4 to 5 inches above the child's abdomen if a gastrostomy is used, or 4 to 5 inches above the child's head if a nasogastric or orogastric tube is used. The food passes slowly through the tube and into the abdomen. Water may be given through the tube after feeding. The pump method is identical to the gravity method except an electric pump is used to move the food from the bag through the feeding tube. Nasogastric and gastrostomy tubes may be left in place and taped to the skin when not in use. Orogastric tubes are usually inserted for each feeding and removed afterward.

The insertion of feeding tubes requires special training. Although parents are frequently trained by a nurse or physician to insert the tube, school districts may require that a licensed healthcare worker (physician or nurse) insert the tube. Teachers and infant specialists should be aware that there are health concerns associated with feeding tubes. There is a risk of infection, particularly at the site of a gastrostomy incision, and there is a risk of aspiration when nasogastric or orogastric feeding tubes are used. Teachers and infant specialists who administer tube feedings should be certain that they receive appropriate training (Heller et al., 2000).

DESIGNING INSTRUCTIONAL PROGRAMS TO PROMOTE INDEPENDENCE

When designing instructional programs to promote independence, be certain that short-term objectives are ones that can be accomplished within 3 or 4 months. In formulating the objectives to foster independence, remember the following pointers: 1) The performance conditions of the objective should be stated as *independent performance conditions*. If adult reminders or prompts do not typically precede the behavior, they should not be included in the conditions of the objective. 2) Whenever possible, the response specified in the objective should be stated as a *general case response*. 3) If the desired response is too difficult for the child to perform independently, consider teaching a *functionally equivalent response* or a response that requires partial participation. Another option is to provide adaptations or environmental modifications that make the task easier or provide assistance to the child. 4) State the criterion for the objective at a level that allows or results in independent performance. It may be necessary to observe others performing the skill to determine the accuracy, fluency, or other response characteristic that best represents the independent performance criterion.

Instructional Context

An instructional context that supports and facilitates independence should also be described in the instructional plan. The instructional context specifies where, when, and under what conditions instruction occurs. The following situational variables should be considered to promote independence:

- Conduct instruction in natural settings in which the skill would typically occur, preferably in more than one natural setting. This will facilitate generalization.

- Use naturally occurring routines and activities as instructional situations rather than setting aside a particular time for instruction. Teaching during naturally occurring routines and activities will help the child recognize when the skill is needed and what purpose it serves.

- Construct skill sequences and conduct instruction with more than one skill at a time. Skill sequences teach relationships between behaviors.

- Use EMT procedures and identify child responses that signal the *occasion for instruction*. Using child-determined occasions for instruction is responsive to the interests of the child and provides meaningful and motivating situations for learning.

Contextual strategies to promote independence include environmental supports and instructional techniques that eliminate a child's overreliance on an adult to accomplish his or her goals.

Prompting Techniques

It is also critical to select prompting techniques that encourage independence. The following considerations should be addressed:

1. Use *least intrusive procedures*, that is, procedures that do not interfere any more than necessary with the naturally occurring events or interactions. The more instruction interferes with the natural situation, the less likely the child is to maintain or generalize the response.

2. Select *naturalistic teaching procedures*, such as EMT and time delay. These procedures help children respond independently to the natural prompts present in the environment.

3. Include *generalization techniques* such as sufficient exemplars, common stimuli, or mediation strategies among the prompting and facilitation techniques. In addition to naturalistic teaching procedures, instructional plans should include multiple approaches to facilitate generalization. Independence is greatly enhanced when responses are generalized.

4. If independent performance of the response seems too difficult for the child (the skill is complex, or the skill includes a physical response beyond the child's current abilities), develop *environmental prompts* or *modifications*

to make independence a realistic goal. The environmental prompts or modifications may be permanent additions to the environment, or they may be faded as part of the instructional plan.

5. Use *prosthetic devices, special equipment, or therapeutic positioning and handling techniques* to facilitate independent responding when the child has physical or sensory disabilities. Sometimes these accommodations alone will result in independent responding; other times instruction in using the accommodations will be required.

6. Consider the use of *peer assistance* to help the child with special needs respond independent of adult assistance. Peer assistance is well suited to group activities and free-play situations.

After prompting and facilitation strategies have been described, the instructional plan must indicate consequences appropriate to the child's response. There are two specific recommendations for promoting independence that apply to this section of the instructional plan.

First, develop *minimally intrusive* corrections; that is, use corrections that interfere as little as possible. As in the recommendations for prompting and facilitation techniques, the less noticeable the correction, the more likely the child will generalize and perform the skill independently. Second, use *naturally occurring reinforcers and corrections* whenever possible. If children learn to recognize and use natural contingencies, they will rely less on instructional support and adult assistance. Pairing instructional consequences with natural ones, or exaggerating the natural ones, are simple ways to help children notice the natural consequences.

These recommendations summarize teaching strategies to consider in planning individualized instruction to promote independence. The examples of instructional plans throughout this chapter illustrate the recommendations. As emphasized in this chapter, independence is not merely a goal that we *hope* to achieve; it is a goal to actively address through effective intervention strategies.

SUMMARY

This chapter discussed independent skills for meaningful participation in natural settings. Instructional procedures should be least intrusive, naturalistic, incorporated into daily routines, and designed to facilitate generalization. When a child's age or disability limits the extent to which independence can be achieved, goals for functional independence may be appropriate. Functional independence is accomplished by teaching the child equivalent responses or by providing adaptive strategies. Equivalent responses are those that accomplish the same function or purpose of a target behavior. If a child is unable to perform a target behavior due to a disability or delay, it is sometimes possible to teach an alternative and equivalent response. Adaptive strategies include functionally equivalent responses as well as the use of assistive technology, adaptive equipment, and materials. Although independence may seem very difficult for some children to accomplish, particularly if they have multiple or severe challenges, functional independence can almost always be achieved with a bit of creativity and problem solving.

STUDY QUESTIONS

1. Describe appropriate *independent behavior* for 1-, 3-, and 5-year-olds associated with playtime, mealtime, and bath time.
2. Discuss specific strategies that can be incorporated into *systematic instructional plans* to help children achieve independence.
3. Define *critical function, functionally equivalent response,* and *functional independence.*
4. What is *assistive technology*? Why are *services* included in the definition of assistive technology?
5. Describe how the following strategies can assist children to achieve functional independence: individualized participation, environmental prompts, learning centers, peer assistance, and prosthetic devices and adaptive equipment.
6. Discuss the effects of damage to the central nervous system on muscle tone, reflexes, postural reactions, and motor milestones.
7. What is the purpose of positioning and carrying techniques?
8. Compare and contrast *static* and *dynamic* positioning.
9. Identify and discuss three examples of *functionally equivalent* gross motor responses for children with physical disabilities.
10. Describe the relationship of fine motor development to gross motor development.
11. Identify and discuss three examples of functionally equivalent fine motor responses for children with fine motor needs.
12. Discuss the primary function of communication.
13. List and describe Dunst et al.'s (1987) five phases in the development of *environmental control skills.*
14. Describe how you might use the following strategies to help an infant acquire environmental control skills: enhance sensitivity, increase opportunities, structure

predictable routines, augment input, and modify the environment.

15. Consider the example of a 4-year-old boy who is reliably using one-word line drawings on his communication board to make requests and to refuse or terminate something. Write a set of three communication objectives illustrating how you could increase the complexity of this child's communication skills.

16. Identify and discuss three examples of functionally equivalent communication responses for children with communication needs.

17. Describe and contrast a task analysis and a partial participation task analysis.

18. What is the *rapid method* of toilet training? Discuss the pros and cons of teaching independent toileting through this method.

19. Discuss the relationship between physical skills (gross and fine motor) and mealtime skills.

REFERENCES

American Heart Association (AHA). (2004). *Relief of choking in children.* Retrieved November 15, 2004, from http://www.americanheart.org/presenter.jhtml?identifier=3025002

Azrin, N. (1989). *Toilet training in less than a day.* New York, NY: Pocket Books.

Azrin, N.H., & Besalel, V.A. (1979). *A parent's guide to bedwetting control: A step-by-step method.* New York, NY: Simon & Schuster.

Azrin, N.H., Sneed, T.J., & Foxx, R.M. (1973). Dry-bed: A rapid method of eliminating bedwetting (enuresis) of the retarded. *Behavior Research and Therapy, 11,* 427–434.

Azrin, N.H., Sneed, T.J., & Foxx, R.M. (1974). Dry-bed training: Rapid elimination of childhood enuresis. *Behavior Research and Therapy, 12,* 147–156.

Bly, L. (1983). *The components of normal movement during the first year of life and abnormal motor development.* Chicago: Neurodevelopmental Treatment Association.

Bricker, D. (Ed.). (2002). *Assessment, evaluation, and programming system (AEPS®) for infants and children: Vol. 2. AEPS® Test for Birth to Three Years and Three to Six Years* (2nd ed.). Baltimore, MD: Paul H. Brookes Publishing Co.

Carr, E.G., & Durand, V.M. (1985). Reducing behavior problems through functional communication training. *Journal of Applied Behavior Analysis, 18,* 111–126.

Copeland, M., Ford, L., & Solon, N. (1976). *Occupational therapy for mentally retarded children.* Baltimore, MD: University Park Press.

Dunst, C.J., Lesko, J.J., Holbert, K.A., Wilson, L.L., Sharpe, K.L., & Liles, R.F. (1987). A systematic approach to infant intervention. *Topics in Early Childhood Special Education, 7*(2), 19–37.

Erwin, E.J., Brotherson, M.J., Palmer, S.B., Cook, C.C., Weigel, C.J., & Summers, J.A. (2009). How to promote self-determination for young children with disabilities Evidenced-based strategies for early childhood practitioners and families. *Young Exceptional Children, 12*(2), 27–37.

Farlow, L.J., & Snell, M.E. (2006). Teaching basic self-care skills. In M.E. Snell & F. Brown (Eds.), *Instruction of students with severe disabilities* (6th ed., pp. 328–374). Upper Saddle River, NJ: Prentice-Hall.

Heller, K.W., Forney, P.E., Alberto, P.A., Schwartzman, M.N., & Goeckel, T.M. (2000). *Meeting physical and health needs of children with disabilities: Teaching student participation and management.* Belmont, CA: Wadsworth.

Hill, J.L. (1999). *Meeting the needs of students with special physical and health care needs.* Upper Saddle River, NJ: Merrill/Prentice Hall.

Illingworth, R.S. (1983). *The development of the infant and young child: Abnormal and normal* (8th ed.). New York, NY: Churchill Livingstone.

Individuals with Disabilities Education Improvement Act (IDEA) of 2004, PL 108-446, 20 U.S.C. §§ 1400 et seq.

Johnson-Martin, N.M., Attermeier, S.M., & Hacker, B.J. (2004). *The Carolina Curriculum for infants* and *toddlers with special needs* (3rd ed.). Baltimore, MD: Paul H. Brookes Publishing Co.

Kaiser, A.P. (1993). Parent-implemented language intervention. In A.P. Kaiser & D.B. Gray (Eds.), *Enhancing children's communication: Vol. 2. Research foundations for intervention* (pp. 63–84). Baltimore, MD: Paul H. Brookes Publishing Co.

Kaiser, A., Hendrickson, J., & Alpert, K. (1991). Milieu language teaching: A second look. In R. Gable (Ed.), *Advances in mental retardation and developmental disabilities* (Vol. 1, pp. 63–92). London: Kingsley.

McCormick, L. (2003). Language intervention in the inclusive preschool. In L. McCormick, D.F. Loeb, & R.L. Schiefelbusch (Eds.), *Supporting children with communication difficulties in inclusive settings: School-based language intervention* (2nd ed., pp. 333–366). Boston, MA: Allyn & Bacon.

McCormick, L., & Wegner, J. (2003). Supporting augmentative communication. In L. McCormick, D.F. Loeb, & R.L. Schiefelbusch (Eds.), *Supporting children with communication difficulties in inclusive settings: School-based language intervention* (2nd ed., pp. 435–459). Boston, MA: Allyn & Bacon.

McWilliam, R.A. (1996). Implications for the future of integrating specialized services. In R.A. McWilliam (Ed.), *Rethinking pull-out services in early intervention: A professional resource* (pp. 343–372). Baltimore, MD: Paul H. Brookes Publishing Co.

McWilliam, R.A., & Casey, A.M. (2008). *Engagement of every child in the preschool classroom.* Baltimore, MD: Paul H. Brookes Publishing Co.

Noonan, M.J., & Siegel, E.B. (2003). Special needs of students with severe disabilities and autism. In L. McCormick, D.F. Loeb, & R.L. Schiefelbusch (Eds.), *Supporting children with communication difficulties in inclusive settings: School-based language intervention* (pp. 409–433). Boston, MA: Allyn & Bacon.

Pellegrino, L. (2002). Cerebral palsy. In M.L. Batshaw (Ed.), *Children with disabilities* (5th ed., pp. 443–466). Baltimore, MD: Paul H. Brookes Publishing Co.

Phillips, C.L., & Vollmer, T.R. (2012). Generalized instruction following with pictorial prompts. *Journal of Applied Behavior Analysis, 45*(1), 37–54.

Ratliffe, K.T. (1998). *Clinical pediatric physical therapy: A guide for the physical therapy team.* St. Louis: Mosby.

Sadao, K.C., & Robinson, N.B. (2010). *Assistive technology for young children: Creating inclusive learning environments.* Baltimore, MD: Paul H. Brookes Publishing Co.

Sandall, S., Hemmeter, M.L., Smith, B.J., & McLean, M.E. (2005). *DEC recommended practices: A comprehensive guide for practical application in early intervention/early childhood special education.* Longmont, CO: Sopris West.

Snell, M.E. (1987). *Systematic instruction of persons with severe handicaps.* Columbus, OH: Merrill.

Stokes, T.F., & Baer, D.M. (1977). An implicit technology of generalization. *Journal of Applied Behavior Analysis, 10,* 349–367.

Stoneman, Z., & Rugg, M.E. (2004). Partnerships with families. In S.R. Hooper & W. Umansky (Eds.), *Young children with special needs* (4th ed., pp. 90–117). Upper Saddle River, NJ: Pearson Education.

Technology-Related Assistance for Individuals with Disabilities Act of 1988, PL 100-407, 29 U.S.C. §§ 2201 *et seq.*

Thompson, T., & Hanson, R. (1983). Overhydration: Precautions when treating urinary incontinence. *Mental Retardation, 21,* 139–143.

White, O.R. (1980). Adaptive performance objectives: Form versus function. In W. Sailor, B. Wilcox, & L. Brown (Eds.), *Methods of instruction for severely handicapped students* (pp. 47–69). Baltimore, MD: Paul H. Brookes Publishing Co.

14

Transitions

Linda McCormick

.... **FOCUS OF THIS CHAPTER** ....

- Major transitions for infants and young children with disabilities
- An ecological transition framework
- Legal mandates related to transition
- Strategies for successful transition

Life is a sequence of transitions or turning points, which are always marked by greater vulnerability than are other times. Even positive transitions that represent achievement of desired goals are stressful. The stress and vulnerability inherent in transitions may not be avoidable, but they can be minimized. The concept of transition in the field of special education was popularized initially as a response to the need to facilitate movement of secondary students from school into postschool environments (Wehman, Moon, & McCarthy, 1986). It soon became evident that the concerns and processes associated with transition have far broader application than postsecondary adjustment.

Transitions that involve young children are not single events but rather processes that occurs over many months of planning and continuing follow up. The number of people and agencies involved makes the process exceedingly complicated. For service providers working with infants and young children and their families, the goal is to minimize the stress by providing a seamless system of services with continuity and smooth movement between and among programs.

Transitions may be horizontal or vertical (Kagan, 1992). Vertical transitions involve changes in programs across time or as there is a need for different or expanded services. For example, a family may move from a hospital neonatal intensive care unit (NICU) to an early intervention program to an inclusive preschool program, and eventually to kindergarten with special education and related services support. Horizontal transitions involve changes in programs across a day or week. For example, the child and family may be involved in multiple activities simultaneously with different support services and in different locations. The child may participate in an inclusive preschool program in the morning, followed by special therapy services in a separate classroom in the afternoon and, later in the afternoon, child care in another environment.

MAJOR TRANSITIONS FOR INFANTS AND YOUNG CHILDREN WITH DISABILITIES

The major transitions for infants and young children with disabilities and their families are from the NICU to the home and a community program (follow-up clinic, public or private health care services, an early intervention [EI] program, public or private child care), to preschool, and then, at age 5, to kindergarten.

Hospital to Home and Community Services

The family assumes responsibility for the day-to-day care of their infant at home when they leave the hospital. This requires enormous adjustments in the routines of any family. These adjustments are many times multiplied when the infant is at risk of, or already has, special health care needs. In the hospital NICU the infant was cared for by a team of highly skilled physicians, nurses, social workers, and other support staff. It is not difficult to understand why the parents feel overwhelmed and abandoned when they prepare to take their infant home. They are doing their best to cope with 1) understanding their infant's condition, 2) basic caregiving responsibilities, 3) self-esteem and confidence issues, and 4) decisions about services (Hanline & Deppe, 1990).

The issues that are foremost for families are those related to understanding their infant's condition (e.g., prematurity, sensory impairment, motor impairment). Compounding their nervousness and apprehension are worries about the their infant's future and feelings of shock, sadness, anger, grief, disappointment, and guilt. They struggle to come to some understanding of the etiology of their infant's condition, a developmental prognosis, and the infant's chances for survival. Major goals for early intervention personnel at this point are to help parents 1) establish and maintain contacts with other families of infants with special needs, 2) locate and obtain respite care and child care services (if needed), and 3) locate community-based family support services.

Second, although parents eagerly anticipate discharge from the NICU, they are understandably anxious about the responsibilities of day-to-day care of a very small infant facing numerous challenges. Many infants are still on a ventilator, gastrointestinal tube feeding, or an apnea monitor when they are discharged from the hospital. In addition, infants with special needs are often fussy and irritable.

The third concern that parents face is their own self-esteem and confidence. A premature birth shatters any assumption of controlling the outcomes of pregnancy. The sense of having lost control is heightened during the infant's stay in the NICU, because parents are not able to make decisions about the day-to-day care of their child. They do not have a chance to gain confidence in their capabilities as caregivers. Early intervention service providers let parents know that they understand the need to regain some control of their lives. As part of the transition process they encourage and support the parents to make decisions regarding their family and their child.

Finally, the parents must begin to consider how and when they want to participate in community-based support services. This is an emotion-laden issue in that it requires the parents to "go public." They must come to terms with the possibility of developmental delay and the fact that there will be a need to allow unfamiliar professionals to enter their lives.

Early Intervention Services to Preschool

Similar to the hospital-to-home and community services transition, the transition from Part C infant services to Part B preschool services is stressful and complicated. At the broadest level, one element of the problem is that these are two distinctly different programs. Recall from Chapter 3 that these programs have different eligibility criteria and different program features. IDEA assigns responsibility for infant and toddler programs to a governor-identified lead agency (which may or may not be the state education agency) while preschoolers are always served by the state education agency.

From the initial stages of planning until the preschooler is actually enrolled and attending the new program or programs, this transition brings a whole new set of issues in addition to new roles and responsibilities. The most salient issues associated with this transition are continuity of services, adapting to change, and adjusting to new program expectations. Issues in relation to transition planning at this point are most challenging for families from culturally and linguistically diverse groups who must now deal with new rules and different professionals.

The program change when their child is 36 months old is especially problematic for those families who did not enter the Part C system when their child was an infant. If they did not begin receiving services until their child was an older toddler they realize that in a very short time, just as they are beginning to adjust to the services, they will need to transfer to a new program. Over the years there has been a great deal of discussion as to ways to amend IDEA to address the issues associated with creating this unnecessary transition in the middle of the early childhood period. However, the problem inherent in having two service deliveries system remains. On the positive side, this transition differs from the other transitions in early childhood in that there are specific federal and state requirements to guide the process. These are described later in the chapter.

Preschool to Kindergarten

Federal and state legislation requires transition plans for children moving from Part C infant and toddler programs into Part B preschool programs. The change in service delivery—and those who deliver it—is unfortunate because this transition is particularly complex for young children with special needs and their families. While there is no such mandate for transition planning for children moving from preschool into kindergarten or first grade classrooms, there have been many studies identifying strategies (described later in the chapter) to support young children as they move from Part B services to typical education settings. These can be helpful in guiding families at this stage, although, again, families are faced with learning new rules and regulations and how to interact with new teachers, new service personnel, and new agencies. There are changes in classroom characteristics (e.g., higher child-to-staff ratios and more large-group instruction) and teacher expectations (e.g., more autonomy and academic skill acquisition).

AN ECOLOGICAL TRANSITION FRAMEWORK

Ecological theory (Bronfenbrenner, 1979), which we have promoted throughout this text as the most appropriate model for viewing development processes and outcomes and guiding assessment and curriculum decisions, is also a useful framework for transition planning. Recall that the ecological model posits multiple layers of influence (the environmental context) on the developing child. The basic premise is that we cannot understand the developing child without reference to the characteristics of his or her environmental context. There is always a dynamic interplay between the child and his or her family and other contextual influences such as school and program, neighborhood, church, and so forth. Over time these *reciprocal interactions* affect and are affected by one another.

The ecological model highlights the importance of the various elements of the child's ecological context: those elements that are closest to the child such as the family, school or program, and neighborhood as well as elements in the larger ecological context such as laws, cultural values, and social customs. It also calls attention to unique characteristics of individual children such as temperament, type of disability, and so on (Bronfenbrenner & Morris, 2006). Researchers at the National Early Childhood Transition Center have used ecological theory as the conceptual foundation that informs their transition framework (Rous, Hardin, Hallam, McCormick, & Jung, 2007). Similar to other processes (assessment and curriculum development) that are predicated on ecological theory, this framework has immense value for planning because it goes beyond a child-centered perspective to consideration of 1) program factors (e.g., the transition procedures, relationship between programs and teachers); 2) classroom or teacher characteristics (e.g., program location, classroom climate, teacher–child relationship); 3) family characteristics (e.g., family strengths, support systems); and 4) child characteristics (e.g., ability level, age at transition, friendships). These variables are undoubtedly significant for all children but especially for children with more significant needs.

In summary, an ecological framework argues for attention to the context of the transition, the available supports as well as the barriers. It goes beyond consideration of academic achievement alone as the criterion for the success of transition to a thoughtful review of the influence of contextual factors such as the adequacy of communication between sending and receiving providers or the accommodations and the supports used in the receiving environment to support the child's participation in classroom routines and activities.

LEGAL MANDATES RELATED TO TRANSITION

Recall from Chapter 1 that there are two parts of IDEA that have requirements regulating services for children from birth to age 6: Part C authorizing services for infants and toddlers (birth to 3) and Part B authorizing services for young children (3 to 6) and school-age children. IDEA requires state and local agencies that provide services to infants and toddlers under Part C to plan for transition of all of the children and families that they serve either to an early childhood program under Part B or another appropriate program. Head Start also has specific requirements related to transition planning. The Head Start Program Performance Standards provide expectations, guidance, and support to ensure a smooth transition into and out of Early Head Start and Head Start programs.

There are two parts of the IDEA requirements related to transition (CONNECT, 2012). One part is the assurances that each state must give to the federal government in order for the state agency to receive the financial assistance necessary to operate their Part C infant/toddler programs. The state agency pledges to do the following:

- Ensure a smooth transition from their early intervention services to preschool, school, or other appropriate services
- Describe how it will include toddlers' families in the transition plans
- Describe how it will coordinate with Early Head Start, early education and child care programs, and Part C services
- Ensure notification of the state and local agency where the child resides that the child will be eligible for Part B services
- Convene a conference with the family and the local education agency at least 3 months and no more than 9 months before the child is eligible for preschool services to discuss services the child may receive

- Assure that if the child may not be eligible for preschool services a conference will be convened to discuss options for services the child may receive
- Develop an individualized education program (IEP) for the child before he or she transitions to a Part B preschool program

The second part of the IDEA requirements related to transition has to do with services and supports that are to be provided at the local level. The four requirements are as follows: 1) the parents will be members of the individualized family service plan (IFSP) team, 2) assessment and services will be provided by an interdisciplinary team, 3) there will be a service coordinator from the profession "most immediately relevant" to the infant/toddler's or family's needs, and 4) the IFSP will contain a transition plan with the steps to be taken to support transition to preschool or other appropriate services.

As noted above, the Head Start Performance Standards also have requirements for transitions into and out of Head Start Programs, including not only Head Start but also Early Head Start, home or other child care settings, elementary schools, and Title I preschool programs. These include both procedural (transfer of records, communication, planning meetings, staff training) and planning requirements (a transition meeting).

Because there are no legal mandates for planning the transition from hospital to home and community programs or from preschool to kindergarten; services for the latter vary enormously across states and across agencies and programs within a state. (Sometimes there is absolutely no transition planning and support for 5-year-olds.) The next section provides strategies to guide all three early childhood transitions.

STRATEGIES FOR SUCCESSFUL TRANSITION

Transition strategies fall into two broad categories (with some overlap): 1) strategies involving communication and collaboration across agencies and programs and 2) strategies focused on preparing the child, the family, and the receiving program. The focuses are minimizing disruptions for the child and the family, sustaining the child's developmental progress, and identifying and implementing needed adaptations and supports in the receiving environment.

Hospital to Home and Community

As noted above, the goals for early intervention personnel in the hospital-to-home transition are to help parents 1) establish and maintain contacts with other families of infants with special needs, 2) locate and obtain respite care and child care services (if needed), and 3) locate community-based family support services. The majority of families receive predischarge hospital training from the hospital NICU staff. This training focuses on the infant's special nutritional needs, operation of specific equipment, and proper positioning. The NICU staff also provide the family with information about the range of available EI programs in the community and the referral process. When possible, one or more of the family's EI service providers (possibly the service coordinator) usually participates in this training with the parents.

To be most effective, training to prepare families for discharge begins shortly after the infant is admitted to the NICU. There should be considerable repetition of all the information because parents are feeling so stressed at this time that they may not recall information unless it is repeated often during the time their child is in the hospital. Similarly, they should have many opportunities to practice the procedures that they will need to follow when they take the infant home. There are many resources for parents (DVDs, web sites books, pamphlets) that clearly describe their child's condition and the procedures they will need to implement at home. These will be available in different formats and the preferred language of the family.

Many hospitals use a discharge information and planning form to encourage and support communication and the sharing of information and needs between families and professionals. It describes the infant's current and future care needs in detail, with space provided for the parents to identify areas of need and topics they would like to have addressed. The meetings in which this form is completed provide a setting for parents to ask specific questions about developmental issues (e.g., rate of developmental milestones), caregiving and expectations for the future.

Once the infant is home, the focus of EI support services shifts to 1) helping the parents implement the procedures recommended by the NICU and other medical personnel, 2) answering questions not answered prior to discharge, 3) assisting parents to understand and respond to the infant's social and communication cues, 4) monitoring the infant's developmental progress, and 5) ensuring that the infant's health care needs are met. As many infants will continue to require care from medical professionals, the EI care coordinator may need to continue to be available as a liaison among the family, the NICU staff, and community health care providers.

Communication with other families is most helpful during this entire process but especially when the family takes their infant home. Because they can really understand what a family is going through, parents who have experienced the same medical issues can provide invaluable support during this period, as can parent groups and online support communities. These parents share their knowledge about life with a preterm infant, community services, and disability and offer much-needed reassurances. A number of national and Internet parent-to-parent groups are also available to help parents grow in confidence and ability to meet their family's changing needs and those of their child.

Early Intervention Services to Preschool

When the child and family transition from early intervention services to preschool, the goal of the team (EI and preschool service providers and the family) is to avoid interruptions and duplications of services. Guidelines for this process are provided in the *DEC Recommended Practices* (Sandall, Hemmeter, Smith, & McLean, 2005). The major recommendations are as follows:

- *Plan ahead to allow adequate time to prepare the child and the family.* Begin planning when the child is 2 years, 6 months old to ensure that the plan is completed by the time he or she is 2 years, 9 months of age.

- *Provide the family with information in their preferred language.* Provide a detailed description of all aspects of the process, including their role in the process, and explain available service options.

- *Arrange visits to available programs.* Schedule opportunities for the family to talk to other families and the service providers during or after the visit.

- *Identify existing and needed transition skills.* Once a receiving program has been identified, make a list of skills that will help the child adjust to the new setting.

- *Teach skills for the next environment.* Arrange activities that will help the child acquire skills and learn the routines that will help him or her adjust in the next environment.

There are very specific guidelines as to the skills and information that EI providers need and the procedures that they need to put in place. EI providers must be knowledgeable about following elements of the transition process: time lines, sending-program responsibilities, available service options and other resources in their community, and the essential of details their program's interagency transition agreements. The transition process will entail months of communication, many reciprocal visits between the EI professionals and early childhood education and early childhood special education professionals, and systematic preparation of the child.

A major goal of proactive planning where the family is concerned is to ensure that they are fully informed of their legal rights and responsibilities and that they have information regarding the preschool classrooms in their district. They should be provided the relevant facts about related services, IEP development, child development expectations, preschool curriculum, and community services. As team members and partners in the transition process, it is especially important for them to be aware of the differences in service delivery between the EI services and the preschool program (in expectations, procedures, and activities) and know that these differences are being addressed as part of the planning process. These differences are stressful for all families: They are especially difficult for families from culturally and linguistically diverse groups. Transition planning meetings will consider 1) a projected date for the transition; 2) what decisions need to be made, when they should be made, and who will make them; 3) eligibility variables; 4) information about available placement options; and 5) how the child will be prepared for the changes.

The skill areas most likely to impede participation when children transition from a home-based EI program to a center-based preschool program are 1) playing with peers (individually and in a group) and 2) following directions, routines, and rules (notably, safety rules). Long before transition to the new placement actually occurs, an EI service provider and one or more family members visit the new program to learn about its rules and observe the daily schedule. Following the steps of the ecological assessment process (described in Chapter 5), it is correct they note expectations of the receiving program and the skills that will help the child participate in routine activities. Additionally, they help the receiving program plan whatever adaptations and supports (if any) will be needed.

The ecological assessment process or whatever means of information gathering is used will suggest possible adaptations to facilitate and support the child with disabilities. Decisions as to when and how to modify and adapt activities to make them individually appropriate for the child with disabilities should be guided by the following caveats (McCormick & Feeney, 1995):

- Activity expectations should be modified only if it is clear that the child cannot participate even partially or at a less sophisticated level without some modification.

- If it is necessary to arrange an alternative activity, that activity should be as rich varied, and rewarding as the original activity.

- Care should be taken in the rare instance when an alternative activity must be arranged that it does not promote dependence or call undue attention to the child.

- Give the highest priority to activities and materials that encourage and support age-appropriate social and communication skills.

Guidelines for transition from both the Division for Early Childhood of the Council for Exceptional Children and the National Association for the Education of Young Children specifically highlight the importance of communication and cooperation among staff of the sending and receiving programs in order to assess family concerns, preferences, and expectations of the transition process. Lack of continuity between home and school values and expectations is confusing to families, resulting in less involvement and, ultimately, increased stress.

Preschool to Kindergarten

Collaboration and coordination among service providers and administrators is essential for a smooth transition from preschool to kindergarten. Unfortunately, many of the most effective transition practices such as home visits require service providers to commit time outside of general work hours, something that is often very difficult for already overworked kindergarten teachers.

The earliest work in planning for the transition of children with disabilities from preschool to kindergarten began in the early 1980s. Vincent et al. (1980) used the term *survival skills* for the list of 84 needed behaviors generated by a survey of kindergarten teachers. These were the behaviors the teachers thought that kindergarteners should demonstrate when they entered kindergarten. The assumption underlying this study was that identifying and then teaching these skills to young children with disabilities would increase their potential for a successful transition to general education kindergarten.

McCormick and Kawate (1982) expanded this research in Hawaii. Kindergarten and first-grade teachers were provided with the list of skills generated by Vincent et al. and asked to rate their importance on a five-point scale. The behaviors that were rated as "very important" or "absolutely essential" fell into seven broad categories:

- Working independently (five items)
- Participating with the group (six items)
- Following routines (six items)
- Practicing self-help skills (e.g., taking care of toileting needs) (four items)
- Following directions (three items)

- Practicing social/play skills (five items)
- Communicating functionally (two items)

These skills were then compared with items on nine traditional assessment instruments often used with children this age. What researchers found was that the traditional assessment procedures were assessing very few of the behaviors that teachers considered important to participation in their classrooms. Other research surveying both preschool and kindergarten teachers confirmed the finding that teachers consider skills related to independence and participation more important than skills related to academic readiness (numbers, colors, shapes, etc.) (Hains, Fowler, Schwartz, Kottwitz, & Rosenkoetter, 1989). Kindergarten teachers expect children to be able to work independently, participate in group activities, follow directions, comply with classroom rules, and use a variety of materials.

Development of the Skills for School Success curriculum built upon these findings (Rule, Fiechtl, & Innocenti, 1990). Nine activity areas were identified:

- "Entry routines": hanging up coat, selecting toy, and playing until the teacher indicates movement to the next activity
- "Sequence tasks": independently completing a series of tasks announced daily
- "Pledge of Allegiance"
- "Group circle activities": discussion of the calendar, weather, etc.
- "Individual tasks"
- "Large group activities using commercially available curricula"
- "Workbook tasks"
- "Quiet time activities": child-selected and child-guided activities
- "Transition activities": getting coat and materials to take home, lining up, and walking in line

Each of these activity areas was analyzed into component skills and tasks with criteria that reflect the speed and accuracy with which the behaviors are performed by most children in a typical classroom. These skills were taught to 18 preschool children with disabilities in two child care centers. Most of the children mastered all of the activities and, most important, the follow-up data suggested that they used them in their kindergarten placement.

Le Ager and Shapiro (1995) used the term *template matching* for the process of extended systematic analysis and comparison of child behaviors and environmental variables across settings. In template matching, a "behavioral profile" is developed that includes information about environmental variables in the sending and receiving educational settings and the performance of persons within those environments. (The ecological assessment process described in Chapter 5 is a template-matching approach.)

In the Le Ager and Shapiro study, templates were developed to evaluate the differences between the sending (preschool) and the receiving (kindergarten) environments. Rather than a specific "survival skills curriculum," the focus was on altering activities and teacher behaviors in the preschool environment to align with activities and teacher behaviors in the kindergarten environment. This intervention was effective. At follow-up, kindergarten children who had been involved in the template-matching intervention exhibited fewer competing behaviors and participated more independently in the kindergarten setting than peers in a control group.

While we have highlighted the value of the information that can be gained by observing the child's receiving classroom, there is an important caveat that must be set forth where skills and expectations for the next environment are concerned. These skills must not at any time be viewed as prerequisites for placement in the general education setting. The goals and objectives generated by observations of the next environment and ecological assessment can aid the preparation of children for transition. However, the lack of these skills should never, under any circumstances, be used to argue that a child is not ready for transition to kindergarten.

SUMMARY

There are multiple factors that influence the transition process for young children with disabilities during the early childhood years. The many transitions (from hospital to home, from early intervention services to preschool, and from preschool to kindergarten) involve complex interactions among the children, families, service providers, and programs. For all children, those with disabilities and typically developing children, positive transition outcomes seem to depend on two factors: 1) frequent and positive communication between sending and receiving programs and 2) teaching children the skills they will need in the next educational setting. Successful transitions are one element in the delivery of high-quality early education services for children with disabilities and their families. One of the basic premises of this chapter is that a valuable framework for planning the transition process is provided by the ecological model—which rests on the contention that developmental processes and outcomes are a function of the developing organism (the child) and characteristics of the environment.

STUDY QUESTIONS

1. Discuss the variables involved in *transitions*.

2. Describe the issues that families face in the course of the major transitions of infants and young children with disabilities.

3. How does transition planning within the framework of the *ecological model* differ from traditional transition planning efforts?

4. Contrast the IDEA Part C and Part B requirements related to transition.

5. Describe goals and strategies for service providers at each of the major transitions of early childhood.

6. Compare the identification of "survivor skills" efforts with the more recent *template matching* procedures.

REFERENCES

Bronfenbrenner, U. (1979). *The ecology of human development: Experiments by nature and design.* Cambridge, MA: Harvard University Press.

Bronfenbrenner, U., & Morris, P.A. (2006). The bioecological model of human development. In W. Damon & R.M. Lerner (Eds.), *Handbook of child psychology: Vol. 1. Theoretical models of human development* (6th ed., pp. 793–828). New York, NY: John Wiley.

CONNECT (The Center to Mobilize Early Childhood Knowledge). (2012). *Policy advisory: The law governing transition of young children* (Rev. ed.). Chapel Hill, NC: The University of North Carolina, FPG Child Development Institute, Author.

Hains, A.H., Fowler, S.A., Schwartz, I. S., Kottwitz, E., & Rosenkoetter, S. (1989). A comparison of preschool and kindergarten teacher expectations for school readiness. *Early Childhood Research Quarterly, 4*(1), 75–88.

Hanline, M.F., & Deppe, J. (1990). Discharging the premature infant: Family issues and implications for intervention. *Topics in Early Childhood Special Education, 9*(4), 15–25.

Kagan, S.L. (1992). *Sticking together: Strengthening linkages and the transition between early childhood education and early elementary school.* Washington, DC: U.S. Department of Education.

Le Ager, C., & Shapiro, E.S. (1995). Template matching as a strategy for assessment of and intervention for preschool students with disabilities. *Topics in Early Childhood Special Education, 15*(2), 187–218.

McCormick, L., & Feeney, S. (1995). Modifying and expanding activities for children with disabilities. *Young Children, 50*(4), 10–17.

McCormick, L., & Kawate, J. (1982). Kindergarten survival skills: New directions for preschool special education. *Education and Training of the Mentally Retarded, 17,* 247–252.

Rous, B., Harbin, G., Hallam, R., McCormick, K.M., & Jung, L.A. (2007). The transition process for young children with disabilities: A conceptual framework. *Infants and Young Children, 20*(2), 135–148.

Rule, S., Fiechtl, B.J., & Innocenti, M.S. (1990). Preparation for transition to mainstreamed post-preschool environments: Development of a survival skills curriculum. *Topics in Early Childhood Special Education, 9*(4), 78–90.

Sandall, S., Hemmeter, M.L., Smith B.J., & McLean, M.E. (Eds.). (2005). *DEC-recommended practices: A comprehensive guide for practical application in early intervention/early childhood special education.* Missoula, MT: Division for Early Childhood.

Vincent, L.J., Salisbury, C., Walter, G., Brown, P., Gruenewald, L.J., & Powers, M. (1980). Program evaluation and curriculum development in early childhood special education: Criteria of the next environment. In W. Sailor, B. Wilcox, & L. Brown (Eds.), *Methods of instruction for severely handicapped students* (pp. 308–328). Baltimore, MD: Paul H. Brookes Publishing Co.

Wehman, P., Moon, M.S., & McCarthy, P. (1986). Transition from school to adulthood for youth with severe handicaps. *Focus on Exceptional Children, 18*(5), 1–11.

Index

Tables and figures are indicated by *t* and *f*, respectively.

AAC devices, *see* Augmentative and alternative communication (AAC) devices
A-B-C records of challenging behavior, 241, 242, 243*f*
ABI, *see* Activity-based interventions
Acceptance, social, 284–285
Access, as feature of inclusion, 16–17
Accommodations
  assessment, 62
  general suggestions for, 167*t*
Acculturation, professional, 32
Activities
  affection, 288–289
  child directed, 182
  high probability (high-*p*), using as reinforcers, 212
  listing on ecological assessment, 104
  in positive behavior support (PBS) plans, 249–251
  scheduling, 165–166
  social integration, 290–291
Activity-based intervention (ABI), 155–156, 156*t*
ADA, *see* Americans with Disabilities Act (ADA) of 1990 (PL 101-336)
Adaptations
  designing instructional programs to promote independence, 323–325
  for functional independence, 301–306
  independence in fine motor skills, 308–309
  instructional planning, 108, 108*t*
  overview, 299–300
  physical development intervention procedures, 306–308
  teaching independent behaviors, 300–301
  see also Environmental control skills; Self-help skills
Adapted participation, 272

Adaptive equipment, 304
Affection activities, 288–289
Affective interventions, 286–287
Age-appropriate behaviors, 54
Age-appropriate skills, naturalistic curriculum model, 81–83
Alternative assessments, 62
Alternative communication modes, 313
Alternative teaching approach, 40
American contributions to field, 4–6
Americans with Disabilities Act (ADA) of 1990 (PL 101-336), 12–13
Amplification devices, 168
Anecdotal records, 112
Annual goals statement, 61
Anticipated corrects, 125
Arena assessment, 41
Asian families, 33
Assessment
  accommodations, 62
  authentic, 52–55
  categories of, 48–49
  cultural issues, 35
  Individuals with Disabilities Education Act (IDEA) of 1990 (PL 101-476), 48
  in naturalistic curriculum model, 80
  purposes of planning, monitoring, and, 100
  traditional, 52
Assistance procedures for group instruction, 275
Assistance strategies, in systematic instruction
  cues, 124
  errorless procedures, 124–125
  fading prompts and cues, 126–127
  graduated guidance, 123–124
  overview, 120
  prompt hierarchies, 122–123
  prompting, 120–122, 125–126

346 • Index

Assistive technology (AT)
  access, 162
  devices, 304
  general discussion, 17–18, 303
  services, 304
Attentional interactions, 310
Attentional prompts, for children with autism, 210–211
Atypical muscle tone, 305
Atypical reflexes, 305
Audio devices, recording instructions on, 192
Auditory prompts, 122
Augmentative and alternative communication (AAC) devices, 304
Augmentative communication, 215–216, 313
Authentic assessment, 52–55
Autism, 51t
  augmentative communication, 215–216
  cues, 213–214
  direct instruction, 210–212
  discrete trial training (DTT), 217
  fading instructional prompts, 214
  floortime, 218–219
  general case instruction, 213
  group instruction, 214–215
  instructional procedures for children with, 216
  learning characteristics of children with, 206–210
  model programs for children with, 220–225
  naturalistic instruction, 212–213
  overview, 205–206
  peer-mediated intervention, 220
  Picture Exchange Communication System (PECS), 219–220
  positive behavior support (PBS) model, 216
  visual supports, 220
  see also Small-group instruction
Auxiliary aids and services, 12

Backward chaining, 130–131, 131f, 321
Basic interpersonal communicative skills (BICS), 193
Bedwetting, 318
Behavior problems, see Challenging behavior
Behavioral chaining, 253–254
Behavioral curriculum model, 78–80, 80t
Behavioral expectations, listing on ecological assessment, 104
Behaviorally based practices, 209
BICS, see Basic interpersonal communicative skills

Blindness, 51t, 169–170
Blocked schedules, 124–125
Bloom, Benjamin, 6
Books, reading in class, 286–287
Buddy skills training package, 292

Call-and-response rhythm, 183
CALP, see Cognitive/academic language proficiency
Can Do scores, ecological assessment, 104, 106
Carrying procedures, 306–307
CC skills, see Complex thinking skills
Challenging behavior
  in children with autism, 208–209
  functional assessment, 239–242
  hypothesis development and verification, 242–245
  levels of intervention for, 234–235
  overview, 233–234
  see also Positive behavior support (PBS)
Changing criterion design, 129
Child-centered planning, 54, 101–102
Child-directed activities, 182
Choice
  core value of special education policy, 32, 33
  decreasing challenging behavior through, 249
Choice-making opportunities, 152
Choking, 322–323
Choosing Options and Accommodations for Children (COACH), 101
Choral responding, 273–274
Circle of communication, 218
Classrooms
  competitive structures in, 186
  environmental-structuring strategies, 286
  layout of, 163
  routines, listing on ecological assessment, 104
  social acceptance and rejection in, 284–285
  social interventions, 285–288
COACH, see Choosing Options and Accommodations for Children
Cognition, instructional conversation (IC) model, 184–186, 188–189t
Cognitive tempo, 185
Cognitive/academic language proficiency (CALP), 193
Collaboration imperative, 18–19
Collaborative team model, 40, 41, 42
Collectivist cultures, 29
Communication
  augmentative, 215–216

of children with autism, 206–207
collaborative team model, 42–43
in partnerships, 38
see also Communication skills
Communication boards, 313, 314f
Communication skills
augmenting input, 312
communication responses, 315t
critical functions, 315t
enhancing sensitivity, 311
environmental modifications for, 312
expanding initial environmental control skills, 312–315
functionally equivalent responses, 315t
general discussion, 309–311
increasing opportunities for use of, 311–312
structuring predictable routines, 312
Community services, transition from hospital to, 332–333, 336–337
Compensations, 306
Competence, social, 284–285
Competitive classroom structures, 186
Complex thinking (CC) skills, 181
Comprehensible input, for English Language Learners (ELLs), 193–194
Comprehensive treatment models, 208–209
Content of communication, focusing on for English Language Learners (ELLs), 191
Content of instruction, naturalistic curriculum model, 80–84
Context, teaching in, for English Language Learners (ELLs), 192
Context for instruction, naturalistic curriculum model, 84–85
Contextual influences on challenging behavior, 239, 244–245
Contextualization, 180–181
Contingencies, group, 274
Contingency interactions, 310
Contingent arrangement of reinforcement, 139
Continuous monitoring of progress, 20
Continuous staff development, 41–42
Continuum of interventions, 20
Controlling prompts, 121, 124, 158
Cooperative learning groups, 277–278
Cooperative learning methods, for English Language Learners (ELLs), 194
Coping strategies, teaching, 194–195
Core values, 32–33
Correction procedures, 120, 125
Co-teaching model, 39–40
Crisis management plans, 247
Crisis plans, positive behavior support (PBS), 236–237

Criterion-referenced tests, 52–53, 54, 55t
Critical function, 301–302, 315t
Cross-cultural competence
cultural values in parenting, 30–31
cultural values of professional fields, 31–34
culturally appropriate intervention practices, 34–37
functional assessment interviews, 241
general discussion, 13–14, 28–29
Cues
fading, 126–127
general discussion, 124
prompting appropriate behavior with, 249–250
using with children with autism, 213–214
Cultural relativity, 102
Culturally relevant instruction
culturally compatible education, 178–182
English as a second language (ESL), 189–190
overview, 177–178
strategies for culturally and linguistically responsive intervention, 195–197
supporting English Language Learners (ELLs), 190–195
see also Instructional conversation model
Culture
consideration in positive behavior support (PBS) plans, 246–247
diversity in United States, 28
general discussion, 13–14
influence on learning, 88
parenting values, 30–31
of professional fields, 31–34
see also Cross-cultural competence
Curriculum models
behavioral model, 78–80, 80t
defined, 76
developmental model, 77, 80t
developmental-cognitive model, 77, 80t
overview, 76–77
see also Naturalistic curriculum model
Curriculum-referenced tests, 52–53, 54, 55t

Daily activities, listing on ecological assessment, 104
Daily routines, teaching independent behaviors with, 301
DAP, *see* Developmentally appropriate practices

Data collection
　cultural issues with assessment and, 35
　ecological assessment, 108–110
　interpreting data, 143–144
　systematic instruction, 140–144, 143f
Data collection matrix, 109, 109f
Data-based decision making, 20, 140
Data-based monitoring, positive behavior support (PBS) plans, 253–255
Deafblindness, 51t
Deafness, 51t, 168–169
Decision making, data-based, 20
Denver Model, 225
Developmental, Individual-Difference, Relationship-Based (DIR) intervention model, 218, 222
Developmental curriculum model, 77, 80t
Developmental delay, 10–11, 51t
Developmental-cognitive curriculum model, 77–78, 80t
Developmentally appropriate practices (DAP), 83
Developmentally Appropriate Treatment for Autism (Project DATA), 222–223
Diagnosis, 49
Differentiated interactions, 311
DIR, see Developmental, Individual-Difference, Relationship-Based (DIR) intervention model
Direct instruction
　in behavioral model, 78
　for children with autism, 210–212
　discrete trial training (DTT), 217
　general discussion, 119–120
Direct threat, 13
Direct verbal prompts, 121
Discourse structures, 183
Discrete trial instruction, 119–120
Discrete trial training (DTT), 217, 223
Discriminative stimulus, 158
Distributing time delay procedures, 157–160
Diversity in United States, 28
Division for Early Childhood of the Council for Exceptional Children, 16
Drinking skills, 318–323
　intervention plan for, 323f
　typical development of, 319–321t
DTT, see Discrete trial training
Duration, measurement of, 67, 141
Dyadic training, 292
Dynamic positioning, 307

Early childhood education (ECE), relationships with early childhood special education (ECSE) teachers, 39–40

Early childhood special education (ECSE)
　American contributions to, 4–6
　European contributions to, 2–4
　historical contributions to, 7t
　overview, 2
　relationships with early childhood education (ECE) teachers, 39–40
　transactional perspectives, 6
Early Education Programs for Children with Disabilities, 8
Early intervention (EI)
　American contributions to, 4–6
　European contributions to, 2–4
　historical contributions to, 7t
　Individuals with Disabilities Education Act (IDEA) of 1990 (PL 101-476), 10
　transactional perspectives, 6
　transition planning, 21–22
　transition to preschool from, 333–334, 337–339
Early Start Denver Model, 225
Ease of integration, indicator of high-quality goals and objectives, 65
Eating skills, 318–323
　intervention plan for, 323f
　typical development of, 319–321t
Echolalia, 219
Ecological assessment
　authentic assessment, 53
　behavioral expectations, listing, 104
　Can Do scores, 104, 106
　daily activities and classroom routines, listing, 104
　data collection, 108–110
　general discussion, 15, 102–104
　goals and objectives, 106–107
　instructional planning, 107–108
　naturalistic curriculum model, 83–84, 89
　Needs to Learn scores, 104, 106
Ecological inventory, 15
Ecological model, 6
Ecological theory, 102
　see also Ecological assessment
Ecological transition framework, 334–335
ECSE, see Early childhood special education
Education for All Handicapped Children Act of 1975 (PL 94-142), 9
Education of the Handicapped Act Amendments of 1986 (PL 99-457), 9
EI, see Early intervention
Elaboration, 192
Electronic portfolios, 110–111
Eligibility determination, 49–50, 51t
ELLs, see English Language Learners

ELO, *see* Embedded learning opportunity
Embedded intervention/instruction, 155–156
Embedded learning opportunity (ELO), 119, 156
Embedded routines, prompting appropriate behavior with, 249–250
Embedding and distributing time delay procedures, 157–160
Emotional disturbance, 51*t*
EMT, *see* Enhanced milieu teaching
Encoded interactions, 311
Encouragement
 of appropriate behavior, positive behavior support (PBS) plans, 248–251
 environmental arrangements, 129–131
 guidelines for effective, 131–132
 overview, 127
 positive reinforcement, 127–128
 procedures for group instruction, 275–276
 shaping and selecting reinforcement, 128–129
Engaged time, 139
English as a second language (ESL)
 capitalizing on all communication skills, 191
 cooperative learning methods, 194
 focusing on content, 191
 providing relaxed environments and comprehensible input, 193–194
 stages in learning, 189–190
 teaching coping strategies, 194–195
 teaching in context, 192
 see also English Language Learners (ELLs)
English Language Learners (ELLs)
 capitalizing on all communication skills, 191
 cooperative learning methods, 194
 focusing on content, 191
 overview, 190–191
 providing relaxed environments and comprehensible input, 193–194
 recommendations and strategies for supportive environments, 196*t*
 teaching coping strategies, 194–195
 teaching in context, 192
Enhanced milieu teaching (EMT)
 environmental arrangement strategies, 151–152
 general discussion, 87
 incidental teaching procedure, 154–155
 mand-model procedure, 153–154
 modeling, 152–153
 overview, 150–151
 promoting social behaviors with, 289–290, 291*t*
 responsive interaction strategies, 151
 teaching communication skills, 314
 teaching independent behaviors, 301
 time delay procedure, 154
Enrichment model, 77
Environmental arrangements, 127, 129–131, 151–152
Environmental control skills
 augmenting input, 312
 in developmental-cognitive curriculum model, 78
 enhancing sensitivity, 311
 environmental modifications for, 312
 expanding initial, 312–315
 general discussion, 309–311
 increasing opportunities for use of, 311–312
 structuring predictable routines, 312
Environmental modifications
 developing environmental control skills, 312
 promoting independence, 301, 324–325
Environmental prompts, teaching functional independence with, 302
Environmental-structuring strategies, 286
E-portfolios, 110–111
Equipment, 165
Equity, 32, 33–34
Errorless instruction, 140
Errorless procedures, 124–125
ESL, *see* English as a second language
European contributions to field, 2–4
Evaluation, 50, 88–89
Evidence-based practice, *see* Practices
Exemplar training, 301
Exosystem, 103
Expansion, 192
Expectations for activities, listing, 104
Expected outcomes, individualized family service plan (IFSP), 58–59
Explicit social-skills interventions
 individual or small-group lessons, 290
 peer-mediated interventions, 291–295
 social integration activities, 290–291
Extinction, 128
Eye contact, 183–184, 211

Face-to-face communication, in cooperative learning groups, 277
Facilitating group participation, 271–274
Facilitation techniques, 308
Facilitative interpersonal factors, 38
Fading instructional prompts, 126–127, 214

Families
  cultural values in parenting, 30–31
  individualized family service plan (IFSP), 55–57
  involvement in assessment and planning stage, 49
  partnerships with, 37–38
  support from parents of children with autism, 209
  system-level supports, 18–19
  see also Transitions
Family-centered practices, 14, 30, 37–38
FAPE, *see* Free appropriate public education
FBA, *see* Functional behavioral assessment
Feeding techniques, 321
Feeding tubes, 323
Fidelity, implementation, 20
Field dependence versus field independence, 184–185
Fine motor skills, independence in, 308–309, 310t
Fixed interval schedule, 128
Fixed ratio schedule, 128
Flexible prompt fading, 123–124
Floortime, 218–219
Fluency, measuring instructional progress by, 141
Fluid intake techniques for toileting, 318
Focused contrasts, 192
Formative evaluation, 50
Forward chaining, 130–131, 131f
Foster parents, 48
Free appropriate public education (FAPE), 9
Free-play sessions, 287
Frequency, measurement of, 66, 141
Friendship activity interventions, 288–289
Full physical assistance prompts, 121
Functional analysis, 245
Functional assessment
  of challenging behavior, 239–242
  positive behavior support (PBS), 237
Functional behavioral assessment (FBA), 21
Functional communication training, 252
Functional independence
  adaptations for, 301–304
  in basic physical skills, 305–306
Functionality, 54, 64, 65
Functionally equivalent response, 302, 315t, 323
Functions for challenging behavior, 238, 243–244

Gaining attention, 238
Gavage feedings, 323

General case instruction, 135, 213
General case response, 323
Generality, as indicator of high-quality goals and objectives, 65
Generalization
  assessment of, 88, 93
  of behavior changes, supports for, 253–255
  enhancing with group instruction, 276–277
  formulating general case objectives, 133–135
  general case instruction, 135
  other procedures, 135–138
  promoting in children with autism, 207, 208, 212–213
  promoting independence, 301, 324
  train sufficient exemplars, 133–135
  types of, 132–133
Generalization probes, 142
Gestural prompts, 121
Goals
  communication, 313
  ecological assessment, 106–107
  for environmental control skills, 311
  individualized education program (IEP), 61
  measurability issues, 68–71
  naturalistic curriculum model, 89
  rating quality of, 65t
  selecting based on criterion- and curriculum-referenced test results, 54, 55t
  selection of, in behavioral model, 79
  writing high-quality, 64–68
Goldfarb, William, 5
Graduated guidance, 123–124
Graphing methods, 143, 144f
Gross motor skills, independence in, 305–308, 309t
Group responding, 273–274
Groups
  affection activities, 288–289
  for children with autism, 214–215
  contingencies, 274
  participation skills, 267–269, 271–274
  process, in cooperative learning groups, 277
  size of, 165
  see also Small-group instruction
Guidance, graduated, 123–124
Guided learning, 86

Handicapped Children's Early Education Assistance Act (PL 90-538), 7–8
Hard of hearing, modifying instructional methods for, 168–169

Head Start, 8–9
Health impairments, 51*t*, 171
Hearing aids, 168
Hearing impairments, 51*t*, 168–169
Heterogeneous groups, 266
Hierarchical relationship, indicator of high-quality goals and objectives, 65–66
Hierarchies, prompt, 122–123
High-probability (high-*p*) request sequences, 160–162, 212, 250
Historical contributions to early intervention concepts
  American contributions, 4–6
  European contributions, 2–4
  overview, 2
  summary of, 7*t*
Home, transition from hospital to, 332–333, 336–337
Homogeneous groups, 265–266
Horizontal transitions, 332
Hospital, transition to home and community services from, 332–333, 336–337
Hunt, J. McVicker, 5–6
Hypotheses about challenging behavior, development of, 242–245

IC model, *see* Instructional conversation model
IDEA, *see* Individuals with Disabilities Education Act
IEP, *see* Individualized education program
IFSP, *see* Individualized family service plan
Implementation fidelity, 20
Impulsive learning styles, 185
Incidental teaching procedure, 154–155
Inclusion
  access, 16–17
  Americans with Disabilities Act (ADA) of 1990 (PL 101-336), 12–13
  myths countering, 15–16
  participation, 18
  system-level supports, 18–19
Independence
  adaptations for functional, 301–304
  designing instructional programs to promote, 323–325
  in fine motor skills, 308–309
  functional, in basic physical skills, 305–306
  physical development intervention procedures, 306–308
  teaching independent behaviors, 300–301
  see also Environmental control skills; Self-help skills
Independent performance conditions, 323
Indirect verbal prompts, 121
Indiscriminable contingencies, 137, 139*f*
Individual accountability, in cooperative learning groups, 277
Individualism, 32, 33
Individualistic cultures, 29
Individualized education program (IEP)
  Individuals with Disabilities Education Act (IDEA) requirements for, 56*t*
  planning, 59–64
Individualized family service plan (IFSP)
  developing, 56–57
  Education of the Handicapped Act Amendments of 1986 (PL 99-457), 9
  general discussion, 55–56
  guidelines for development of, 60*t*
  Individuals with Disabilities Education Act (IDEA) requirements for, 56*t*
Individualized instruction, 108
Individualized participation, teaching functional independence with, 302
Individuals with Disabilities Education Act (IDEA) of 1990 (PL 101-476)
  eligibility categories, 51*t*
  general discussion, 9–12
  individualized education program (IEP) requirements, 56*t*
  individualized family service plan (IFSP) requirements, 56*t*
  transition requirements, 335–336
Individuals with Disabilities Education Act (IDEA) of 2004 (PL 108-446), 48, 303
Input, augmenting communicative, 312
Instructional context, 324
Instructional conversation (IC) model
  characteristics of, 188–189*t*
  cognition, 184–186
  for English Language Learners (ELLs), 190–191
  implementing, 181
  motivation, 186–187
  overview, 182
  social organization, 186–187, 189
  sociolinguistics, 182–184
Instructional feedback, using with progressive time delay, 125
Instructional methods, naturalistic curriculum model, 85–88
Instructional planning, ecological assessments, 107–108, 107*f*
Instructional plans
  for children with autism, 213
  incorporating generalization procedure, 135, 136*f*

Instructional plans—continued
    naturalistic curriculum model, 89–91, 90f, 92
    for teaching communication skills, 314–315, 314f
Instructional positive reinforcement, 128
Instructional procedures
    implementation of systematic instruction, 138, 139–140
    monitoring systematic instruction, 140–144
    overview, 117–118
    systematic instruction in natural settings, 118–120
    see also Encouragement; Generalization; Prompting
Instructional process, supporting with groups, 274–277
Instructional programs, designing to promote independence, 323–325
Instructional progress, measuring, 141
Instructional prompts, 120–121
Instructional situation, 129
Instructional techniques, in behavioral model, 79
Instructional universe, 133–134
Instructions, recording on audio devices, 192
Integrated therapy, 155–156, 305–309
Intellectual disability, 51t
Interaction, peer, see Peer interaction
Interaction in groups, 266, 272, 273, 273f
Interdependence, 272
Interdisciplinary model, 41
Interspersed requests, 250
Interval, measurement of instructional progress, 141
Intervention planning, 50
Intervention practices, culturally appropriate, 34–37
Interventions, continuum of, 20
Interviews
    cultural issues, 35
    for functional assessment of challenging behavior, 240–241, 240t
Introduction to novelty, 87
Intrusive programs, 221
Itard, Jean-Marc, 2–3
Itinerant teacher model, 40

Joint attention, 206, 285
Joint functioning, 41
Joint productive activity, 179–180

Kindergarten, transition from preschool to, 334, 339–340
Kirk, Samuel, 5

Languages
    accommodations, 195–197
    assessment in primary, 49
    impairments, 51t
    see also English as a second language (ESL)
Latency, measurement of, 67, 141
Layout of classrooms, 163
LEAP, see Learning Experiences and Alternative Program for Preschoolers and Their Parents
Learning centers, teaching functional independence with, 302
Learning Experiences and Alternative Program for Preschoolers and Their Parents (LEAP), 221–222
Learning style, 184
Least intrusive procedures, 300, 324
Least restrictive environment (LRE)
    Education for All Handicapped Children Act of 1975 (PL 94-142), 9
    Individuals with Disabilities Education Act (IDEA) of 1990 (PL 101-476), 11
Least-to-most prompt hierarchies, 123
Legislation
    Americans with Disabilities Act (ADA) of 1990 (PL 101-336), 12–13
    Education for All Handicapped Children Act of 1975 (PL 94-142), 9
    Education of the Handicapped Act Amendments of 1986 (PL 99-457), 9
    Handicapped Children's Early Education Assistance Act, 7–8
    Head Start, 8–9
    Individuals with Disabilities Education Act (IDEA) of 1990 (PL 101-476), 9–12
    overview, 6, 7
    related to transitions, 335–336
    timeline of, 8t
Limited motor abilities, modifying instructional methods for children with, 171, 172–173t
Line graphs depicting child progress, 143, 144f
Linguistic accommodations, 195–197
Listening, importance in partnerships, 38
Literacy development, 180
Lovaas, Ivar, 217
Lovaas Institute, 223–224
LRE, see Least restrictive environment

Macroculture, 31
Macrosystem, 103
Magnitude, measurement of, 67
Maintaining variables, 238–239
Mand-model procedure, 153–154

MAPS, *see* McGill Action Planning System
Materials
  enhancing motivation with, 130
  environmental arrangement strategies, 151–152
  selecting for environments, 163–165
  toy rotation plans, 164–165
McGill Action Planning System (MAPS), 54, 101
Mealtime skills, 318–323
  intervention plan for, 323*f*
  typical development of, 319–321*t*
Measurability
  indicator of high-quality goals and objectives, 66
  issues with objectives, 64–68
Measuring instructional progress, 141–142
Mediate generalization, 137
Mesosystem, 103
Mexican families, study of view of hospital practices, 30–31
Microculture, 31–32
Microsystem, 103
Mild physical disabilities
  motor interventions for, 306
  toileting skills, 317
Milestones, 305
Milieu teaching, 154–155, 212–213
Minimally intrusive corrections, 325
Model prompts, 121
Modeling
  in culturally diverse classrooms, 182
  general discussion, 152–153
  peer, 275
Modifications
  environmental, 301, 312, 324–325
  general suggestions for, 167*t*
  specialized instruction procedures, 167–173
Monitoring
  in assessment and planning stage, 50
  of progress, 20, 92–93
  purposes of assessment, planning, and, 100
  results of positive behavior support (PBS) plans, 255
  systematic instruction, 140–144
  time delay trials, 159
Montessori, Maria, 3
Most-to-least prompt hierarchies, 123
Motivation
  instructional conversation (IC) model, 186–187, 188–189*t*
  pivotal response treatment model, 225
  see also Encouragement
Motor interventions, 305–309

Motor skills
  fine, independence in, 308–309, 310*t*
  gross, independence in, 305–308, 309*t*
Movement prompts, 121
Multidisciplinary model, 41
Multiple disabilities, 51*t*
Muscle tone, atypical, 305
Musical Chairs, 288–289

National Association for the Education of Young Children, 16
National Research Council, 209
Natural environments
  clarification of term, 48
  skills for participating in, 83–84
  systematic instruction in, 118–120
Natural maintaining contingencies, 136
Natural prompts, 120
Naturalistic assessment, 53
Naturalistic curriculum model
  assessment in, 80
  content of instruction, 80–84
  context for instruction, 84–85
  cultural relevance, 88
  evaluation methods, 88–89
  implementing, 89–93
  instructional methods, 85–88
  overview, 76
  traditional curriculum models, 76–80, 80*t*
Naturalistic instruction
  activity-based intervention (ABI), 155–156
  arranging physical and social environments, 162–166
  for children with autism, 212–213
  embedding and distributing time delay procedures, 157–160
  enhanced milieu teaching (EMT), 150–155
  high-probability (high-*p*) request sequences, 160–162
  modifications and accommodations for, 167–173
  promoting independence, 301, 324
Naturalistic peer interaction interventions, 288–290
Naturally occurring reinforcers and corrections, 325
Needs to Learn scores, ecological assessment, 104, 106
Nighttime toilet training, 318
Nocturnal enuresis, 318
Nonintrusive programs, 221
Norm-referenced tests, 52
Notecards for observational assessments, 241, 242*f*

Novelty, introduction to, 87
Number, measurement of, 66

O&M specialists, Orientation and mobility specialists
Objectives
  ecological assessment, 106–107
  formulating general case, 133–135
  individualized education program (IEP), 61
  measurability issues, 68–71
  naturalistic curriculum model, 89
  promoting independence, 323–324
  rating quality of, 65t
  small-group instruction, 267–268
  writing high-quality, 64–68
Observational assessment of challenging behavior, 240, 241–242
Observational learning, 275
Occasions for instruction, 324
One teaching, one supporting approach, 40
Online support communities, 337
Opportunities for communication, increasing, 311–312
Organizing small-group instruction, 269–271
Orientation and mobility (O&M) specialists, 170
Orthopedic impairments, 51t
Outcome statements, individualized family service plan (IFSP), 58–59
Overhydration, 318
Overlapping speech, 182–183

Pacing, quick, 271
Parallel talk, 288
Parallel teaching approach, 40
Parents
  cultural values, 30–31
  floortime sessions, 218
  foster, 48
  guided discussions about stories read in class, 287
  importance of involvement according to Individuals with Disabilities Education Act (IDEA), 48
  partnerships with, 37–38
Partial participation, 272
Partial participation task analysis, 316
Partial physical assistance prompts, 121
Participation
  general discussion, 18
  in groups, 267–269, 271–274
  individualized, teaching functional independence with, 302
  structures, 183

Partnerships
  general discussion, 37
  with other professionals, 38–40
  with parents and other family members, 37–38
PATHS, *see* Promoting Alternative Thinking Strategies
PBS, *see* Positive behavior support
PECS, *see* Picture Exchange Communication System
Peer assistance, promoting independence through, 303, 325
Peer interaction
  classroomwide interventions, 285–288
  explicit social-skills interventions, 290–295
  in groups, 272, 273, 273f
  naturalistic peer interaction interventions, 288–290
  overview, 283–284
  social acceptance and rejection in classroom settings, 284–285
Peer modeling, 275
Peer tutoring, 275
Peer-mediated interventions, 220, 291–295
Percentages, 70
Periodic attention, 271
Permanent product measures, 141
Personal-futures planning, 54
Person-centered planning, 54
Photographs of group projects, 111–112
Physical and social environments, arranging, 162–166
Physical development
  difficulties, 305–306
  intervention procedures, 306–308
  modifying instructional methods for children with impairments, 171, 172–173t
Piaget, Jean, 3–4
Picture Exchange Communication System (PECS), 216, 219–220
Picture schedules, 220
Pivotal response treatment model, 224–225
PL 90-538, *see* Handicapped Children's Early Education Assistance Act
PL 94-142, *see* Education for All Handicapped Children Act of 1975
PL 99-457, *see* Education of the Handicapped Act Amendments of 1986
PL 100-407, *see* Technology-Related Assistance for Individuals with Disabilities Act of 1988
PL 101-336, *see* Americans with Disabilities Act (ADA) of 1990

PL 101-476, *see* Individuals with Disabilities Education Act (IDEA) of 1990
PL 108-146, *see* Individuals with Disabilities Education Act (IDEA) of 2004
Planning
 child-centered, 101–102
 cultural competency, 36
 general discussion, 55
 individualized education program (IEP), 59–64
 individualized family service plan (IFSP), 55–57
 measurability issues with objectives, 68–71
 portfolio assessment, 110–113
 purposes of assessment, monitoring, and, 100
 service coordinator responsibilities, 57–59
 writing high-quality goals and objectives, 64–68
 see also Ecological assessment
Play possibilities, social integration activities, 291
Play-based assessment, 53
Portfolio assessment, 110–113
Positioning procedures, 306–307, 307t, 321
Positive behavior support (PBS)
 for children with autism, 216
 components of plans, 245–246
 crisis management plans, 247
 cultural considerations, 246–247
 data-based monitoring, 253–255
 example of plan, 259–261
 functional assessment of behavior, 239–242, 240t
 general discussion, 20–21
 hypothesis development and verification, 242–245
 levels of, 234–235
 supports to encourage appropriate behavior, 248–251
 supports to maintain and generalize behavior changes, 253–255
 supports to prevent challenging behavior, 248
 supports to teach effective replacement behaviors, 251–253
 tertiary level, 235–239
Positive interdependence, in cooperative learning groups, 277
Positive reinforcement, 127–129
Positive social comments, 250
Postural reaction deficits, 305–306
Postural stability, 308, 309

Practical and naturalistic considerations, 142
Practices
 for children with autism, 209–210
 culturally competent and relevant services, 13–14
 ecological assessment, 15
 family-centered intervention, 14
 inclusion, 15–19
 overview, 13
 positive behavior support (PBS), 20–21
 response to intervention (RTI), 19–20
 transition planning, 21–22
Pragmatics, 219, 312
Predictable routines
 association with appropriate behavior, 250–251
 developing environmental control skills, 312
 importance to children with autism, 208
Preferences of children, decreasing challenging behavior through, 249
Prepared environment, 3
Preschool
 transition from early intervention services to, 333–334, 337–339
 transition to kindergarten from, 334, 339–340
Present-levels statement, 60
Preteaching, 251
Primary level of positive behavior support (PBS), 234
Priming, 251
Proactive instruction of socially appropriate replacement behavior, 251–253
Problem behavior, *see* Challenging behavior
Problem solving, data-based, 20
Professionals
 acculturation, 32
 cultural values of fields, 31–34
 expertise, 38
 partnerships with, 38–40
Program common stimuli technique, 136, 301
Progress, continuous monitoring of, 20
Progressive schedules, 124
Project DATA, *see* Developmentally Appropriate Treatment for Autism
Project TEACCH, *see* Treatment and Education of Autistic and Related Communication—Handicapped Children
Promoting Alternative Thinking Strategies (PATHS), 287
Prompt hierarchies, 122–123

Prompt sequence, 122
Prompting
　appropriate behavior, 249–250
　for children with autism, 210–211
　cues, 124, 213–214
　environmental, teaching functional independence with, 302
　errorless procedures, 124–125
　fading procedures, 126–127
　graduated guidance, 123–124
　guidelines for effective, 125–126
　peer tutoring, 275
　promoting independence, 324–325
　prompt hierarchies, 122–123
　types of, 120–122
Prostheses, 304
Public policy
　Americans with Disabilities Act (ADA) of 1990 (PL 101-336), 12–13
　Education for All Handicapped Children Act of 1975 (PL 94-142), 9
　Education of the Handicapped Act Amendments of 1986 (PL 99-457), 9
　Handicapped Children's Early Education Assistance Act, 7–8
　Head Start, 8–9
　Individuals with Disabilities Education Act (IDEA) of 1990 (PL 101-476), 9–12
　overview, 6, 7
　timeline of legislation, 8t
Punishment for challenging behavior, 236

Qualitative data, 109
Quality of goals and objectives, 64–68, 65t
Quantitative data, 109
Quick pacing, 271

Rapid method, 318
Rate, measurement of, 66–67, 141
RBI, see Routines-based intervention
Reasonable modifications, 12
Reciprocal interactions, 334
Recording instructions on audio devices, 192
Redirection, in positive behavior support (PBS) plans, 253
Reflective learning styles, 185
Reflexes, atypical, 305
Reinforcement
　for children with autism, 211–212
　contingent arrangement of, 139
　high-probability (high-*p*) activities, using as, 212
　instructional positive, 128
　naturally occurring reinforcers and corrections, 325
　positive, 127–129
　reinforcers, selecting, 158
　selective, 128–129
　shaping and selecting, 128–129
　social, 211
　of successive approximations, 128–129
Reinforcer surveys, 211
Rejection, social, 284–285
Relationship-oriented communication skills, 42–43
Relaxed environments, for English Language Learners (ELLs), 193–194
Replacement behaviors, teaching in positive behavior support (PBS) plans, 251–253
Research-based practice, see Practices
Response class, 132
Response generalization, 132, 134
Response to intervention (RTI), 19–20
Responsive interaction strategies, 151
Responsive intervention, strategies for culturally and linguistically, 195–197
Responsivity to multiple cues, pivotal response treatment model, 225
Role release, 42
Routines
　importance to children with autism, 208
　in positive behavior support (PBS) plans, 249–251
　predictable, developing environmental control skills with, 312
　teaching independent behaviors, 301
Routines-based intervention (RBI), 155–156
RTI, see Response to intervention

Sameness, importance to children with autism, 207
Scheduling activities, 165–166
Scheduling matrix, naturalistic curriculum model, 91–92, 91f
Screening, 49
Seamless system of services delivery, 21–22
Secondary level of positive behavior support (PBS), 234–235
Selective attention, 272
Selective reinforcement, 128–129
Self-help skills
　general discussion, 315–316
　mealtime skills, 318–323
　participation intervention plan for, 317f
　toileting, 316–318
Self-initiation, pivotal response treatment model, 225
Self-management, pivotal response treatment model, 225

Self-prompting, 301
Self-regulating challenging behavior, 244
Self-reinforcing challenging behavior, 244
Semantics, 312, 313
Sensitivity to environmental control skills, 311
Sensitivity training, 292
Sensory impairments, 168–171
Service coordinator responsibilities, 57–59, 58t
Severe physical disabilities
    motor interventions for, 306–308
    toileting skills, 318
Shaping and selecting reinforcement, 128–129
Signaling devices for toilet training, 318
Sizes of groups, 265
Skeels, Harold, 4–5
Skills
    for children with autism, 208
    embedding, 269–270, 270t
    group-participation, 267–269, 268t, 271–274
    needed for preschool to kindergarten transition, 339–340
    sequencing, 270–271
    social competence, 284–285
    social interaction, 266
    see also Generalization
Skills for School Success curriculum, 340
Small-group instruction
    characteristics of, 265–267
    cooperative learning groups, 277–278
    facilitating group participation, 271–274
    group-participation skills and objectives, 267–268
    organizing, 269–271
    overview, 263–264
    rationale for, 264–265
    supporting instructional process with groups, 274–277
    teaching group-participation skills, 269
Small-group lessons, explicit social-skills interventions, 290
Small-group social organization, 187
Social acceptance and rejection in classroom settings, 284–285
Social coaching, 295
Social competence, 284–285
Social competence curriculum, 287–288
Social density, 165
Social development component, of developmental-cognitive curriculum model, 78
Social environments, arranging, 162–166
Social integration activities, 290–291
Social interaction skills, 266

Social judgment, 237–238
Social narratives, combining with peer-mediated interventions, 292–293
Social organization, instructional conversation (IC) model, 186–187, 188–189t, 189
Social reinforcement, 211
Social skills
    of children with autism, 206–207
    classroom-wide interventions, 285–288
    explicit social-skills interventions, 290–295
    naturalistic peer interaction interventions, 288–290
    overview, 283–284
    social acceptance and rejection in classroom settings, 284–285
Social validity, 54
Sociolinguistics, instructional conversation (IC) model, 182–184, 188–189t
Songs, in friendship activities, 288
Spatial density, 165
Spatial prompts, 121
Special education services statement, 61–62
Specialized instruction procedures
    activity-based intervention (ABI), 155–156
    arranging physical and social environments, 162–166
    enhanced milieu teaching (EMT), 150–155
    high-probability (high-*p*) request sequences, 160–162
    modifications and accommodations for, 167–173
    overview, 150
    time delay procedures, 157–160
Specific learning disabilities, 51t
Speech or language impairments, 51t
Speech volume, 183
Spitz, Rene, 5
Standardized procedures, 52
State motivation, 186–187
Static positioning, 307
Station teaching approach, 40
Stimulus class, 132
Stimulus generalization, 132, 134
Stimulus shaping and fading procedures, 125, 126f
Storytimes, 286–287
Strategy-use training, 292
Structured free-play sessions, 287
Student-directed activities, 182
Style of presentation, 130
Summative evaluation, 50
Support communities for parents, 337

Support plans, positive behavior support (PBS), 237
Supported routines, 251
Supportive teaching, for children with autism, 208
Supports
  to encourage appropriate behavior, in positive behavior support (PBS) plans, 248–251
  in individualized education programs (IEPs), 61–62
  instructional planning, 108, 108t
  to maintain and generalize behavior changes, in positive behavior support (PBS) plans, 253–255
  to prevent challenging behavior, in positive behavior support (PBS) plans, 248
  to teach effective replacement behaviors, in positive behavior support (PBS) plans, 251–253
Survival skills, 268, 268t, 339
Symbol use, 285
Symbolic interactions, 311
Syntax, 312–313
Systematic instruction
  implementation of, 138, 139–140
  monitoring, 140–144
  in natural settings, 118–120
  overview, 117–118
  teaching independent behaviors, 300–301
  see also Encouragement; Generalization; Prompting
System-level supports, 18–19

Tactile prompts, 121
Task analysis, 130, 130t
Task cues, 158
Task simplification, 251
Task-oriented communication skills, 42
Teaching independent behaviors, 300–301
Team teaching, 40
Teaming, 40–43
Technology, 165
Technology-Related Assistance for Individuals with Disabilities Act of 1988 (PL 100-407), 303
Temperament, suiting instructional methods to, 86
Template matching, 340–341
Tertiary level of positive behavior support (PBS), 235–239
Tests
  criterion-referenced, 52–53, 54, 55t
  curriculum-referenced, 52–53, 54, 55t
  norm-referenced, 52
Theory of mind, 207
Therapeutic feeding techniques, 322
Time delay procedures
  embedding and distributing, 157–160
  general discussion, 124–125
  steps in, 154
Time sampling, 141
Timed toileting, 317
Toileting, 316–318
Tool skills, 208
Topography, measurement of, 67
Total-task approach, 130, 131f
Toys
  rotation plans, 164 165
  selecting, 164
Traditional assessment, 52
Traditional behavioral approaches versus positive behavior support (PBS), 235–236, 236t
Train sufficient exemplars, 133
Training parents for infant discharge, 336–337
Train-loosely technique, 137–138, 138f
Trait motivation, 186–187
Transactional perspectives, 6
Transdisciplinary model, 41
Transitional movements, 305
Transitions
  between activities, 166, 166t
  for children with autism, 209
  early intervention services to preschool, 333–334, 337–339
  ecological transition framework, 334–335
  hospital to home and community services, 332–333, 336–337
  legal mandates related to, 335–336
  overview, 331–332
  planning, 21–22
  preschool to kindergarten, 334, 339–340
  strategies for successful, 336–341
Traumatic brain injury, 51t
Treatment and Education of Autistic and Related Communication—Handicapped Children (Project TEACCH), 223
Triangulation, 110
Triggers for challenging behavior, 239, 244–245
Turn taking, 285, 293
Tutoring, peer, 275

UDL, *see* Universal design for learning
Unison responding, 273–274
Unit approach, 266

United States, cultural diversity in, 28
Universal design for learning (UDL)
　access, 162–163
　general discussion, 17
Universal screening, 19
Universally potent features, 189

Variable interval schedule, 128
Variables that trigger challenging behavior, 239
Verbal praise, 211
Verbal thinking, 184
Vertical transitions, 332
Violations of expectations, 87

Visual impairments, 51t, 169–170
Visual supports, for children with autism, 220
Visual thinking, 184
Visual/pictorial prompts, 122
Volume, speech, 183

Wait time, 182
Waited corrects, 125

Young Autism Project, 223–224

Zones, 166